Lecture Notes in Computer Science 8545

Commenced Publication in 1973
Founding and Former Series Editors:
Gerhard Goos, Juris Hartmanis, and Jan van Leeuwen

Sébastien Ourselin   Marc Modat (Eds.)

Biomedical Image Registration

6th International Workshop, WBIR 2014
London, UK, July 7-8, 2014
Proceedings

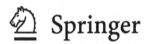 Springer

Volume Editors

Sébastien Ourselin
Marc Modat
University College London, Centre for Medical Imaging
Front Engineering Building, Malet Place, London WC1E 6BT, UK
E-mail: {s.ourselin; m.modat}@ucl.ac.uk

ISSN 0302-9743   e-ISSN 1611-3349
ISBN 978-3-319-08553-1   e-ISBN 978-3-319-08554-8
DOI 10.1007/978-3-319-08554-8
Springer Cham Heidelberg New York Dordrecht London

Library of Congress Control Number: Applied for

LNCS Sublibrary: SL 6 – Image Processing, Computer Vision, Pattern Recognition, and Graphics

Typesetting: Camera-ready by author, data conversion by Scientific Publishing Services, Chennai, India

Printed on acid-free paper

Springer is part of Springer Science+Business Media (www.springer.com)

Preface

WBIR 2014 was the sixth international Workshop on Biomedical Image Registration. It was held at University College London, UK, July 7–8, 2014. This scientific event aims to bring together leading researchers in the area of biomedical image registration to present and discuss recent developments in the field.

The previous workshops were held in Bled, Slovenia (1999), at the University of Pennsylvania, USA (2003), at the University Medical Center Utrecht, The Netherlands (2006), in Lubeck, Germany (2010), and at the University of Vanderbilt, Nashville, USA (2012).

The WBIR 2014 proceedings, published in the Lecture Notes in Computer Science series, contain the latest original research results selected through a rigorous peer-review process. Every full paper (8 to 10 pages in length) was reviewed in a double-blind process by three members of the international Program Committee, composed of 44 renowned scientists in the field of medical image registration. The result of this selection process is a set of 24 articles from 14 countries and 4 continents. A total of 16 papers were selected for oral presentation and 8 as posters, all presented during a single track oral and poster session.

The conference program has been greatly enhanced by our four invited speakers, Professors J. Ashburner (University College London, UK), D. Rueckert (Imperial College London, UK), and Doctors T. Kadir (Mirada Medical, UK), and Stéphane Nicolau (IRCAD, France). All four presented exciting state-of-the-art advances during their keynote lectures covering the main aspect of the scientific remit of our conference.

We warmly thank the members of our Program Committee and all the participants of the event, who made this conference an exciting place to share the latest discoveries in this fascinating research area.

July 2014   Sébastien Ourselin
                                                                             Marc Modat

Organization

The 6th International Workshop on Biomedical Image Registration (WBIR 2014) was organized at University College London

Conference Chairs

General Chair   Sébastien Ourselin, University College London, UK

Program Chair   Marc Modat, University College London, UK

Program Committee

Paul Aljabar	King's College London, UK
John Ashburner	University College London, UK
Brian Avants	University of Pennsylvania, USA
Nathan Cahill	Rochester Institute of Technology, USA
Gary Christensen	University of Iowa, USA
Olivier Commowick	Inria, France
Christos Davatzikos	University of Pennsylvania, USA
Benoit Dawant	Vanderbilt University, USA
Kai Ding	John Hopkins University, USA
Kaifang Du	UW Health, USA
Stanley Durlemann	Inria, France
James Gee	University of Pennsylvania, USA
Ben Glocker	Imperial College London, UK
Ali Gholipour	Boston Children's Hospital, USA
Mattias Heinrich	University of Lubeck, Germany
Joachim Hornegger	Friedrich-Alexander University Erlangen-Nuremberg, Germany
Stefan Klein	Erasmus MC, The Netherlands
Sebastien Kurtek	The Ohio State University, USA
Marco Lorenzi	Inria, France
Matthew McCormick	Kitware Inc., USA
Jan Modersitski	University of Lubeck, Germany
Kensaku Mori	Nagoya University, Japan
Nassir Navab	Technische Universität München, Germany
Wiro Niessen	Erasmus MC, The Netherlands
Nikos Paragios	Ecole Centrale Paris, France
Xavier Pennec	Inria, France

Fanjo Pernus   University of Ljubljana, Slovenia
Josien Pluim   University Medical Center Utrecht,
                                    The Netherlands
Kilian Pohl   University of Pennsylvania, USA
Joseph Reinhardt   University of Iowa, USA
Torsten Rohlfing   SRI International, USA
Karl Rohr   University of Heidelberg, Germany
Daniel Rueckert   Imperial College London, UK
Julia Schnabel   University of Oxford, UK
Benoit Scherrer   Boston Children's Hospital, USA
Dinggang Shen   The University of North Carolina at
                                    Chapel Hill, USA
Ivor Simpson   University College London, UK
Stefan Sommer   University of Copenhagen, Denmark
Anuj Srivastava   Florida State University, USA
Colin Studholme   University of Washington, USA
Maxime Taquet   Université catholique de Louvain, Belgium
Simon Warfield   Boston Children's Hospital, USA
William Wells   Harvard Medical School and Brigham and
                                    Women's Hospital, USA
Gary Zhang   University College London, UK

Table of Contents

Reconstruction

Interventional Application

Application Specific Measures of Similarity

Poster Session

Fast, Simple, Accurate Multi-atlas Segmentation of the Brain

Sean Murphy[1], Brian Mohr[1], Yasutaka Fushimi[2],
Hitoshi Yamagata[3], and Ian Poole[1]

[1] Toshiba Medical Visualization Systems Europe,
2 Anderson Pl, Edinburgh, EH6 5NP, UK
bmohr@tmvse.com
[2] Department of Diagnostic Imaging and Nuclear Medicine, Kyoto University
Graduate School of Medicine, 54 Shogoin Kawaharacho,
Sakyoku, Kyoto, 606-8507, Japan
[3] Toshiba Medical Systems Corporation,
1385 Shimoishigami, Otawara, 324-8550, Japan

Abstract. We are concerned with the segmentation of structures within the brain particularly the gyri of the cerebral cortex, but also subcortical structures from volumetric T1-weighted MRI images. A fully automatic multi-atlas registration based segmentation approach is used to label novel data. We use a standard affine registration method combined with a small deformation (non-diffeomorphic), non-linear registration method which optimises mutual information, with a cascading set of regularisation parameters. We consistently segment 138 structures in the brain, 98 in the cortex and 40 in the sub-cortex. An overall Dice score of 0.704 and a mean surface distance of 1.106 mm is achieved in leave-one-out cross validation using all available atlases. The algorithm has been evaluated on a number of different cohorts which includes patients of different ages and scanner manufacturers, and has been shown to be robust. It is shown to have comparable accuracy to other state of the art methods using the MICCAI 2012 multi-atlas challenge benchmark, but the runtime is substantially less.

1 Introduction

The aim of this work is to provide fully automated, accurate segmentation of the gyrus regions and substructures in T1 weighted images. Fully automatic segmentation has applications in visualisation, localisation of pathology, navigation, neurosurgery planning, radio-therapy planning and in understanding the morphometry and longitudinal changes of the brain, particularly with respect to neurological conditions like Alzheimer's, schizophrenia and Parkinson's [1,2,3].

The notion of a medical image atlas is introduced in [4]. The atlas can be decorated with a variety of extra information such as points, curves, structures and probabilistic maps. Most schemes for segmenting the brain are based on volumetric registration although a deformable surface model approach is used in [5,6]. Methods based on registration are dependent on the accuracy of that registration.

S. Ourselin and M. Modat (Eds.): WBIR 2014, LNCS 8545, pp. 1–10, 2014.
© Springer International Publishing Switzerland 2014

An extensive evaluation [7], compares the accuracy of 14 non-linear registration algorithms in the context of brain parcellation. The paper concluded that there is a modest correlation between the degrees of freedom of a registration method and its accuracy. It also found that the relative accuracy of methods appeared to be little affected by subject population, labelling protocol and accuracy measurement. This suggests (at least for the evaluated algorithms) that they will generalize well to unseen populations and protocols. The top entrants were SPM (Ashburner, University College London), ART (NITRC, Mass), IRTK (Rueckert, Imperial College London) and SyN (Avants, University of Pennsylvania).

For an example on how to combine segmentation and registration in one complete framework see [8]. This approach shows how to use the expectation maximization algorithm to determine the variance and mean of the MR signals in tissue types/compartments which incorporates priors from probabilistic masks.

In [9], Fischl constructs a probabilistic model of the position of each compartment in the brain. He also constructs a model of the MRI-signal which is assumed to be drawn from a Gaussian distribution where the parameters are free to vary from point to point. These models are constructed by data-mining many samples. The probabilistic model also includes a Markov Random Field component and is used to drive non-linear registration as in [8].

Multi-atlas methods involve performing multiple independent registrations and fusing the results together, typically using per pixel majority voting as discussed in [10]. Many variations on this theme exist. The STAPLE algorithm [11] shows how to solve the segmentation problem while simultaneously evaluating the accuracy of the different raters (atlases). For a comparison between state of the art multi-atlas segmentation techniques see the MICCAI 2012 challenge on multi-atlas labelling [12]. Techniques used included variations of the expectation maximisation algorithm, variations of the STAPLE algorithm, patch based label fusion, trained classification methods, different registration approaches including log domain diffeomorphic demons, spline based methods and dense deformation field methods. The winning entry from the University of Pennsylvania performed affine registration using FLIRT, followed by non-rigid registrtion using AIR of the novel image to all atlases, followed by a label fusion algorithm and a corrective learning approach using AdaBoost classifier with a mixture of spatial, appearance and contextual features within a 5 x 5 x 5 window [13]. In section 3, we numerically compare our technique to those in the challenge by evaluating on the same training and test sets.

In the following sections we describe our method in chronological order, followed by a results section which is broken into three subsections, followed by a conclusions section.

2   Method

We also propose a multi-atlas based solution. The algorithm is outlined in figure 1, with details given in the following sub-sections. We first affinely register all available atlases (27) by maximising mutual information (MI) over the set of rigid body transformations using simulated annealing at a reduced scale of 8, and then over a 9 parameter search space which includes axis aligned scales using Powell's method [14] at a scale of 4. A specified number of these atlases (possibly all atlases) are selected to proceed to the non-linear registration phase by performing hierarchical clustering on the resultant transformations and selecting the most consistent subset. The selection trades runtime for accuracy. The multi-scale non-linear registration phase optimises MI over the set of dense displacement fields by gradient descent, with a semi-numerical expression for the gradient. Finally the results from these atlases are used to construct a per compartment probability map which are used as priors in the expectation maximisation (EM) fitting of a per compartment Gaussian intensity model. The final segmentations are arrived at by maximum a posteriori (MAP) classification.

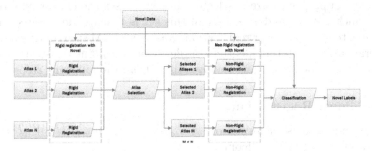

Fig. 1. Proposed workflow

2.1   Affine Registration

Affine registration between each atlas and the novel dataset is achieved by initially optimizing MI computed from a joint histogram using simulated annealing [15] over the class of rigid body transformations. The rotation is parameterised in terms of roll, pitch and yaw Euler angles around the center of the atlas volume. The novel and atlas volumes are both downscaled with anti-aliased smoothing by a factor of 8 prior to registration. The joint histogram is computed by sparsely sampling from the volumes. The transformation which aligns the center of the two volumes with no relative scaling or rotation is used to initialise the search. The simulated annealing optimizer has the effect of restarting in several locations, which avoids local minima and provides robustness. This is then followed by a search over the set of 9-parameter transformations which includes axis aligned scaling, using Powell's method at a reduced scale of 4.

2.2   Atlas Clustering

Clustering of the atlases with respect to the computed affine transformation is used to reduce the runtime of the algorithm by reducing the number of non-linear registrations to atlas volumes. Our method requires that a number of anatomical landmarks are manually marked on the *atlas* datasets. The novel volume is affinely registered to all atlas volumes. The distance metric $d(A, B)$ for atlases A and B is defined in 1, as the sum of the distances between corresponding landmarks.

$\|\cdot\|$ is the Euclidean norm, T_A and T_B are the affine transformations to the novel image

$$d(A, B) = \sum_i \|T_A(\mathbf{x}_{A,i}) - T_B(\mathbf{x}_{B,i}))\| \quad (1)$$

from atlas A and B respectively, and $\mathbf{x}_{A,i}$ and $\mathbf{x}_{B,i}$ are the positions of predetermined anatomical landmarks, indexed by i, in atlases A and B respectively. In this way the pre-defined landmark positions $\mathbf{x}_i$, which have been identified offline by a clinician, are transformed to the novel coordinate system using the affine transformation T for each atlas.

The distance metric is used to populate a square matrix with dimensions of the number of atlases (in this case 28). Hierarchical clustering, [16], is used to identify the atlases which perform consistent registrations. The most consistent cluster of the appropriate size is selected. In some cases the cluster may be too large, in which case a random subset of this set is taken. The selected atlases will continue to the non-linear registration, voting, and EM steps outlined below. Thus overall, atlas clustering identifies outliers from the affine registration stage, presumes these to be errors, and removes them from the following steps.

2.3   Non-linear Registration

This stage finds a dense deformation field W (not necessarily diffeomorphic), parameterised as vectors on a Cartesian grid, which maximises (locally)

$$W = \arg\max_{W'} \text{MI}(R, W'[T]) \quad (2)$$

the MI between the floating volume T and the reference R. The deformation-field is initialised from the affine phase and evolved to convergence, using a gradient ascent optimiser, with the deformation-field at iteration i given by:

$$W_{i+1} = E * (W_i + kV * F_i) \quad (3)$$

$$F = \frac{\partial \text{MI}(R, W[T])}{\partial W} \quad (4)$$

Convolution kernels V and E enforce the viscous fluid and elastic constraints, respectively; both modelled by Gaussian filters ($*$ is the convolution operator). F_i is the current force-field, calculated as the multivariate derivative of the MI with respect to the components of the deformation at each point as described in [17]. k is a free constant which controls the rate of ascent. It is beneficial to use a decreasing cascade of k's and of fluid regularisation parameters. Both these parameters are reduced geometrically when temporary convergence of MI is detected, with a lower bound on the fluid regularisation.

The non-linear registration algorithm is multi-scale where results from lower scales are used as the input to finer scales. The down scale factors used here are 4, 2 and 1. For this application, no elastic constraints are used. The registration is restricted to the domain of the brain in the atlas dataset dilated by 5 voxels.

2.4   Expectation-Maximization (EM)

The T1 weighted signal of each voxel x, in a given compartment, c, is assumed to be drawn from a Gaussian distribution: $P(x|c) = \mathcal{N}(x|\mu_c, \sigma_c^2)$. The parameters of each Gaussian distribution, the mean μ_c and variance σ_c^2, are unknown.

The compartment/class, c, of each voxel is also unknown and is modelled as a per voxel distribution $\rho_{c,i} = p(c|i, x)$ where i denotes the voxel. The Gaussian parameters and voxel classifications can be estimated by maximizing the joint probability density function of the entire image, using the EM algorithm [18] with sufficient independency assumptions. This iterative algorithm uses gradient descent to converge to a locally maximal configuration. The votes from each of the atlases can be used to inform this process as in [19,20], by constructing a probability mask for each compartment which takes the form of a prior $p(c|i)$. The variables in the algorithm at iteration t are denoted as $\rho_{c,i}^{(t)}$, $\mu_c^{(t)}$ and $\sigma_c^{2(t)}$. In this scheme background is also included as a class.

$$\rho_{c,i}^{(0)} = p(c|i) \tag{5}$$

$$\mu_c^{(t)} = \frac{\sum_i x_i \rho_{c,i}^{(t)}}{\sum_i \rho_{c,i}^{(t)}} \tag{7}$$

$$\rho_{c,i}^{(t+1)} = \frac{\mathcal{N}(x_i|\mu_c^{(t)}, \sigma_c^{2(t)})p(c|i)}{\sum_c \mathcal{N}(x_i|\mu_c^{(t)}, \sigma_c^{2(t)})p(c|i)} \tag{6}$$

$$\sigma_c^{2(t)} = \frac{\sum_i (x_i - \mu_c^{(t)})^2 \rho_{c,i}^{(t)}}{\sum_i \rho_{c,i}^{(t)}} \tag{8}$$

3 Results

The method has been evaluated in three ways. Firstly, on a unaltered subset of the OASIS database as discussed in section 3.1, using a leave one out strategy. Secondly, on data derived from the MICCAI multi-atlas labelling challenge, using a classic training/test split in section 3.2. Evaluating on this group allows for a like for like comparison to other entrants in the challenge. Thirdly, the results have been qualitatively evaluated on a broad range of private T1 weighted images from different cohorts, scanner manufacturers and geographic locations as discussed in 3.3.

Table 1. Top: 98 detected cortical structures. Middle: 40 detected subcortical structure. Bottom: 12 annotated anatomical landmarks. All identifiers have a left and right variant with the exception of those marked with *.

inferior temporal gyrus	cuneus	postcentral gyrus
superior parietal lobule	precuneus	frontal operculum
superior occipital gyrus	gyrus rectus	central operculum
occipital fusiform gyrus	frontal pole	parietal operculum
inferior occipital gyrus	temporal pole	supramarginal gyrus
anterior cingulate gyrus	planum polare	medial orbital gyrus
transverse temporal gyrus	lingual gyrus	middle frontal gyrus
posterior cingulate gyrus	angular gyrus	parahippocampal gyrus
supplementary motor cortex	occipital pole	middle temporal gyrus
precentral gyrus medial segment	fusiform gyrus	medial frontal cortex
postcentral gyrus medial segment	entorhinal area	lateral orbital gyrus
superior frontal gyrus medial segment	anterior insula	superior frontal gyrus
orbital part of the inferior frontal gyrus	subcallosal area	middle occipital gyrus
opercular part of the inferior frontal gyrus	planum temporale	middle cingulate gyrus
triangular part of the inferior frontal gyrus	precentral gyrus	anterior orbital gyrus
	posterior insula	superior temporal gyrus
	calcarine cortex	posterior orbital gyrus

Lateral Ventricle	CSF*	Hippocampus
Cerebral Exterior	Vessel	Optic Chiasm*
Cerebellum Exterior	Putamen	Inf Lat Vent
Cerebral White Matter	Caudate	4th Ventricle*
Cerebellum White Matter	Pallidum	3rd Ventricle*
Cerebellar Vermal Lobules I-V*	Amygdala	Accumbens Area
Cerebellar Vermal Lobules VIII-X*	Ventral DC	Basal Forebrain
Cerebellar Vermal Lobules VI-VII*	Brain Stem*	Thalamus Proper

Frontal Horn of the Lateral Ventricle	Floor of the Maxillary Sinus	Pineal Gland*
Optic Nerve Attachment Point	Pituitary Gland (Base)*	
Superior Aspect of Eye Globe	Centre of Eye Globe	

3.1   OASIS

28 datasets were manually segmented from the OASIS database [21] by Neuro-morphometrics (NMM)[1]. The patients range in age from 30 to 96, with approximately four patients from each decade: 12 male and 16 female. The patients are all right-handed. NMM clinicians have annotated 138 structures in all. A complete list of the cortical and subcortical regions defined can be found in table 1. Each dataset was additionally annotated with up to 12 key anatomical landmarks as specified in 1. These are not detected in the novel dataset, but are used during the clustering stage. The OASIS volumes have been anonymised digitally by removing the face, and the signal to noise ratio has been improved by averaging together several repeated scans. Not every structure has been labelled in every dataset because it may not have been present.

We performed a leave-one-out cross validation and evaluated two accuracy metrics: Dice coefficient, see 9, and mean surface distance in millimetres, see 10.

$$\frac{2|X \cap Y|}{|X| + |Y|} \quad (9) \qquad\qquad \frac{1}{|S_X|} \sum_{i \in S_X} \arg\min_{j \in S_Y} \|i - j\| \quad (10)$$

$\|\cdot\|$ is the Euclidean norm. X and Y are the ground truth and generated segmentations, respectively, and S_X and S_Y the corresponding set of points on the surface of these. Table 2 shows the mean over all compartments and all volumes, for both of these statistics. Structures which are not present in the ground truth in all datasets do not contribute to the average Dice or surface distance as in [12]. Figure 2 shows the effect of the number of atlases used on the accuracy.

Table 2. Mean Dice and mean surface distance for 28 oasis datasets for all structures, for the cortex and for the non-cortex

	Overall	Cortical	Non-Cortical
Mean Dice	0.704	0.689	0.745
Surface Distance (mm)	1.094	1.119	1.026

3.2   MICCAI Multi-atlas Labelling Challenge

A separate set of 35 datasets were manually segmented from the OASIS database [21] by NMM for the purpose of the challenge. The patients ranged in age from 18 to 90. 15 datasets were used for training and the remaining 20 were used for testing. These volumes were pre-processed using bias-field correction and aligned manually to the AC-PC axis using translation and rotation. Because of this, the initial affine registration problem is somewhat easier than might be expected on truly novel data. A more realistic representation of the expected score can be seen on the pure OASIS dataset in section 3.1. Nonetheless, this set is interesting because it was used in the MICCAI multi-atlas labelling challenge [12]. Held in 2012, this challenge made the training set available and invited entrants to submit their methods and results to be independently evaluated on the test

---

[1] http://www.neuromorphometrics.com/

Table 3. The results of the MICCAI multi-atlas segmentation challenge [12]. Shown is the mean overall Dice, the mean Dice in the cortical areas, the mean Dice in the non-cortical areas and also estimated runtimes. The score and ranking of our method (TMVSE_BGM) was retrospectively calculated and is shown in the table in bold.

Overall Rank	Team Name	Reg Method	Mean Dice Overall	Mean Dice Cortical	Mean Dice Non-Cortical	Runtime Estimate (mins)
1	PICSL_BC	*ANTS*	0.7654	0.7388	0.8377	> 1200
2	NonLocalSTAPLE	*ANTS*	0.7581	0.7318	0.8296	> 1200
3	MALP_EM	*Nifti-Seg*	0.7576	0.7328	0.8252	> 50 (5 on GPU)
4	PICSL_Joint	*ANTS*	0.7499	0.7216	0.8271	> 1200
5	MAPER	*Nifti-Seg*	0.7413	0.7144	0.8144	> 50 (5 on GPU)
6	STEPS	*Nifti-Seg*	0.7372	0.7107	0.8095	> 50 (5 on GPU)
7	SpatialSTAPLE	*ANTS*	0.7372	0.7093	0.8130	> 1200
8	CIS_JHU	*LDDMM*	0.7357	0.7131	0.7971	10 - 450
8.5	**TMVSE_BGM**		**0.7346**	**0.7183**	**0.7807**	**> 5**
9	CRL_Weighted_STAPLE_ ANTS+Baloo	*ANTS*	0.7344	0.7122	0.7950	> 1200
10	CRL_Weighted_STAPLE_ ANTS	*ANTS*	0.7308	0.7066	0.7966	> 1200
11	CRL_STAPLE_ANTS+Baloo	*ANTS*	0.7290	0.7064	0.7919	> 1200
12	CRL_STAPLE_ANTS	*ANTS*	0.7280	0.7033	0.7951	> 1200
13	CRL_Probabilistic_STAPLE_ANTS+Baloo	*ANTS*	0.7251	0.7009	0.7911	> 1200
14	CRL_MV_ANTS+Baloo	*ANTS*	0.7247	0.6966	0.8012	> 1200
15	CRL_MV_ANTS	*ANTS*	0.7243	0.6951	0.8035	> 1200
16	DISPATCH	*Nifti-Seg*	0.7243	0.6965	0.8000	> 50 (5 on GPU)
17	CRL_Probabilistic_STAPLE_ANTS	*ANTS*	0.7223	0.6972	0.7907	> 1200
18	SBIA_SimRank+NormMS+WtROI	*DRAMMS*	0.7212	0.6940	0.7953	> 240
19	SBIA_BrainROIMaps_MV_IntCorr	*DRAMMS*	0.7193	0.6933	0.7904	> 240
20	SBIA_BrainROIMaps_JaccDet_IntCorr	*DRAMMS*	0.7186	0.6913	0.7927	> 240
21	BIC-IPL-HR	*ANIMAL*	0.7173	0.6888	0.7948	> 168
22	SBIA_SimMSVoting	*DRAMMS*	0.7172	0.6898	0.7918	> 240
23	UNC-NIRAL	*ANTS*	0.7171	0.6869	0.7992	> 1200
24	SBIA_SimRank+NormMS	*DRAMMS*	0.7162	0.6884	0.7919	> 240
25	BIC-IPL	*ANIMAL*	0.7107	0.6829	0.7864	> 168

set. Since all methods were trained and evaluated on the same set, it provided a rare opportunity for the quantitative comparison between various methods. We have retrospectively trained and tested on this data in the same way. The results in table 3 show that are results are comparable to the state of the art in the field. The average Dice was calculated as described in section 3.1. The runtimes per registration are estimated from the specified registration methods cited in [12]. The methods used were "Nifty-Seg", see [22] which reported approximately 3.3 minutes on the CPU, or 20 seconds on a GPU, "ANTS-SyN" [23] which is reported to have runtimes in the order of 80 minutes[7], "DRAMMS" which reports to have a runtime of approximately 20% of ANTS (16 minutes) in [24], "LDDMM" which is reported to have a runtime in the range 40 secs to 30 minutes, on a high end server, depending on required accuracy [25] and "ANIMAL" with a reported time of 11.2 minutes. TMVSE registration (CPU based) has a runtime of 20 seconds on architecture comparable to that specified in [7]. Since all registrations are independent, multiplying by 15 gives the estimated runtime.

3.3 Subjective Evaluation

The results on 90 other T1 MR brain datasets have also informally examined. These datasets had no pre-processing applied to them and are representative of what might be expected when the method is applied to novel data. The

Fig. 2. The average dice achieved as a function of the number of atlases used, for both the random and clustering strategy. For the random strategy, the requested number of atlases are chosen at random. For the clustering strategy the most consistent cluster of atlases of the requested size are used.

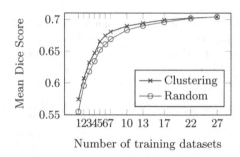

Number of training datasets

datasets covered a range of different cohorts, acquisition parameters, acquisition directions, slice spacing, venders (Siemens, GE, Philips and Toshiba), resolutions, ages, pathologies and geographic locations. No major failure cases were reported, which suggests a robustness of the affine registration phase. In one case, a volume was segmented correctly even though only the left side of the patients head was present in the volume. Subjectively, the method appears to perform better on high resolution data. Examples of these results can be seen in figure 3.

It has been reported that the location of structures are mostly correct although there are often multiple errors per patient, which is typical of other competing approaches. Both under and over segmentation is observed. Segmentations are often noisy, although this can be corrected by post-processing. The multi-atlas approach boosts overall classification/Dice accuracy but it can sometimes come at the cost of unrealistic resultant segmentation shapes. Structures that are topologically inconsistent (not simply connected) with the ground truth have been observed in some cases. The method makes no explicit provision for pathological tissue types. When presented with pathology the method will label it as one (or more) of the known nearby compartments. This has been observed in at least one patient which a large tumour.

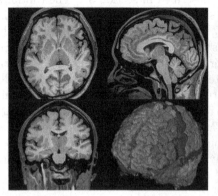
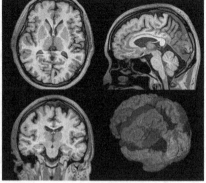

Fig. 3. 2 fully automatic results. 3D T1 Weighted images. Acquired: August 2012 on Toshiba's Titan 3T scanner, Kyoto. Resolution: 512×512. Voxel size: $0.49mm \times 0.49mm \times 0.6mm$.

4 Conclusions

A fast and simple method for segmenting structures in the brain is presented. The speed comes from its algorithmic simplicity. The cost of this simplicity is a loss in some advantageous properties that are afforded by the more complex methods like LDDMM and ANTS such as **a)** guaranteed, efficient invertibility, **b)** symmetry: invariance to the order of source and target or **c)** the natural emergence of a mathematical metric and associated space. However it seems that this simplicity does not imply low segmentation accuracy in a multi-atlas setting as shown by the comparable performance to other state-of the art techniques. The simplicity translates to favourable runtimes, with the next fastest CPU based non-rigid registration method in the MICCAI challenge taking an estimated 10 times longer which is useful for time critical applications such as image-guided intervention or for processing large numbers of datasets. We acknowledge that these are rough runtime estimates since they were not directly measured and had to be inferred, but they serve as reasonable order of magnitude estimates. We also acknowledge that our results are retrospective, having had time to optimize performance with sight of other methods and results from the challenge.

Acknowledgements. The authors would like to acknowledge Neuromorphometrics contribution to the project in the form of fully annotated datasets. We would also like to thank the commitee and entrants of the MICCAI 2012 grand challenge on multi-atlas labeling.

References

1. Petrella, J.R., Coleman, R.E., Doraiswamy, P.M.: Neuroimaging and early diagnosis of Alzheimer disease: a look to the future. Radiology 226, 315–336 (2003)
2. Andreasen, N.C., Olsen, S.A., Dennert, J.W., Smith, M.R.: Ventricular enlargement in schizophrenia: relationship to positive and negative symptoms. The American Journal of Psychiatry 139, 297–302 (1982)
3. Hutchinson, M., Raff, U.: Structural Changes of the Substantia Nigra in Parkinson's Disease as Revealed by MR Imaging. Imaging 21, 697–701 (2000)
4. Mazziotta, J., Toga, A., Evans, A., Fox, P., Lancaster, J.: A probabilistic atlas of the human brain: theory and rationale for its development the international consortium for brain mapping (ICBM). Neuroimage 2(2PA), 89–101 (1995)
5. MacDonald, D., Kabani, N., Avis, D., Evans, A.C.: Automated 3-D extraction of inner and outer surfaces of cerebral cortex from MRI. NeuroImage 12(3), 340–356 (2000)
6. Patenaude, B., Smith, S.M., Kennedy, D.N., Jenkinson, M.: A Bayesian model of shape and appearance for subcortical brain segmentation. NeuroImage 56(3), 907–922 (2011)
7. Klein, A., Andersson, J., Ardekani, B., Ashburner, J., et al.: Evaluation of 14 nonlinear deformation algorithms applied to human brain MRI registration. NeuroImage 46(3), 786–802 (2009)
8. Ashburner, J., Friston, K.: Multimodal image coregistration and partitioning–a unified framework. NeuroImage 6(3), 209–217 (1997)

9. Fischl, B.: Automatically Parcellating the Human Cerebral Cortex. Cerebral Cortex 14(1), 11–22 (2004)
10. Rohlfing, T., Brandt, R., Menzel, R., Maurer, C.R.: Evaluation of atlas selection strategies for atlas-based image segmentation with application to confocal microscopy images of bee brains. NeuroImage 21, 1428–1442 (2004)
11. Warfield, S.K., Zou, K.H., Wells, W.M.: Simultaneous Truth and Performance Level Estimation (STAPLE): An Algorithm for the Validation of Image Segmentation 23(7), 903–921 (2004)
12. Landman, B., Warfield, S.: MICCAI 2012 workshop on multi-atlas labeling.. Challenge and Workshop on Multi-Atlas Labeling . . . (2012)
13. Wang, H., Das, S.R., Suh, J.W., Altinay, M., Pluta, J., Craige, C., Avants, B., Yushkevich, P.A.: A learning-based wrapper method to correct systematic errors in automatic image segmentation: consistently improved performance in hippocampus, cortex and brain segmentation. NeuroImage 55(3), 968–985 (2011)
14. Powell, M.: An efficient method for finding the minimum of a function of several variables without calculating derivatives. The Computer Journal 7(2), 155 (1964)
15. Kirkpatrick, S., Gelatt, C.D., Vecchi, M.P.: Optimization by simulated annealing. Science 220, 671–680 (1983)
16. Ward Jr., J.H.: Hierarchical grouping to optimize an objective function. Journal of the American Statistical Association (1963)
17. Crum, W.R., Hill, D.L.G., Hawkes, D.J.: Information theoretic similarity measures in non-rigid registration. In: Taylor, C.J., Noble, J.A. (eds.) IPMI 2003. LNCS, vol. 2732, pp. 378–387. Springer, Heidelberg (2003)
18. Moon, T.: The expectation-maximization algorithm. IEEE Signal Processing Magazine 13 (1996)
19. Ashburner, J., Friston, K.J.: Unified segmentation. NeuroImage 26, 839–851 (2005)
20. Murgasova, M., Rueckert, D., Edwards, D., Hajnal, J.: Robust segmentation of brain structures in MRI. In: 2009 IEEE International Symposium on Biomedical Imaging: From Nano to Macro (1), pp. 17–20 (June 2009)
21. Marcus, D.S., Wang, T.H., Parker, J., Csernansky, J.G., Morris, J.C., Buckner, R.L.: Open Access Series of Imaging Studies (OASIS): cross-sectional MRI data in young, middle aged, nondemented, and demented older adults. Journal of Cognitive Neuroscience 19(9), 1498–1507 (2007)
22. Modat, M., Ridgway, G.R., Taylor, Z.A., Lehmann, M., Barnes, J., Hawkes, D.J., Fox, N.C., Ourselin, S.: Fast free-form deformation using graphics processing units. Computer Methods and Programs in Biomedicine 98(3), 278–284 (2010)
23. Avants, B., Tustison, N., Song, G., Cook, P.: A reproducible evaluation of ANTs similarity metric performance in brain image registration. Neuroimage 54(3), 2033–2044 (2011)
24. Ou, Y., Ye, D.H., Pohl, K.M., Davatzikos, C.: Validation of DRAMMS among 12 popular methods in cross-subject cardiac MRI registration. In: Dawant, B.M., Christensen, G.E., Fitzpatrick, J.M., Rueckert, D. (eds.) WBIR 2012. LNCS, vol. 7359, pp. 209–219. Springer, Heidelberg (2012)
25. Ceritoglu, C., Tang, X., Chow, M., Hadjiabadi, D., Shah, D., Brown, T., Burhanullah, M.H., Trinh, H., Hsu, J.T., Ament, K.A., Crocetti, D., Mori, S., Mostofsky, S.H., Yantis, S., Miller, M.I., Ratnanather, J.T.: Computational analysis of LDDMM for brain mapping. Frontiers in Neuroscience 7, 151 (2013)

Fast Multidimensional B-spline Interpolation Using Template Metaprogramming

Wyke Huizinga[1], Stefan Klein[1], and Dirk H.J. Poot[1,2]

[1] Biomedical Imaging Group Rotterdam, Depts. of Radiology & Medical Informatics,
Erasmus MC, Rotterdam, The Netherlands
[2] Quantitative Imaging Group, Dept. of Imaging Physics,
Faculty of Applied Sciences, Delft University of Technology, Delft, The Netherlands

Abstract. B-spline interpolation is a widely used interpolation technique. In the field of image registration, interpolation is necessary for transforming images to obtain a measure of (dis)similarity between the images to be aligned. When gradient-based optimization methods are used, the image gradients need to be calculated as well, which also accounts for a substantial share of computation time in registration. In this paper we propose a fast multidimensional B-spline interpolation algorithm with which both image value and gradient can be computed efficiently. We present a recursive algorithm for the interpolation which is efficiently implemented with template metaprogramming (TMP). The proposed algorithm is compared with the algorithm implemented in the Insight Toolkit (ITK), for different interpolation orders and image dimensions. Also, the effect on the computation time of a typical registration problem is evaluated. The results show that the computation time of B-spline interpolation is decreased by the proposed algorithm from a factor 4.1 for a 2D image using 1st order interpolation to a factor of 19.9 for 4D using 3rd order interpolation.

Keywords: B-spline interpolation, template metaprogramming, computation time, image registration.

1 Introduction

Due to the discrete nature of images that are stored in a computer, interpolation is necessary for calculating intensity values of points that are off the voxel grid. During image registration, iteratively many points are interpolated. Besides the interpolation of points, the gradient of the image is also required when a gradient-based optimization method is used [1]. The computation time of an image registration procedure therefore strongly depends on the efficiency of the interpolation algorithm.

A widely used interpolation technique is B-spline interpolation. We propose an algorithm for B-spline interpolation and gradient evaluation. In our work we exploit the separability of the B-spline polynomial, which was shown by [2], and derive a recursive algorithm for interpolation in images of any dimension. The

S. Ourselin and M. Modat (Eds.): WBIR 2014, LNCS 8545, pp. 11–20, 2014.

proposed method is effectively implemented using template metaprogramming (TMP). In TMP, templates are used to let the compiler generate efficient assembly code. Language features such as for loops and if-statements can be replaced by template specialization and recursion, allowing elimination of run-time flow control instructions [3]. The computation time and complexity of proposed algorithm was evaluated and compared to the B-spline interpolation algorithm that is used in ITK version 4.4.1.

A previously published method to speedup B-spline interpolation is based on creating an approximation of the B-spline weights in a look-up table [4]. Although we do not use this method, it is fully compatible and could be used to achieve even further speedup at the cost of introducing approximation errors. In this paper we propose a non-approximated B-spline interpolation algorithm, which is especially effective for multidimensional images (dimension ≥ 2).

In Section 2.1 a direct implementation of B-spline interpolation is shown and in Section 2.2 the recursive formulation is derived. Section 2.3 presents the extension to computing gradients. In Section 2.4 we explain how the recursive formulation is efficiently implemented with TMP. Section 2.5 compares the algorithmic complexity of the direct and the recursive implementation, Section 3 explains the experiments that are performed and Section 4 shows the results of these experiments. Finally we draw a conclusion in Section 5.

2   Method

All algorithms and equations in this paper are written using one-based counting, which means that the initial element of a sequence is assigned the index 1. Let $S_{\boldsymbol{k}}$ be a discrete image of dimension D, with $\boldsymbol{k}$ an integer index vector. B-spline interpolation for a point $\boldsymbol{x} \in \mathbb{R}^D$ is defined by [5]

$$s(\boldsymbol{x}) = \sum_{\boldsymbol{k} \in \boldsymbol{\mathcal{Z}}^n} \beta^n(\boldsymbol{x} - \boldsymbol{k}) c_{\boldsymbol{k}}, \tag{1}$$

where $s(\boldsymbol{x})$ is the interpolated intensity value, β^n is the B-spline polynomial of order n that is non-zero in support region $\boldsymbol{\mathcal{Z}}^n$ and $c_{\boldsymbol{k}}$ are the B-spline coefficients which are specified on the image grid. The multidimensional B-spline polynomial can be written as

$$\beta^n(\boldsymbol{x}) = \prod_{i=1}^{D} \beta^n(x_i). \tag{2}$$

The higher n, the larger $\boldsymbol{\mathcal{Z}}^n$ and generally, the higher the interpolation accuracy. The support region $\boldsymbol{\mathcal{Z}}^n$ is the set of $(n+1)^D$ points in the image grid that are taken into account in the interpolation at $\boldsymbol{x}$. The positions of these grid points depend on $\boldsymbol{x}$. Let $\mathcal{Z}_d^n$ be the region of support in dimension d, which is given by [5]

$$\mathcal{Z}_d^n = \left\{ \left\lceil x_d - \frac{n+1}{2} \right\rceil + i \right\} \text{ for } i \in \{0, \ldots, n\} \tag{3}$$

The B-spline coefficients $c_{\boldsymbol{k}}$ are defined such that $s(\boldsymbol{k}) = S_{\boldsymbol{k}}$ and they are precomputed by filtering $S_{\boldsymbol{k}}$ [5,1]. In this work the computation of the coefficients is not considered. We focus on the efficient evaluation of Eq. (1).

2.1   Direct Implementation

A direct implementation of Eq. (1) is given by

$$s(\boldsymbol{x}) = \sum_{k_1 \in \mathcal{Z}_1^n} \sum_{k_2 \in \mathcal{Z}_2^n} \cdots \sum_{k_D \in \mathcal{Z}_D^n} \left[\beta^n(x_1 - k_1)\beta^n(x_2 - k_2)\ldots\beta^n(x_D - k_D) \right] c_{\boldsymbol{k}}, \quad (4)$$

where in each dimension the sum runs over all elements in $\mathcal{Z}_d^n$. The part of Eq. (4) between the square brackets is computed before the multiplication with $c_{\boldsymbol{k}}$. Since each $\beta(x_i - k_i)$ is required many times (depending on D), probably all implementations first compute the $\beta^n(x_i - k_i)$ terms and store these into temporary variables, in order to quickly access these in the evaluation of the sum.

2.2   Recursive Implementation

From Eq. (4) one can immediately see that it can be rewritten into [2]:

$$s(\boldsymbol{x}) = \sum_{k_1 \in \mathcal{Z}_1^n} \beta^n(x_1 - k_1) \sum_{k_2 \in \mathcal{Z}_2^n} \beta^n(x_2 - k_2) \ldots \sum_{k_D \in \mathcal{Z}_D^n} \beta^n(x_D - k_D)c_{\boldsymbol{k}}. \quad (5)$$

To derive a recursive formulation of Eq. (5) we first change the notation of $c_{\boldsymbol{k}}$. The coefficients $c_{\boldsymbol{k}}$, which are accessed by a D-dimensional point $\boldsymbol{k}$, are vectorized into $\tilde{c}_\kappa$ with $\kappa = \boldsymbol{\alpha} \cdot \boldsymbol{k}$, where α_d contains the step in linear index κ due to a unit step in dimension d in the coefficient image $c_{\boldsymbol{k}}$. The recursive interpolation function $V(d, \boldsymbol{x}, \kappa)$ for dimension index d is given by:

$$V(d, \boldsymbol{x}, \kappa) = \begin{cases} \sum_{k_d \in \mathcal{Z}_d^n} \beta^n(x_d - k_d)V(d - 1, \boldsymbol{x}, \kappa + \alpha_d k_d) & \text{for } d \geq 1 \\ \tilde{c}_\kappa & \text{for } d = 0 \end{cases} \quad (6)$$

where the interpolated intensity value at $\boldsymbol{x}$ equals

$$s(\boldsymbol{x}) = V(D, \boldsymbol{x}, 0). \quad (7)$$

Pseudo-code implementing Eq. (6) is shown in Alg. 1(a).

2.3   Gradient Evaluation

Often, the image gradient is necessary in image registration methods. The gradient at a sampled point $s(\boldsymbol{x})$ is given by:

$$\nabla s(\boldsymbol{x}) = \begin{pmatrix} \partial s(\boldsymbol{x})/\partial x_1 \\ \partial s(\boldsymbol{x})/\partial x_2 \\ \vdots \\ \partial s(\boldsymbol{x})/\partial x_D \end{pmatrix} =$$

$$\begin{pmatrix} \sum_{k_1 \in \mathcal{Z}_1^n} \sum_{k_2 \in \mathcal{Z}_2^n} \cdots \sum_{k_D \in \mathcal{Z}_D^n} \frac{\partial \beta^n}{\partial x_1}(x_1 - k_1)\beta^n(x_2 - k_2)\ldots\beta^n(x_D - k_D)c_{\boldsymbol{k}} \\ \sum_{k_1 \in \mathcal{Z}_1^n} \sum_{k_2 \in \mathcal{Z}_2^n} \cdots \sum_{k_D \in \mathcal{Z}_D^n} \beta^n(x_1 - k_1)\frac{\partial \beta^n}{\partial x_2}(x_2 - k_2)\ldots\beta^n(x_D - k_D)c_{\boldsymbol{k}} \\ \vdots \\ \sum_{k_1 \in \mathcal{Z}_1^n} \sum_{k_2 \in \mathcal{Z}_2^n} \cdots \sum_{k_D \in \mathcal{Z}_D^n} \beta^n(x_1 - k_1)\beta^n(x_2 - k_2)\ldots\frac{\partial \beta^n}{\partial x_D}(x_D - k_D)c_{\boldsymbol{k}} \end{pmatrix}. \quad (8)$$

The partial derivative $\partial s/\partial x_i$ can be evaluated more efficiently by a recursive algorithm than evaluating all sums of $\partial s/\partial x_i$ explicitly. The recursive algorithm is given by:

$$G_i(d, \boldsymbol{x}, \kappa) = \begin{cases} \displaystyle\sum_{k_d \in \mathcal{Z}_d^n} \beta^n(x_d - k_d)G_i(d-1, \boldsymbol{x}, \kappa + \alpha_d k_d) & \text{for } d \geq 1 \text{ and } d \neq i \\ \displaystyle\sum_{k_d \in \mathcal{Z}_d^n} \frac{\partial\beta^n}{\partial x_d}(x_d - k_d)G_i(d-1, \boldsymbol{x}, \kappa + \alpha_d k_d) & \text{for } d = i \\ \tilde{c}_\kappa & \text{for } d = 0, \end{cases} \quad (9)$$

with

$$\frac{\partial s(\boldsymbol{x})}{\partial x_i} = G_i(D, \boldsymbol{x}, 0). \quad (10)$$

2.4 Efficient Implementation Using TMP

The recursive algorithm of Eq. (6) can be efficiently implemented using TMP. Both D and n are set as template arguments, causing the compiler to un-roll the

---

Algorithm 1. Pseudo code of recursive (a) and TMP implementation (b) of B-spline interpolation

---

(a) In the actual implementation, the B-spline weights $\beta^n(x_d - k_d)$ are precomputed and accessed in the INTERPOLATE function.

```
function V = INTERPOLATE(d, x, κ)
    if d == 0 then
        return c̃κ
    else
        V = 0
        for kd ∈ Zd^n do
            V = V + INTERPOLATE(d − 1, x, κ + αd kd)β^n(xd − kd)
        end for
        return V
    end if
end function

s(x) = INTERPOLATE(D, x, 0)
```

(b) In the actual implementation, the B-spline weights $\beta^n(x_d - k_d)$ are precomputed and accessed in the INTERPOLATE function.

```
template< d, n > class TMP
function V = INTERPOLATE(x, κ)
    V = 0
    for kd ∈ Zd do
        V = V + TMP< d − 1, n >::INTERPOLATE(x, κ + αd kd)β^n(xd − kd)
    end for
    return V
end function

//Template specialization for d = 0

template< n > class TMP< 0, n >
function V=INTERPOLATE(x, κ)
    return c̃κ
end function

s(x) = TMP< D, n >::INTERPOLATE(x, 0)
```

Algorithm 2. Pseudo code of TMP implementation that computes the value and gradient

In the actual implementation, the B-spline weights $\beta^n(x_d - k_d)$ and the B-spline derivative weights $\frac{\partial \beta^n}{\partial x_d}(x_d - k_d)$ are precomputed and accessed in the INTERPOLATE function.

```
template< d, n > class TMP
function [V, G] = INTERPOLATE(x, κ)
    V = 0
    G = 0_d //Zero vector of size d
    for k_d ∈ Z_d^n do
        Ṽ, G̃ = TMP< d − 1, n >::INTERPOLATE(x, κ + α_d k_d)
        V = V + Ṽ β^n (x_d − k_d)
        for i = 1 to d − 1 do
            G_i = G_i + G̃_i β^n (x_d − k_d)
        end for
        G_d = G_d + Ṽ (∂β^n/∂x_d)(x_d − x_k)
    end for
    return V, G
end function

//Template specialization for d = 0

template< n > class TMP< 0, n >
function [V, G] = INTERPOLATE(x, κ)
    V = c̃_κ
    G = [] //A vector of length 0
    return V, G
end function
```

$$s(\boldsymbol{x}), \nabla s(\boldsymbol{x}) = \text{TMP}< D, n >::\text{INTERPOLATE}(\boldsymbol{x}, 0)$$

---

entire weighted sum for the relatively low n and D, which are typically encountered in image interpolation. This leads to efficient assembly code and reduced run-time of the interpolation algorithm. Alg. 1(b) shows the TMP implementation of the recursive formulation in Eq. (6).

A TMP implementation for calculation both the value and the gradient is presented in Alg. 2. For efficient implementation of Eq. (9) one should note that $G_i(d, \boldsymbol{x}, \kappa)$ is identical for all $i > d$, and thus only needs to be evaluated once for all $i > d$, allowing a reduction in computational complexity. Also note, by comparing to Eq. (6), that $V(d, \boldsymbol{x}, \kappa)$ for $i > d$ is equivalent to $G_i(d, \boldsymbol{x}, \kappa)$ and thus $s(\boldsymbol{x}) = G_i(D, \boldsymbol{x}, 0)$ for $i \geq D + 1$. Therefore, by simultaneously evaluating the value and gradient, the intermediate values $V(d, \boldsymbol{x}, \kappa)$ can be used instead of $G_i(d, \boldsymbol{x}, \kappa)$ for $i > d$, as shown in Alg. 2.

The proposed algorithm thus consists in the combination of 1) the recursive algorithm that reduces the number of arithmetic operations, and 2) the efficient implementation using TMP. Note that our actual implementation differs slightly from Alg. 2 to handle edge cases identical to the ITK reference algorithm, by precomputing $\alpha_d k_d$ for all $k_d \in \mathcal{Z}_d^n$ with $d \in \{1, \ldots, D\}$ and adjusting this for the edge cases.

2.5   Complexity Analysis

The reference algorithm with which the proposed algorithm is compared is the algorithm which is used in ITK version 4.4.1. This algorithm uses the direct implementation, see Sec. 2.1. A way to compare the computational complexity irrespective of the actual implementation is by counting the number of arithmetic operations, that is the floating point additions and multiplications.

The reference algorithm (Eq. (4)) sums over $\mathbf{Z}^n$, consisting of $(n+1)^D$ points. In this sum are $D+2$ arithmetic operations. Thus, the number of arithmetic operations is given by:

$$A_V^{\text{ref}}(D,n) = (n+1)^D \left[D+2\right] \tag{11}$$

where the superscript 'ref' indicates the reference algorithm and the subscript V indicates the evaluation of the value. As the proposed algorithm is recursive, the number of arithmetic operations for the proposed algorithm can most easily be counted with a similar recursion. The recursive algorithm sums over $\mathbf{Z}_d^n$, consisting of $n+1$ points. In this sum, there are 2 arithmetic operations and the recursion, in which D is reduced by 1. Therefore, the number of arithmetic operations equals:

$$A_V^{\text{prop}}(D,n) = \begin{cases} (n+1)\left[2 + A_V^{\text{prop}}(D-1,n)\right] & \text{for } D \geq 1 \\ 0 & \text{for } D = 0, \end{cases}$$
$$= \frac{(n+1)\left[2(n+1)^D - 2\right]}{n}. \tag{12}$$

In big-O notation the complexity can be expressed as $A_V^{\text{ref}}(D,n) \in O(Dn^D)$ and $A_V^{\text{prop}}(D,n) \in O(n^D)$. The reference method for computing both the value and the gradient performs all operations D times (once for each element of the gradient). Within the sum over $\mathbf{Z}^n$, a sum over all dimensions is included with a conditional for multiplying with either $\beta^n(x_d - k_d)$ or with $\frac{\partial \beta^n}{\partial x_d}(x_d - k_d)$. The number of arithmetic operations as a function of D and n for the reference algorithm evaluating the value and gradient is equal to:

$$A_{VG}^{\text{ref}}(D,n) = D(n+1)^D \left[D+3\right]. \tag{13}$$

For the proposed algorithm computing both value and gradient, the sum over $\mathbf{Z}_d^n$ includes $2D+2$ arithmetic operations and the recursion. Therefore, the number of arithmetic operations of the proposed algorithm is equal to:

$$A_{VG}^{\text{prop}}(D,n) = \begin{cases} (n+1)\left[2D + 2 + A_{VG}^{\text{prop}}(D-1,n)\right] & \text{for } D \geq 1 \\ 0 & \text{for } D = 0, \end{cases}$$
$$= \frac{2(n+1)\left[(2n+1)(n+1)^D - n(D+2) - 1\right]}{n^2}. \tag{14}$$

In big-O notation the complexity can be expressed as: $A_{VG}^{\text{ref}}(D,n) \in O(D^2 n^D)$ and $A_{VG}^{\text{prop}}(D,n) \in O(n^D)$.

3   Experiments

Three experiments are performed to compare both the interpolated values and computation times of the reference and proposed algorithm. The three experiments are:

1. Evaluating the difference between both algorithms after interpolation and gradient calculation of an image to validate the accuracy of the recursive algorithm.
2. Computing the ratio of the computational complexity and run-time of both algorithms using value and gradient calculation for different image dimensions D and interpolation orders n.
3. Computing the run-time of an image registration using both algorithms for different interpolation orders.

For the first experiment a 2D standard normal distributed noise image of size 100 in each dimension is interpolated after a rotation of 10 degrees. To evaluate the accuracy of the recursive algorithm the root-mean-square difference (RMSD) of the resulting interpolated images and the gradient magnitude images are reported.

For the second experiment, standard normal distributed noise images of size 100 in each dimension are created. In each measurement the image is rotated around a predefined axis and translated in the direction of the axis of rotation. Each timing measurement is repeated 35 times, in which the rotation angle is changed from $10°$ to $350°$ in steps of $10°$ and the translation is kept constant at half a voxel in the direction of the axis of rotation. The mean and standard deviation of these measurements are calculated. The output image was interpolated on a grid of size 50 in each dimension with identical voxel spacing, centered on the original image, to avoid boundary effects. Before measuring the computation times, 10 dummy transformations are applied to the image to reach a steady state prior to evaluating the computation times and prevent loading data and filling the cache memory from taking part in the computation time evaluation.

For the third experiment two 3D CT lung images images are registered. The fixed image was of size $115\times157\times129$ and the moving image was of size $115\times166\times131$. The voxel spacing of both images was $1.4\times1.4\times2.5$ mm^3. The registrations were performed with Elastix, an open source image registration package based on ITK [6]. In this registration experiment, in which the images where affinely registered, an adaptive stochastic gradient descent optimizer [7] was used. The default settings for an affine registration were used: four resolutions, 250 iterations per resolution and 2048 samples per iteration. A mean squared difference measure was used as a dissimilarity measure. For each algorithm and for each interpolation order the registration was repeated 50 times to obtain a mean and standard deviation of the run time. Before measuring, one dummy registration was performed.

All experiments were performed on an Intel®Core™2.7 GHz CPU under a Ubuntu 12.04 64-bit operating system. The used compiler was the GNU Compiler Collection (GCC) version 4.6.3.

4 Results

The RMSD of the interpolated 2D noise image was equal to $2.34 \cdot 10^{-16}$. The RMSD of the gradient magnitude difference was $4.08 \cdot 10^{-16}$. This difference is

Table 1. Ratios of computational complexity and run-times with respect to the case $D = 2$ and $n = 1$. The ratios in this table are for the algorithms calculating the value only (Alg. 1(b)). (a) # algorithmic operations reference, (b) # algorithmic operations proposed, (c) run-time reference and (d) run-time proposed.

(a)	$A_V^{ref}(D,n)\big/A_V^{ref}(2,1)$			(b)	$A_V^{prop}(D,n)\big/A_V^{prop}(2,1)$		
n \ D	2	3	4	n \ D	2	3	4
1	1.00	2.5	6.00	1	1.00	2.33	5.00
2	2.25	8.44	30.38	2	2.00	6.50	20.00
3	4.00	20.00	96.00	3	3.33	14.00	56.67
(c)	$R_V^{ref}(D,n)\big/R_V^{ref}(2,1)$			(d)	$R_V^{prop}(D,n)\big/R_V^{prop}(2,1)$		
n \ D	2	3	4	n \ D	2	3	4
1	1.01 ± 0.18	1.10 ± 0.13	1.59 ± 0.19	1	1.00 ± 0.03	1.05 ± 0.04	1.27 ± 0.02
2	1.11 ± 0.17	1.78 ± 0.22	4.11 ± 0.50	2	1.08 ± 0.04	1.37 ± 0.05	2.07 ± 0.08
3	1.29 ± 0.16	3.02 ± 0.37	11.01 ± 1.35	3	1.22 ± 0.09	1.76 ± 0.04	3.71 ± 0.14

Table 2. Ratios of computational complexity and run-times with respect to the case $D = 2$ and $n = 1$. The ratios in this table are for the algorithms calculating both value and gradient (Alg. 2). (a) # algorithmic operations reference, (b) # algorithmic operations proposed, (c) run-time reference and (d) run-time proposed.

(a)	$A_{VG}^{ref}(D,n)\big/A_{VG}^{ref}(2,1)$			(b)	$A_{VG}^{prop}(D,n)\big/A_{VG}^{prop}(2,1)$		
n \ D	2	3	4	n \ D	2	3	4
1	1.00	3.60	11.20	1	1.00	2.57	5.86
2	2.25	12.15	56.70	2	1.93	6.64	21.00
3	4.00	28.80	179.20	3	3.14	13.71	56.29
(c)	$R_{VG}^{ref}(D,n)\big/R_{VG}^{ref}(2,1)$			(d)	$R_{VG}^{prop}(D,n)\big/R_{VG}^{prop}(2,1)$		
n \ D	2	3	4	n \ D	2	3	4
1	1.00 ± 0.07	1.52 ± 0.07	2.88 ± 0.13	1	1.00 ± 0.03	1.17 ± 0.04	1.65 ± 0.04
2	1.23 ± 0.06	3.08 ± 0.14	10.80 ± 0.48	2	1.21 ± 0.05	1.71 ± 0.05	3.21 ± 0.11
3	1.66 ± 0.11	6.15 ± 0.28	32.20 ± 1.44	3	1.53 ± 0.05	2.70 ± 0.14	6.53 ± 0.23

only due to numerical differences. Since floating point additions and multiplications are non-associative, the reordering of the summations might introduce small round-off differences.

Table 1 shows how the number of arithmetic operations $A_V(D,n)$ and the run-time $R_V(D,n)$ of the interpolation depend on D and n. The values in the table are for the algorithms computing the value only. The table shows the ratios for $D \in \{2 \ldots 4\}$ and $n \in \{1 \ldots 3\}$ with respect to the case $D = 2$ and $n = 1$. The results in this table show that the proposed algorithm is less dependent on D and n than the reference algorithm. The same can be concluded for the results in Tab. 2, showing the ratios for the algorithms calculating both value and gradient. Note that for both Tab. 1 and Tab. 2 the numbers in (a) are higher than the numbers in (c) and the numbers in (b) are higher than the numbers in (d). This is because besides the interpolation, other operations are performed by both algorithms in the measured run-time, such as transforming $\boldsymbol{x}$, calculating the B-spline weights, and several bounds checks.

Table 3. Ratios of the reference algorithm / proposed algorithm (a) # algorithmic operations value, (b) # algorithmic operations value and gradient, (c) run-time value ratio and (d) run-time value and gradient.

(a)	$A_V^{\text{ref}}(D,n)\big/A_V^{\text{prop}}(D,n)$			(b)	$A_{VG}^{\text{ref}}(D,n)\big/A_{VG}^{\text{prop}}(D,n)$		
n \ D	2	3	4	n \ D	2	3	4
1	1.33	1.43	1.60	1	1.43	2.00	2.73
2	1.50	1.73	2.03	2	1.66	2.61	3.86
3	1.60	1.90	2.26	3	1.82	3.00	4.55

(c)	$R_V^{\text{ref}}(D,n)\big/R_V^{\text{prop}}(D,n)$			(d)	$R_{VG}^{\text{ref}}(D,n)\big/R_{VG}^{\text{prop}}(D,n)$		
n \ D	2	3	4	n \ D	2	3	4
1	3.26 ± 0.44	3.38 ± 0.11	4.01 ± 0.07	1	4.05 ± 0.25	5.27 ± 0.12	7.05 ± 0.10
2	3.31 ± 0.34	4.18 ± 0.16	6.40 ± 0.24	2	4.12 ± 0.14	7.29 ± 0.10	13.63 ± 0.33
3	3.42 ± 0.21	5.52 ± 0.11	9.53 ± 0.37	3	4.37 ± 0.23	9.24 ± 0.41	19.94 ± 0.52

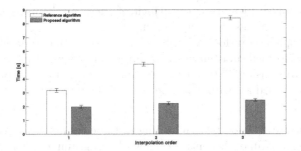

Fig. 1. Run time of registration using B-spline interpolation with the reference and the proposed algorithm

The ratios of the reference to the proposed algorithm are shown in Tab. 3. In this table, (a) and (b) show the ratios of the number of arithmetic operations and (c) and (d) the ratios of the run-times. In all cases the proposed algorithm has a lower run-time and the difference increases for increasing D and increasing n. Note that the values in Tab. 3(a) are lower than the values in Tab. 3(c) and the values in Tab. 3(b) are lower than the values in Tab. 3(d). The obtained acceleration is thus larger than predicted. This indicates that besides the reduction of the number of arithmetic operations in the proposed algorithm, the overhead such as address computations and flow control operations have also decreased, which shows the effect of TMP.

Figure 1 shows the computation time of a registration of two 3D images for $n \in \{1 \ldots 3\}$ for both algorithms. For all n the proposed algorithm is faster than the reference algorithm, and for increasing n the difference increases. The results also show that with the reference algorithm, the computation time of the registration depends more on the choice of interpolation order, than with the proposed algorithm. It was verified that the resulting transformation was identical in all cases, thus the proposed algorithm only influences the computation time.

5   Conclusion

The proposed algorithm decreases the computation time of B-spline interpolation substantially, while providing identical results as the reference algorithm. The improvement of the proposed algorithm over the reference algorithm increases with increasing dimension D and interpolation order n. The registration experiment shows that the proposed interpolation algorithm significantly decreases the computation time of image registration algorithms that use B-spline interpolation.

The exact mechanisms that explain the reduction in computation time achieved with TMP may depend on the compiler that is used. These mechanisms could comprise a reduction in the number of jumps in the code, more efficient access of the cache memory, reduction in memory latency, etc. Future research could therefore investigate the compiler dependency of the proposed method, and analyze in more detail which of these mechanisms is mainly responsible for the reduction in computation time.

Since the B-spline transformation [8] uses the same mathematical equations to obtain a transformed coordinate, in the future we will aim to develop a similar recursive algorithm using TMP for the implementation of the B-spline transformation. The proposed algorithm will be made publicly available in ITK.

Acknowledgments. The research leading to these results has received funding from the European Union Seventh Framework Programme (FP7/2007 – 2013) under grant agreement no. 601055, VPH-DARE@IT.

References

1. Thévenaz, P., Unser, M.: Optimization of mutual information for multiresolution image registration. IEEE Transactions on Image Processing 9(12), 2083–2099 (2000)
2. Thévenaz, P., Blu, T., Unser, M.: Interpolation revisited. IEEE Transactions on Medical Imaging 19, 739–758 (2000)
3. Veldhuizen, T.: Using C++ template metaprograms. C++ Report 7, 36–43 (1995)
4. Sarrut, D., Vandemeulebroucke, J.: B-LUT: Fast and low memory b-spline image interpolation. Computer Methods and Programs in Biomedicine 99, 172–178 (2010)
5. Unser, M.: Splines: A perfect fit for signal and image processing. IEEE Signal Processing Magazine 16, 22–38 (1999)
6. Klein, S., Staring, M., Murphy, K., Viergever, M.A., Pluim, J.: elastix: a toolbox for intensity based medical image registration. IEEE Transactions on Medical Imaging 29(1), 196–205 (2010)
7. Klein, S., et al.: Adaptive stochastic gradient descent optimization for image registration. Int. J. Comput. Vis. 81, 227–239 (2009)
8. Rueckert, D., et al.: Nonrigid registration using free-form deformations: Application to breast MR images. IEEE Transactions on Medical Imaging 18, 712–721 (1999)

SymBA: Diffeomorphic Registration Based on Gradient Orientation Alignment and Boundary Proximity of Sparsely Selected Voxels

Dante De Nigris[1], D. Louis Collins[2], and Tal Arbel[1]

[1] Centre for Intelligent Machines, McGill University, Canada
{dante,tal}@cim.mcgill.ca
[2] Montreal Neurological Institute, McGill University, Canada
louis.collins@mcgill.ca

Abstract. We propose a novel non-linear registration strategy which seeks an optimal deformation that maps corresponding boundaries of similar orientation. Our approach relies on a local similarity metric based on gradient orientation alignment and distance to the nearest inferred boundary and is evaluated on a reduced set of locations corresponding to inferred boundaries. The deformation model is characterized as the integration of a time-constant velocity field and optimization is performed in coarse to fine multi-level strategy with a gradient ascent technique. Our approach is computational efficient since it relies on a sparse selection of voxels corresponding to detected boundaries, yielding robust and accurate results with reduced processing times. We demonstrate quantitative results in the context of the non-linear registration of inter-patient magnetic resonance brain volumes obtained from a public dataset (CUMC12). Our proposed approach achieves a similar level of accuracy as other state-of-the-art methods but with processing times as short as 1.5 minutes. We also demonstrate preliminary qualitative results in the time-sensitive registration contexts of registering MR brain volumes to intra-operative ultrasound for improved guidance in neurosurgery.

Keywords: image registration, pixel selection, diffeomorphism.

1 Introduction

Image registration is a critical component of a wide variety of medical image analysis contexts. Inspired by a wide range of time-sensitive clinical applications (e.g. image-guided interventions), this paper focuses on the domain whereby registration efficiency is required, without the subsequent sacrifice in accuracy. The result is a non-linear registration framework that is applicable to a wide variety of domains —from unimodal to multi-modal image matching —with a similarity metric that is robust to complex image acquisition variability as is typical in real, clinical domains. This include domains where intensity homogeneity within common anatomical regions is violated, as is typical in imaging modalities such as ultrasound (US). This severely compromises traditional similarity metrics that

S. Ourselin and M. Modat (Eds.): WBIR 2014, LNCS 8545, pp. 21–30, 2014.

either rely on either direct intensity matches between structures in both images (e.g. SSD) or on derived functional matches (e.g. NCC, MI)[1].

In this work, we propose a new, non-linear image registration framework that pursues high computational efficiency, without compromising accuracy. Rather than perform intensity matching, the technique focuses on matching detected boundaries from both images. Specifically, the method first performs the inference of boundaries in each image, and then seeks a diffeomorphism that optimally maps boundaries across images based not on intensities but rather on image gradient orientations, similar to [2,3]. Gradient orientations are robust and informative features which are of a more geometric nature and can be easily compared. We extend the gradient orientation alignment metric by also evaluating the distance to the nearest inferred boundary. Hence, our proposed metric seeks to both maximize gradient orientation alignment and minimize the distance to the nearest boundary. Computational complexity is significantly reduced given the aggressive voxel selection restricted to boundary locations, similar to [2].

Experimental results demonstrate the computational gains of the method in the context of a non-linear registration of inter-patient MR brain volumes derived from the publicly available CUMC12 dataset[1]. In particular, by evaluating the image similarity solely on identified image boundaries, the number of voxels selected and evaluated is reduced to 6% of the total number of voxels found in the full image, and the subsequent processing time is reduced to 1.5 minutes with registration accuracies that are comparable to that of state-of-the-art methods. The method is applied to the time-sensitive context of registering real clinical, pre-operative patient MR brain volumes to intra-operative ultrasound (iUS) for improved navigation guidance in neurosurgery. We also present preliminary qualitative results based on the publicly available BITE dataset[4] where we demonstrate the method yields successful results in half a minute.

2   Methodology

In this section we describe our proposed approach characterized by the following major components: an inference of the location of boundaries of interest in both images, a local similarity metric based on gradient orientation alignment and distance to the nearest inferred boundary, and a time-constant velocity field optimized in a coarse-to-fine strategy with a gradient ascent technique.

2.1   Boundary Inference

Our approach relies on an initial inference of locations of boundaries of interest. Note that the task of accurately and robustly identifying the location of anatomical boundaries represents a non-trivial challenge by itself. In this work, we choose to not devote an important effort to such task and rather rely on a conventional Canny edge detector for all our experiments. Once the boundary

---

[1] Data was obtained from http://mindboggle.info/data.html

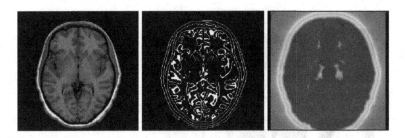

Fig. 1. Illustration of the edges detected on a T1-weighted MR brain volume with a canny-edge detector. The first column shows the MR brain volume. The second column shows the detected boundary locations. The third column shows the distance image (jet colormap) computed from the detected edges.

locations have been identified, we compute a distance map where the euclidean distance to the nearest boundary is evaluated at every voxel. Fig. 1 illustrates the locations that are detected by a Canny edge operator applied to a MR T1-weighted brain volume, as well as the corresponding distance map.

2.2 Similarity Metric

Once a set of boundary locations, Ω, and a corresponding distance map, D, are computed for each image, we define a localized similarity metric which evaluates gradient orientation alignment and euclidean distance to the nearest boundary. For a location, $\mathbf{x}_f$, in the fixed image domain, we can express the metric as,

$$s(\mathbf{x}_f; D_m^\downarrow, \nabla I_m^\downarrow) = \exp\left(-\frac{(D_m^\downarrow(\mathbf{x}_f))^2}{2\sigma^2}\right) \times \left\langle \frac{\nabla I_f(\mathbf{x}_f)}{|\nabla I_f(\mathbf{x}_f)|}, \frac{\nabla I_m^\downarrow(\mathbf{x}_f)}{|\nabla I_m^\downarrow(\mathbf{x}_f)|} \right\rangle^k \quad (1)$$

where ∇I_f is the fixed image gradient, $\nabla I_m^\downarrow = \nabla(I_m \circ \mathbf{T})$ is the image gradient from the moving image deformed by the transformation function $\mathbf{T}$, and $D_m^\downarrow = (D_m \circ \mathbf{T})$ is the distance map obtained from the moving image deformed by $\mathbf{T}$.

The idea of relying on gradient orientation alignment as a cue for similarity has been explored in previous papers, particularly in the context of both rigid[2,1] and nonrigid registration[3]. The metric is characterized by two parameters: the standard deviation, σ, defining the falloff of the Gaussian function evaluating the distance to the closest boundary, and the gradient orientation selectivity, k, defining how gradient orientation alignment is evaluated. For a mono-modal registration contexts, an *odd* integer value of k is reasonable since we expect corresponding gradient orientations across image to be both aligned and with a similar direction. For the multi-modal registration contexts, where corresponding gradient orientations across modalities may be aligned but with an inverse direction, it is more reasonable to use an *even* integer value for k.

In contexts where we expect all boundaries inferred in one image to have a counter-part in the other image, we can define an energy function evaluated over both sets boundary locations,

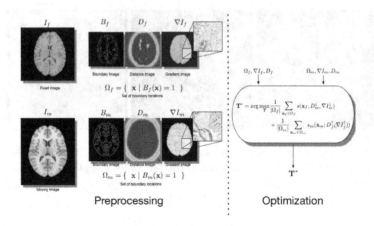

Fig. 2. Algorithmic Outline

$$S(\Psi_f, \Psi_m) = \frac{1}{|\Omega_f|} \sum_{\mathbf{x}_f \in \Omega_f} s(\mathbf{x}_f; D_m^\downarrow, \nabla I_m^\downarrow) + \frac{1}{|\Omega_m|} \sum_{\mathbf{x}_m \in \Omega_m} s(\mathbf{x}_m; D_f^\uparrow, \nabla I_m^\uparrow) \quad (2)$$

where $\Psi = (\nabla I, D, \Omega)$ is a notation convention used to group features of interest inferred from each image. Furthermore, $D_f^\uparrow = D_f \circ \mathbf{T}^{-1}$ and $\nabla I_m^\uparrow = \nabla(I_m \circ \mathbf{T}^{-1})$ are the fixed distance map and gradient image deformed by $\mathbf{T}^{-1}$. Note that the energy function leads to a stronger notion of compromise between the inferences made in each image and that it involves the use of an invertible transformation.

In this work, we rely on a time-constant velocity field for the characterization of a diffeomorphism. Specifically, we obtain the forward-mapping transformation by numerically composing the velocity field from time 0 to time 1 in N steps,

$$\mathbf{T}(\mathbf{x}_f) = \left(\prod_{}^{N} \Phi_{\Delta t} \right)(\mathbf{x}_f) = (\Phi_{\Delta t} \circ \ldots \circ \Phi_{\Delta t})(\mathbf{x}_f) \quad (3)$$

where $\Phi_{\Delta t}(\mathbf{x}_f) = \mathbf{x}_f + \mathbf{v}(\mathbf{x}_f)\Delta t$ and $N \times \Delta t = 1$. The backward-mapping transformation is found by integrating the velocity field in the negative direction.

In our implementation, the composition of the velocity field is performed *on-demand* at every location during the optimization of the metric. As a consequence, the computational cost of the algorithm is proportional to the number of locations evaluated and to the number of time steps, N. Hence, there is significant interest to keep both quantities within a minimum. Additionally our current implementation does *not* involve any explicit regularization penalty, such as the L^2 norm on the velocity field[5].

2.3 Optimization

The energy function is optimized with a gradient ascent approach, where we rely on a finite-difference operator at each location to obtain the metric's derivative.

The learning rate of the gradient ascent is continuously adapted with a "bold driver" strategy[6], and the optimization is stopped when either a minimum rate of change or a maximum number of iterations is reached.

In order to improve computational efficiency and robustness against local extrema, we adopt a coarse-to-fine strategy in which both the resolution of the images being registered and the velocity field is increased from stage to stage. It is important to note that the resolution of the velocity field does not directly correspond to the resolution of the images being registered. In other words, we evaluate a displacement field with a finer voxel resolution than the one found in the velocity field. This corresponds to an implicit regularization of the transformation space effectively constraining the spatial variation of the velocity field.

3   Experiments and Results

3.1   Inter-patient Registration of MR Brain Volumes

We evaluated our proposed approach in the context of the non-linear registration of inter-patient T1-weighted MR brain volumes. In particular, we rely on a public dataset, referred to as the CUMC12 dataset, composed of 12 subjects with corresponding manual segmentations of 128 unique brain regions. The dataset has been used in previous publications[7,8] for the evaluation of non-linear registration techniques and thus allows for direct comparison with previously reported results. The volumes found in the dataset where acquired at the Columbia University Medical Center on a 1.5 T GE scanner. For the purposes of manually segmenting the volumes, the original images were resliced coronally to a slice thickness of 3mm. The resolution of the manual labels is thus slightly coarser than the resolution of the naive MR volumes which have a coronal slice thickness of 1.5mm. The expert labellers followed the Cardviews labeling protocol [9] with the use of the Cardviews software.

Registration performance is evaluated by first applying the estimated non-linear transformation to the expert labels of the moving image, and then comparing such transformed labels with the expert labels of the fixed image (i.e. "ground truth"). We rely on the target overlap measure and the union overlap measure[7] for quantifying the agreement between labels.

We parametrized our approach with four coarse-to-fine registration stages, where at each consequent registration stage we increase the image resolution as well as the resolution of the velocity field being optimized. Registration performance is evaluated across all stages and is summarized in Table 1. Note that the processing time for each stage includes the processing time of the preceding stages. Hence, the complete registration with all four stages takes on average five minutes. Note that the gain in registration accuracy between stage three and four is relatively small, and that the registration with only the first three stages takes on average one and a half minutes. The approach was implemented in C++ and evaluated on a Linux computer with an Intel i7-3770 CPU.

For direct comparison against state-of-the-art registration techniques, we compare the results of our approach, referred to as *SymBA*, with results reported on

Table 1. Registration performance and processing time for each registration stage. Performance is evaluated with the mean target and mean union (Jaccard) overlap measure across cases and regions. Note that the processing time for each stage includes the processing time of the preceding stages.

Stage	Mean Target (%)	Mean Union (%)	Mean Run Time
1	41.45	26.49	20 secs
2	46.76	30.83	35 secs
3	**50.20**	**33.88**	**1 min 30 secs**
4	**51.31**	**34.78**	**5 min**

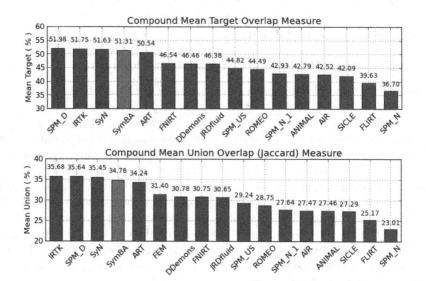

Fig. 3. Mean target and union (Jaccard) overlap across regions and across cases. The proposed approach (in red), *SymBA*, is within the top five techniques.

a previous publication[7] focused on the exhaustive comparison of 14 non-linear registration techniques for MR brain volumes. Fig. 3 shows the compound average of the target overlap and union overlap (Jaccard) across regions and across registration cases. Note that the proposed approach has similar results to the top five techniques, which all have comparable performance. The union overlap results found in Fig. 3 also include the numbers reported on a recently proposed registration technique [8], with an average processing time of 15 minutes, as reported by the authors.

The compound means for each overlap measure are useful criteria for comparing performance across methods, yet they do not describe the variability found across regions. In Fig. 4, we illustrate the mean and standard deviation of the target overlap measure for each region. To minimize visual clutter we only include three techniques: a top ranking method from the top five techniques, *SyN* [5];

our proposed approach, *SymBA*; and an alternative method, *ROMEO*[10]. Note that the performance of our approach tends to tightly match the performance of the top ranking method, and is consistently superior than the poor performing method. However, the processing time of *SyN* was of 38 minutes when ran on the same computer where we ran our technique.

3.2   Registration of MR to Intra-operative Ultrasound

An important motivation for our work lies in improving the registration performance in time-sensitive contexts. Registration of MR to iUS for image guided neurosurgery is a valuable example which requires a technique that addresses widely different image modalities in a short amount of time.

Our proposed approach can provide substantial advantages for this context by focusing solely on anatomical boundaries exposed in the iUS and relying on the fact that brain-shift deformations can be large but are generally characterized by a coherent displacement. Hence, in this context, we evaluate the energy function solely over the boundary locations identified in the iUS. Our method was applied to the 14 real clinical cases available in the BITE public dataset, containing pre-operative MR to iUS registration cases in tumor resection surgeries[8]. The dataset includes a set of homologous landmarks for validation of registration techniques. However, most of the cases presented rigid deformations and tag points were limited, and not informative for the evaluation of detailed non-linear movements (discussed in [1]).

Fig. 5 presents a preliminary qualitative example of the performance of our approach in a case from the dataset. The case was selected based on the apparent prominence of a non-linear deformation around the tumor boundary, which would be of interest for guidance. The improvement brought forward by the non-rigid registration can be clearly observed in the close alignment of the tumor boundary and was obtained with registration time of 30 seconds.

4   Discussion

We have presented a non-linear registration technique which relies on boundary information for improved computational efficiency while yielding accurate results. Our first set of experiments rely on volume overlap measures of manually labelled regions for assessing the accuracy of inter-patient registration of healthy MR volumes. There are a few limitations with such validation strategy. First, is the point that the use of a tissue-overlap "surrogate measure" for validating registration may poorly reflect the true *geometric* performance of registration algorithms. Such critique has been discussed in detail in previous work[11]. However, we should point out that the 128 segmented regions found in the dataset used in this work are anatomical and localized, and thus suffer far less limitations than overlap based measures which evaluate solely the overlap of major healthy tissues (e.g. gray matter). Second, it is also clear that the task of warping one patient's brain to another patient's brain is fundamentally

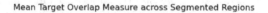

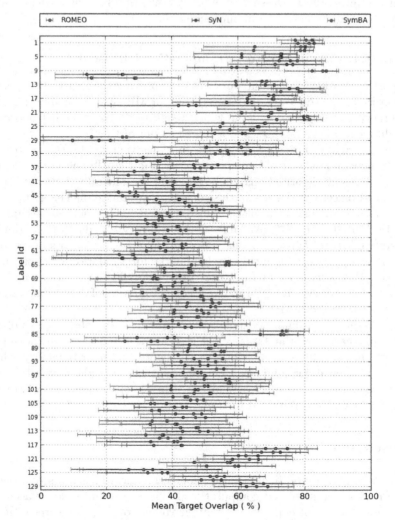

Fig. 4. Mean Target Overlap and Standard Deviation per Region. Registration performance of the proposed method, *SymBA*, is compared against three techniques: a top performing method, *SyN*, and *ROMEO*. Note how the registration performance of the top performing method, *SyN*, closely resembles the performance of our proposed method, and is consistently superior to the low ranking method. *SyN* had an average processing time of 38 minutes, while *SymBA* had an average processing times of 5 minutes, when evaluated on the same machine.

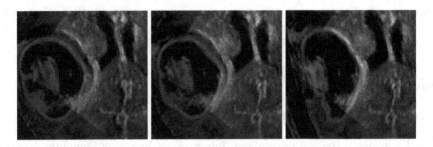

Fig. 5. Registration of a MR volume (grayscale) to an iUS (heat colormap). The first column illustrates the initial (misregistered) position of the MR image. The second column illustrates the MR image after a rigid registration[1]. The third column illustrates the MR image after proposed non-rigid registration.

ill-posed in the sense that there are anatomical variations across patients which simply cannot be recovered by a diffeomorphism. However, one could argue that there are "major" anatomical structures which can indeed be mapped across patients with a diffeomorphism and where a measure of volume overlap is indeed informative. Ultimately, for the purposes of evaluating the performance of our technique, what remains of critical value, is that such validation strategy has been employed for the validation of many other techniques and allows for a direct and fair comparison with previously reported results.

Our approach relies on the inference of boundaries and it is clear that such stage plays a critical role in the overall performance. In this work, we have relied on a Canny edge detector, which can be considered a "conventional" technique for identifying image edges. Future work will look into analyzing the sensitivity of registration performance with regards to variations in the boundary inference stage. Additionally, we believe that by explicitly identifying the boundaries of interest to be aligned, the proposed technique may allow for advantages in various contexts. For example, any context in which prior information can be exploited so as to robustly and accurately identify boundaries of interest may lead to improvement in registration performance. Consider the task of registering to a template for the segmentation of a specific anatomical structure. In such a context, one could rely on the atlas labels to restrict the boundary alignment to locations in the atlas which belong to the region of interest.

5 Conclusion

We have a presented a registration approach which seeks an optimal alignment between explicitly identified image boundaries and yields successful results in short processing times. Performance was evaluated in the context of the registration of inter-patient MR brain volumes, where we demonstrated that our approach can achieve accurate results in processing times as short as 1.5 minutes. We've also shown preliminary results that illustrate the utility of our approach in time-sensitive and challenging contexts such as the registration of MR brain volumes to an iUS for improved guidance in neurosurgery. Further efforts will be pursued in fully characterizing the performance of the proposed approach, particularly in the context of registration MR to iUS.

References

1. De Nigris, D., Collins, D.L., Arbel, T.: Fast rigid registration of pre-operative magnetic resonance images to intra-operative ultrasound for neurosurgery based on high confidence gradient orientations. International Journal of Computer Assisted Radiology and Surgery 8(4), 649–661 (2013)
2. De Nigris, D., Collins, D.L., Arbel, T.: Multi-modal image registration based on gradient orientations of minimal uncertainty. IEEE Transactions on Medical Imaging PP(99), 1 (2012)
3. Haber, E., Modersitzki, J.: Intensity gradient based registration and fusion of multi-modal images. In: Larsen, R., Nielsen, M., Sporring, J. (eds.) MICCAI 2006. LNCS, vol. 4191, pp. 726–733. Springer, Heidelberg (2006)
4. Mercier, L., Del Maestro, R.F., Petrecca, K., Araujo, D., Haegelen, C., Collins, D.L.: Online database of clinical mr and ultrasound images of brain tumors. Medical Physics 39(6) (2012)
5. Avants, B., Epstein, C., Grossman, M., Gee, J.: Symmetric diffeomorphic image registration with cross-correlation: Evaluating automated labeling of elderly and neurodegenerative brain. Medical Image Analysis 12(1), 26–41 (2008)
6. Battiti, R.: Accelerated backpropagation learning: Two optimization methods. Complex Systems 3(4), 331–342 (1989)
7. Klein, A., Andersson, J., Ardekani, B.A., Ashburner, J., Avants, B., Chiang, M.C., Christensen, G.E., Collins, D.L., Gee, J., Hellier, P., et al.: Evaluation of 14 non-linear deformation algorithms applied to human brain mri registration. Neuroimage 46(3), 786–802 (2009)
8. Popuri, K., Cobzas, D., Jägersand, M.: A variational formulation for discrete registration. In: Mori, K., Sakuma, I., Sato, Y., Barillot, C., Navab, N. (eds.) MICCAI 2013, Part III. LNCS, vol. 8151, pp. 187–194. Springer, Heidelberg (2013)
9. Caviness Jr., V.S., Meyer, J., Makris, N., Kennedy, D.N.: Mri-based topographic parcellation of human neocortex: an anatomically specified method with estimate of reliability. Journal of Cognitive Neuroscience 8(6), 566–587 (1996)
10. Hellier, P., Barillot, C., Memin, E., Perez, P.: Hierarchical estimation of a dense deformation field for 3-d robust registration. IEEE Transactions on Medical Imaging 20(5), 388–402 (2001)
11. Rohlfing, T.: Image similarity and tissue overlaps as surrogates for image registration accuracy: Widely used but unreliable. IEEE Transactions on Medical Imaging 31(2), 153–163 (2012)

Non-rigid Image Registration with Equally Weighted Assimilated Surface Constraint

Cheng Zhang[1], Gary E. Christensen[1], Martin J. Murphy[2], Elisabeth Weiss[2], and Jeffrey F. Williamson[2]

[1] Department of Electrical and Computer Engineering,
University of Iowa, Iowa City, IA, USA
cheng-zhang@uiowa.edu
[2] Department of Radiation Oncology,
Virginia Commonwealth University, Richmond, VA, USA

Abstract. An important research problem in image-guided radiation therapy is how to accurately register daily onboard Cone-beam CT (CBCT) images to higher quality pretreatment fan-beam CT (FBCT) images. Assuming the organ segmentations are both available on CBCT and FBCT images, methods have been proposed to use them to help the intensity-driven image registration. Due to the low contrast between soft-tissue structures exhibited in CBCT, the interobserver contouring variability (expressed as standard deviation) can be as large as 2-3 mm and varies systematically with organ, and relative location on each organ surface. Therefore the inclusion of the segmentations into registration may degrade registration accuracy. To address this issue we propose a surface assimilation method that estimates a new surface from the manual segmentation from a priori organ shape knowledge and the interobserver segmentation error. Our experiment results show the proposed method improves registration accuracy compared to previous methods.

1 Introduction

Rigid image registration has established its role in reducing geometric targeting uncertainty in the external radiation therapy of the prostate cancer [6]. Non-rigid registration has the potential to map the planning data to the treatment images more accurately than the rigid alignment [1] without the need for invasively implanted radio-opaque markers. However, this ability is limited at least by two factors. First, the full knowledge of biomechanical properties is lacking. Therefore assumptions regarding the plausible range of transformation properties, e.g. different parameterizations, elastic or fluid models, maybe inaccurate. This type of registration error was studied in [12] under the Bayesian framework. Another challenge to the prostate CT image registration is the limited intensity contrast among the soft tissue organs (bladder, prostate and rectum). Thus the matching accuracy of solely intensity-driven non-rigid registration is often unsatisfactory, especially at the organ boundaries.

In a typical problem of registering a planning fan-beam CT (FBCT) to an onboard cone-beam CT (CBCT) acquired just before administering a daily treatment, the manual segmentations of the FBCT image set are generally available. The idea has been proposed that these organ segmentations can be exploited in the registration. Some methods

S. Ourselin and M. Modat (Eds.): WBIR 2014, LNCS 8545, pp. 31–40, 2014.

assume the manual segmentations on the CBCT are known [2,8]. And some methods do not make this assumption. They automatically segment and register the organs, either sequentially [18] or iteratively [10].

An interesting problem is: if the segmentations differ significantly between different CBCT observers [11, 16], forcing the registration to match possibly inaccurate segmented surfaces may increase registration error. Zhang et al. [17] suggested using the interobserver segmentation error (ISE) to locally penalize the surface matching. However, this method only works for certain cases. To address the same issue, we propose a different registration algorithm to lower the registration error in a scenario that the manual segmentation is inaccurate.

2   Method

Our registration cost function combines the costs of intensity similarity and surface closeness. In short, we improve the registration accuracy by providing an estimated target surface that is closer to the true segmentation. In this section, we first introduce the method of surface estimation and then the registration algorithm based on it.

2.1   Surface Estimation

Suppose we represent a surface as a parametric surface discretized to N vertices. At the i-th parametric node t_i, let y_i denote the location of the i-th vertex of observed surface (from manual segmentation), which we model as the true vertex $f(t_i)$ location corrupted by the additive noise $\epsilon(t)$,

$$y_i = f(t_i) + \epsilon_i, \quad i = 1, 2, \ldots, N \tag{1}$$

where f is smooth and has a continuous derivative of at least order m, and ϵ_i is a i.i.d Gaussian random variable with zero mean and variance σ^2.

One way to estimate the true surface from a manual segmentation is the prediction based on a shape model (let $\hat{y}_i$ denote the predicted surface). The shape model can be obtained from statistical shape analysis [5]. In our case, a set of high quality prostate segmentations for each patient is available and we chose the Point Distribution Model (PDM) to describe it [3]. Briefly, the PDM of a shape object with N vertices contains M variation modes is given by

$$x = \bar{x} + Pb \tag{2}$$

where $\bar{x}$ is the mean shape, $b = (b^1, b^2, \ldots, b^M)^T$ is a $M \times 1$ vector of Gaussian random variables, $P = (\mathbf{p}^1, \mathbf{p}^2, \ldots, \mathbf{p}^M)$ is a $N \times M$ matrix defining the shape variation directions. Given an observed surface y, the linear regression:

$$\hat{b} = \arg\min_b [\bar{x} + Pb - R(y)]^2 \tag{3}$$

gives a new set of shape coefficients $\hat{b}$, where $R(\bullet)$ is the Procrustes transformation. It follows that we obtain a predicted surface: $\hat{y} = \bar{x} + P\hat{b}$ based on the prior shape knowledge. This idea is illustrated in Fig. 1.

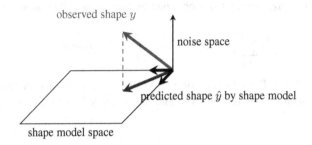

observed shape y

noise space

predicted shape $\hat{y}$ by shape model

shape model space

Fig. 1. Observed shape (red) is projected onto the shape model space, forming a predicted surface (blue)

Eq. (3) can be viewed as a signal-noise filtering problem. Suppose a PDM can capture all shape instances of an object (signal) and the inter-observer segmentation error is the only source of noise. Given a manual segmentation y (corrupted signal), we can fully filter out the inter-observer segmentation error (ISE) by solving Eq. (3) if the ISE is in the null space of the PDM. And the resulting $\hat{y}$ will be close to the signal. The worse case happens when the ISE falls into the same space of the PDM where the noise and signal are undistinguishable. Therefore the recoverability of the PDM against the ISE is affected by the orthogonality between the two. Also, it is compromised by the Procrustes transform since the differences in scale, rotation and translation are removed.

In practice, the predicted surface $\hat{y}$ may not be more accurate than the manual segmentation y everywhere. Thus we seek a way of fusing y and $\hat{y}$ together. In this study we propose the following cost function:

$$C(f) = \sum_{i=1}^{N} \frac{(y_i - f(t_i))^2}{\sigma_i^2} + \sum_{i=1}^{N} \frac{(\hat{y}_i - f(t_i))^2}{\delta_i^2} + \lambda \int_0^1 (f^{(m)}(u))^2 du \qquad (4)$$

where the first term is weighted by the interobserver segmentation error (ISE) σ_i^2, the second one is weighted by the accuracy of prediction δ_i^2, and the third term regularizes the smoothness of f. The pointwise correspondence between y_i, $f(t_i)$ and $\hat{y}_i$ is assumed or can be established using surface registration.

As in [17], a set of multi-observer segmented objects are collected to determine the segmentation error σ_i. By only considering the relative accuracy, Eq. (4) is simplified to:

$$C(f) = \sum_{i=1}^{N} (1 - \alpha_i)(y_i - f(t_i))^2 + \sum_{i=1}^{N} \alpha_i(\hat{y}_i - f(t_i))^2 + \lambda \int_0^1 (f^{(m)}(u))^2 du \quad (5)$$

where $\alpha_i \in [0, 1]$ is the pointwise normalized of ISE balancing the contribution from the model prediction and the current observation at the i-th point. The first two terms of Eq. (5) forms a quadratic function. It is easy to verify that its minimizer is given by

$$\hat{f}_i = (1 - \alpha_i)y_i + \alpha_i \hat{y}_i \qquad (6)$$

Therefore the minimizer of Eq. (5) is obtained by minimizing the following equation

$$\frac{1}{N}\sum_{i=1}^{N}(\hat{f}_i - f(t_i))^2 + \lambda \int_0^1 (f^{(m)}(u))^2 du \tag{7}$$

Inspired by the idea of Data Assimilation (DA) [9], we refer to this process of surface estimation as *Surface Assimilation* (SA) and the estimated surface as the assimilated surface.

2.2 Smoothing Spline Regression

Eq. (7) is actually a Penalized Least Square (PLS) problem. The first part in Eq. (7), represented by the residual sum of squares (RSS), measures the fidelity to the observed signal. The second part measures the smoothness of the estimated signal. The smoothing parameter λ balances these two penalties, which is also known as the bandwidth in some statistics literature. When $\lambda = 0$, Eq. (7) becomes an interpolation problem. When $\lambda \to \infty$, it is close to a linear regression model.

Craven and Wahba [4] shows the minimizer of Eq. (7) is a natural polynomial spline. By limiting the solution f_λ to a reproducing kernel Hilbert space (RKHS), $\mathcal{H}$, with the reproducing kernel denoted by R, this problem can be solved under the framework of smoothing spline regression (SSR) [14]. f_λ contains two parts: one that is not penalized by the smoothness operator in Eq. (7) and one that is orthogonal to the former. Correspondingly, $\mathcal{H}$ can be decomposed into two subspaces: $\mathcal{H} = \mathcal{H}_0 + \mathcal{H}_1$. By Kimeldorf-Wahba representer theorem [14], a closed form of f_λ at a fixed λ is given by:

$$f_\lambda = \sum_{\nu=1}^{P} d_\nu \phi_\nu + \sum_{i=1}^{N} c_i \xi_i \tag{8}$$

where $\phi_1, \ldots, \phi_P$ span $\mathcal{H}_0$ and ξ_i is the i-th representer in $\mathcal{H}_1$.

Different applications require different splines, such as polynomial splines, periodic splines, spherical splines, vector splines (see [15] for more details). For our problem, we chose the periodic splines for closed 2D curve assimilation and spherical splines for closed 3D surface assimilation. We used Generalized Cross Validation (GCV) [14] to automatically estimate the smoothing parameter λ. Although, its optimality is not guaranteed if the segmentation error is correlated with the true boundary location, GCV estimation can still be used as a starting point for searching better λ [14].

2.3 Intensity Image Registration with Assimilated Surface Constraint

Suppose the template and the target images are denoted as $T : \Omega \to \mathbb{R}$ and $S : \Omega \to \mathbb{R}$, respectively, where $\Omega = [0, 1]^3$ is the image domain. Let $X : \mathbb{S}^2 \to \Omega$ be a parametric surface denoting the true ROI in the template space. Let $Y_g : \mathbb{S}^2 \to \Omega$ and $Y : \mathbb{S}^2 \to \Omega$ denote the parametric surfaces of the true and segmented ROI in the target spaces, respectively, and let $F : \mathbb{S}^2 \to \Omega$ be the assimilated surface of Y where $\mathbb{S}^2$ is the unit sphere. The image registration problem can be stated as: Find a dense transformation $h : \Omega \to \Omega$ that maps points in the target image to the corresponding points in the template image. We parameterized h using B-spline representation [13]. The cost function is defined as:

$$C_{\text{Total}}(h) = C_{\text{Intensity}}(h) + \rho C_{\text{Surface}}(h) + \beta\, C_{\text{Smooth}}(h) \tag{9}$$

where ρ and β control the relative contribution of each cost term. $C_{\text{Intensity}}$ is the grayscale similarity between the template and target images. We chose the sum of the squared difference (C_{SSD}) in our phantom experiment and the negative mutual information in FBCT to CBCT registration. C_{Smooth} is the regularization term that penalizes the transformations that are not smooth. In this work we used the bending energy based on the Laplacian operator (C_{LAP}).

C_{Surface} measures the closeness between the template and target surfaces. We define the equally-weighted assimilated-surface constraint (EWAS) as:

$$C_{\text{EWAS}}(h) = \int_0^{2\pi} \int_{-\frac{\pi}{2}}^{\frac{\pi}{2}} \|h(F(u,v)) - X(u,v)\| \, |\sin u| \, du \, dv \tag{10}$$

where u, v are the polar and azimuthal angles, respectively. For evaluation purpose, we designed the following variant of C_{EWFS}: the equally-weighted manual surface constraint (EWMS):

$$C_{\text{EWMS}}(h) = \int_0^{2\pi} \int_{-\frac{\pi}{2}}^{\frac{\pi}{2}} \|h(Y(u,v)) - X(u,v)\| \, |\sin u| \, du \, dv \tag{11}$$

As in [17], we define an uncertainty-weighted manual surface constraint (UWMS) as:

$$C_{\text{UWMS}}(h) = \int_0^{2\pi} \int_{-\frac{\pi}{2}}^{\frac{\pi}{2}} \frac{1}{\omega(u,v)} \|h(Y(u,v)) - X(u,v)\| \, |\sin u| \, du \, dv \tag{12}$$

where $\omega(u,v)$ is the ISE distributed on the surface. Hereafter EWAS refers to equally-weighted assimilated surface constrained image registration.

3 Experiments

We evaluated the proposed algorithm on phantom data set and compare it to three other algorithms (listed in Table 1). For a fair comparison, the balancing parameter ρ_1 in UWMS and ρ in other algorithms satisfies the relation:

$$\rho_1 \int_0^{2\pi} \int_{-\frac{\pi}{2}}^{\frac{\pi}{2}} \frac{1}{\omega(u,v)} |\sin u| \, du \, dv = \rho \tag{13}$$

We used the target registration error (TRE) [7] to evaluate the algorithm performance. The TRE is defined as the geometric discrepancy between two true surfaces after the registration, i.e. the difference between $X(u,v)$ and the deformed true target surface $h(Y_g(u,v))$.

Table 1. Image registration algorithms in the evaluation experiment

Algorithm	Cost function	Transformation	Optimization
SSD	$C_{SSD} + \beta C_{LAP}$	B-splines	Gradient descent
EWMS	$C_{SSD} + \rho C_{EWMS} + \beta C_{LAP}$	B-splines	Gradient descent
UWMS	$C_{SSD} + \rho_1 C_{UWMS} + \beta C_{LAP}$	B-splines	Gradient descent
EWAS	$C_{SSD} + \rho C_{EWAS} + \beta C_{LAP}$	B-splines	Gradient descent

$\rho=5$, $\rho_1=25$ and $\beta=0.005$

3.1 Phantom Experiment

Suppose the template and target spaces are with the dimensions $128 \times 128 \times 128$ mm^3. In the center of template space, we placed an ellipsoid object whose z-axis is not fixed to simulate the possible shape changes of $X(u,v)$:

$$X(u,v) = (a \cos u \cos v, \, a \cos u \sin v, \, b \sin u) \tag{14}$$

where $u \in [-\frac{\pi}{2}, \frac{\pi}{2}]$, $v \in [0, 2\pi)$, $a = 24$ mm to simulate the radius of a regular prostate, b is a Gaussian random variable with 24 mm mean and 4 mm standard deviation. The mean shape of $X(u,v)$ is a sphere with a 24 mm radius.

To simulate the manual segmented surfaces with ISE, we sampled an instance of true surface $Y_g(u,v)$ from Eq. (14) and then generate $Y(u,v)$ as

$$Y(u,v) = (Y_{g1}(u,v), \, Y_{g2}(u,v) + \theta \cos u \sin v, \, Y_{g3}(u,v))$$

where θ is a Gaussian random variable with zero mean and 4 mm standard deviation. For a fixed $Y_g(u,v)$, the shape of $Y(u,v)$ changes only along the y-axis. Under this setting, the segmentation error at the poles is zero and the largest segmentation error occurs at the equator. The surface assimilation algorithm was applied to each instance of $Y(u,v)$ to obtain $F(u,v)$. We illustrate this process in Fig. 2 where a cross-section view is chosen through the poles of the 3D surfaces.

All ROI surfaces are contained within a grayscale background object, representing the surrounding tissue. In the template space $T(x)$, the surrounding tissue is simulated by a vertically elongated ellipsoid rasterized from the surface

$$T(u,v) = (40 \cos u \cos v, \, 40 \cos u \sin v, \, 52 \sin u)$$

In the target space $S(x)$, the surrounding tissue is simulated by a horizontally elongated ellipsoid rasterized from the surface

$$S(u,v) = (40 \cos u \cos v, \, 52 \cos u \sin v, \, 40 \sin u)$$

where we chose 40 mm and 52 mm as the lengths of axes of the background objects to guarantee no surface sample touches them. The shapes of the these grayscale objects are fixed.

We made 400 sets of $X(u,v)$, $Y(u,v)$, $Y_g(u,v)$ and $F(u,v)$, respectively. And in total 400 pairs of images and surfaces registration were done. The TRE results (in five categories) are reported in Table 2. SSD performs worst among all algorithms. EWMS, UWMS and EWAS all improved the TRE and EWAS achieves the best results.

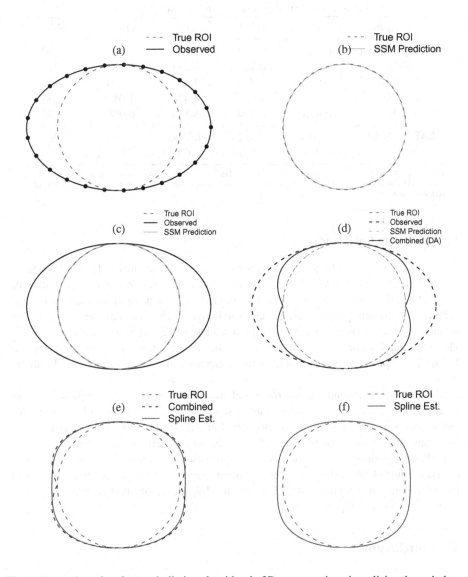

Fig. 2. Illustration of surface assimilation algorithm in 2D cross-section view slicing through the poles of the 3D surfaces. (a) shows a simulated manual segmentation (black) overlying on the true shape (pink). (b) the point distribution model (PDM) predicts where the true boundary is (cyan). (c) shows the true, the observed and the PDM-predicted surfaces together. The latter two are combined into the blue one in (d) for visual comparison. The estimated true shape by the spline regression is shown red in (e) and (f). Comparing (a) and (f) we can see that the assimilated surface is closer to the true one than the original segmentation.

Table 2. The target registration errors of each algorithm

Algorithm	RO	DSC	LDSC	MAD	HD
No Registration	0.835	0.905	2.693	2.364	4.464
SSD	0.631	0.770	1.241	4.182	9.363
EWMS	0.882	0.936	2.867	1.104	2.893
UWMS	0.886	0.938	2.914	1.052	2.811
EWAS	**0.913**	**0.954**	**3.124**	**0.900**	**2.263**
EWAS vs. EWMS	3.51%	1.96%	8.93%	18.5%	21.8%
improves	$(p < 0.001)$	$(p < 0.001)$	$(p < 0.001)$	$(p < 0.001)$	$(p < 0.001)$

RO: Relative Overlap, DSC: Dice Similarity Coefficient, LDSC: Logit Dice Similarity Coefficient, MAD: Mean Absolute Distance (mm), HD: Hausdorff Distance (mm). For RO, DSC and LDSC, higher is better. For MAD and HD, lower is better.

3.2 Real Data Case Study

We applied the proposed registration algorithm to register a pair of 3D FBCT images. The registration between FBCT to CBCT remains to be done. We chose a patient with 9 repeated FBCT scans on different treatment days. The prostate on each scan was contoured consistently by a single expert. The image and its associated manual prostate segmentation at the first day served as the template image $T(x)$ and surface $X(u, v)$. The image and surface of Scan 9 served as the target image $S(x)$ and true surface $Y_g(u, v)$. The prostate segmentations between Scan 1 and 8 were used to train the shape model.

$Y_g(u, v)$ is the ground truth surface and was not involved in the registration cost function. We simulated a possible manual segmentation $Y(u, v)$ with large segmentation error using the ISE model as described previously [17]. We estimated $Y_g(u, v)$ from the given $Y(u, v)$ using the surface assimilation method and obtained $F(u, v)$. For EWAS algorithm, $F(u, v)$ and $X(u, v)$ were used in the cost function. The output transformation deformed $Y_g(u, v)$ and compare with $X(u, v)$. Since all images were from the same imaging modality, C_{SSD} was used in the registration cost function. The results are shown in Fig. 3.

4   Conclusion

We presented a non-rigid image and surface registration algorithm that accommodates the surface segmentation error. Given a noisy surface, we construct a new one by correcting the boundary with large segmentation error using a statistical shape model. This surface estimation problem is solved by the method of smoothing spline regression. Experiments were done for 3D digital phantoms and one real patient case. By comparing the results with previous registration algorithms, our method shows its advantages in matching the images and surfaces.

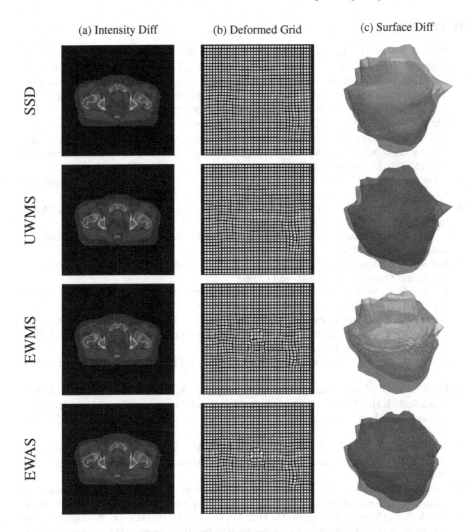

Fig. 3. The registration results of SSD, UWMS, EWMS and EWAS on the patient data. (a) the red-green blended image showing the difference between the template and the deformed target images after registration. (b) the deformed grid visualizing the transformation. (c) the 3D view of the template (pink) and the deformed true target surfaces with EWMS tinted gray and EWAS tinted blue, respectively. We can see that 1) the quality of intensity alignment among the algorithms is close, 2) the quality of local boundary matching around the prostate is different. Large deformation at the center (where the prostate is) can be seen in the deformed grids of EWMS and EWAS. Our results show the deformed surface of EWAS is closer to the template surface.

Acknowledgments. This work was supported by the National Cancer Institute Grant No P01CA116602.

References

1. Balik, S., Weiss, E., Jan, N., Roman, N., Sleeman, W.C., Fatyga, M., Christensen, G.E., Zhang, C., Murphy, M.J., Lu, J., Keall, P., Williamson, J.F., Hugo, G.D.: Evaluation of 4-dimensional computed tomography to 4-dimensional cone-beam computed tomography deformable image registration for lung cancer adaptive radiation therapy. International Journal of Radiation Oncology*Biology*Physics 86(2), 372–379 (2013)
2. Christensen, G., Carlson, B., Chao, K., Yin, P., Grigsby, P., Nguyen, K., Dempsey, J., Lerma, F., Bae, K., Vannier, M., et al.: Image-based dose planning of intracavitary brachytherapy: registration of serial-imaging studies using deformable anatomic templates. International Journal of Radiation Oncology Biology Physics 51(1), 227–243 (2001)
3. Cootes, T., Taylor, C., Cooper, D., Graham, J., et al.: Active shape models-their training and application. Computer Vision and Image Understanding 61(1), 38–59 (1995)
4. Craven, P., Wahba, G.: Smoothing noisy data with spline functions. Numerische Mathematik 31(4), 377–403 (1978)
5. Davies, R.H., Twining, C.J., Taylor, C.J.: Statistical models of shape - optimisation and evaluation. Springer (2008)
6. Dawson, L.A., Sharpe, M.B.: Image-guided radiotherapy: rationale, benefits, and limitations. The Lancet Oncology 7(10), 848–858 (2006)
7. Fitzpatrick, J., West, J., Maurer Jr., C.R.: Predicting error in rigid-body point-based registration. IEEE Transactions on Medical Imaging 17(5), 694–702 (1998)
8. Greene, W., Chelikani, S., Purushothaman, K., Knisely, J., Chen, Z., Papademetris, X., Staib, L., Duncan, J.: Constrained non-rigid registration for use in image-guided adaptive radiotherapy. Medical Image Analysis 13(5), 809–817 (2009)
9. Kalnay, E.: Atmospheric modeling, data assimilation, and predictability. Cambridge University Press (2003)
10. Lu, C., Chelikani, S., Papademetris, X., Knisely, J.P., Milosevic, M.F., Chen, Z., Jaffray, D.A., Staib, L.H., Duncan, J.S.: An integrated approach to segmentation and nonrigid registration for application in image-guided pelvic radiotherapy. Medical Image Analysis 15(5), 772–785 (2011)
11. Remeijer, P., Rasch, C., Lebesque, J.V., van Herk, M.: A general methodology for three-dimensional analysis of variation in target volume delineation. Medical Physics 26(6), 931–940 (1999)
12. Risholm, P., Janoos, F., Norton, I., Golby, A., Wells III, W.: Bayesian characterization of uncertainty in intra-subject non-rigid registration. Med. Image Anal. 17(5), 538–555 (2013)
13. Rueckert, D., Sonoda, L., Hayes, C., Hill, D., Leach, M., Hawkes, D.: Nonrigid registration using free-form deformations: application to breast mr images. IEEE Transactions on Medical Imaging 18(8), 712–721 (1999)
14. Wahba, G.: Spline models for observational data, vol. 59. Society for Industrial Mathematics (1990)
15. Wang, Y.: Smoothing splines: methods and applications. Taylor & Francis US (2011)
16. Wu, J., Murphy, M.J., Weiss, E., Sleeman IV, W.C., Williamson, J.: Development of a population-based model of surface segmentation uncertainties for uncertainty-weighted deformable image registrations. Medical Physics 37(2), 607–614 (2010)
17. Zhang, C., Christensen, G.E., Kurtek, S., Srivastava, A., Murphy, M.J., Weiss, E., Bai, E., Williamson, J.F.: SUPIR: Surface uncertainty-penalized, non-rigid image registration for pelvic CT imaging. In: Dawant, B.M., Christensen, G.E., Fitzpatrick, J.M., Rueckert, D. (eds.) WBIR 2012. LNCS, vol. 7359, pp. 236–245. Springer, Heidelberg (2012)
18. Zhou, J., Kim, S., Jabbour, S., Goyal, S., Haffty, B., Chen, T., Levinson, L., Metaxas, D., Yue, N.J.: A 3d global-to-local deformable mesh model based registration and anatomy-constrained segmentation method for image guided prostate radiotherapy. Medical Physics 37(3), 1298–1308 (2010)

3D Articulated Registration of the Mouse Hind Limb for Bone Morphometric Analysis in Rheumatoid Arthritis

James M. Brown[1,2,3], Amy Naylor[3],
Chris Buckley[3], Andrew Filer[3], and Ela Claridge[1,2]

[1] PSIBS Doctoral Training Centre, University of Birmingham, UK
J.M.Brown.1@cs.bham.ac.uk
[2] School of Computer Science, University of Birmingham, UK
[3] Rheumatology Research Group, School of Immunity and Infection,
University of Birmingham, UK

Abstract. We describe an automated method for building a statistical model of the mouse hind limb from micro-CT data, based on articulated registration. The model was initialised by hand-labelling the constituent bones and joints of a single sample. A coarse alignment of the entire model mesh to a sample mesh was followed by consecutive registration of individual bones and their descendants down a hierarchy. Transformation parameters for subsequent bones were constrained to a subset of vertices within a frustum projecting from a terminal joint of an already registered parent bone. Samples were segmented and transformed into a common coordinate frame, and a statistical shape model was constructed. The results of ten registered samples are presented, with a mean registration error of less than 40 µm ($\sim$ 3 voxels) for all samples. The shape variation amongst the samples was extracted by PCA to create a statistical shape model. Registration of the model to three unseen normal samples gives rise to a mean registration error of 5.84 µm, in contrast to 27.18 µm for three unseen arthritic samples. This may suggest that pathological bone shape changes in models of RA are detectable as departures from the model statistics.

1 Introduction

Rheumatoid arthritis (RA) is an autoimmune disease that affects approximately 1% of the world's population [1]. The autoimmune response mounted by the body gives rise to chronic inflammation of the synovial joints, which can cause active destruction of cartilage and bone. Although the exact cause of RA is unknown, new therapeutic targets may be discovered by investigating genes or processes that exacerbate or ameliorate disease progression. Animal models of inflammatory arthritis are frequently employed for this purpose, in conjunction with imaging techniques which provide data for deriving measures of disease severity [2,3]. Histological scoring is commonly used to ascertain the amount of

S. Ourselin and M. Modat (Eds.): WBIR 2014, LNCS 8545, pp. 41–50, 2014.

bone destruction, whereas x-ray microtomography (micro-CT) provides qualitative assessments of the damage. These commonly used techniques are subjective. In response to the need of the biomedical community we are working towards developing objective and quantitative measures of bone destruction from micro-CT images of the mouse hind limb.

The hypothesis underpinning our work is that shapes of bones affected by a pathology depart from statically normal bone shape variations. When a diseased limb sample is registered with a statistical shape model of a normal limb, any diseased regions will show as gross departures from the model. Such regions can then be characterised as erosions or spurs, and have their morphology and volume assessed. Statistical shape models describe the variation that exists within a set of aligned training shapes described by points. The active shape model (ASM) is commonly used to identify shape instances in medical image data by utilising the variability extracted from the training set by principal component analysis (PCA) [4]. In building such a model, it is necessary to establish point correspondences across the training set. This is often achieved by registering a single reference onto each sample, using algorithms such as iterative closet point (rigid) and B-spline free form deformation (non-rigid). This approach has been employed previously in building shape models of bones for the assessment of morphological variations in the primate humerus and scapula [5].

In our research, registration plays a vital role in both model construction and in abnormality detection. For the construction of a statistical shape model the individual samples must be co-registered in order to remove any differences that are not attributable to shape, such as their position, orientation and size. As the mouse hind limb is composed of multiple bones of various shapes and sizes, registration of a complete sample requires a 3D anatomical model that describes both structure and articulation. Having registered this model onto a series of samples, the pose-normalised bone shapes may be compared. The resulting model is similar to the hip joint model detailed in [6] in which only bone shape variations are modelled statistically, having previously aligned the samples based on known kinematic constraints. Finally, for abnormality detection, a sample in question must be co-registered with the model before establishing whether its shape deformations fall within the bounds defined by the model statistics. The closest work related to the bone pathology detection via model registration detailed the development of a statistical model of the rabbit femur, which was used to segment osteophytes (bone spurs) present in osteoarthritic femurs imaged by micro-CT [7]. Research described in this paper explores the possibility of identifying bone shape changes over the whole mouse hind limb in models of rheumatoid arthritis, such as periarticular bone loss and full thickness cortical bone damage. Although bone damage observed in RA is generally confined to the joints, we consider the entire hind limb in order to examine a variety of mouse models that may develop bone abnormalities elsewhere (e.g. spondyloarthropathy).

2   Method

This section first describes the methodology used to acquire and process the necessary image data used to construct an articulated model of the mouse hind limb. The framework for model-based registration and segmentation of a training set is then described, followed by the construction of a statistical model of non-pathological bone shapes and model validation. Analysis of an abnormal sample is performed by registering the articulated model, and iteratively deforming the mean bone shapes to produce the closest biologically feasible fit, and then assessing departures from the model as a measure of disease severity.

2.1   Image Acquisition and Processing

All experiments were carried out at the University of Birmingham following strict guidelines governed by the "Animal (Scientific Procedures) Act 1986" and approved by the local ethics committee. Female C57Bl/6 mice (Harlan, UK) were housed in individually ventilated cages in groups of 3-6 individuals on a 12 hour light-dark cycle with ad lib access to standard laboratory mouse chow diet and water. For arthritis experiments 200 µl KBxN serum was injected intraperitoneally into 10 week old mice, details of which can be found in [8]. All mice were sacrificed at 12 weeks of age. Both hind limbs were dissected and fixed in formalin over 24 hours in preparation for imaging.

Samples were imaged using a Skyscan1172 micro-CT scanner (Bruker), at a source voltage of 60 kV and source current of 167 µA, with a 0.5mm aluminium filter. Projections were taken every 0.45 degrees at 1000 ms exposure, with an image pixel size of 13.59 µm. Flat field corrections were performed to remove any effects caused by varied pixel sensitivity. Image slices (2000 x 2000 px) were reconstructed using NRecon 1.6.1.5 (Bruker), and beam hardening correction was applied to reduce cupping artefacts. Bone regions were segmented from soft tissue by global thresholding and a 3D surface mesh was computed using the marching cubes algorithm (CTAn 1.12, Bruker). The global threshold value was chosen manually, and kept consistent for all samples. Meshes were resampled using Poisson surface reconstruction to produce a smooth uniformly sampled mesh, and simplified using quadric edge collapse decimation [9]. Any mesh structure due to marrow space is of no interest in itself, and may misguide registration due to its highly variable morphology. Therefore, internal structures were isolated by ambient occlusion, and removed to give a completely hollow surface mesh (MeshLab 1.3.2, open-source).

2.2   Construction of an Articulated Model

To bootstrap the model construction, a single micro-CT scan of a wild-type mouse hind limb was first manually segmented into the constituent bones of interest by outlining individual slices (CTAn 1.12, Bruker). Global thresholding and mesh processing was then performed as described in Section 2.1. Joint positions were approximated by isolating the articulating bone surface, and calculating the mean vertex position. In constructing the model, the leg bones (tibia and fibula) were ignored due to the limited field of view in the micro-CT instrument. Sesamoid bones and claws were ignored as they are irrelevant to pathology detection.

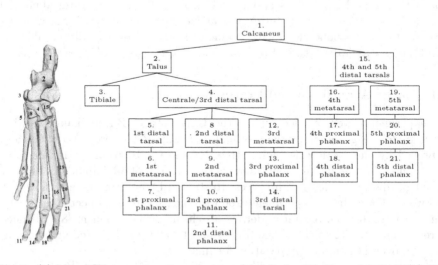

Fig. 1. (a) Micro-CT reconstruction of mouse hind limb with bones labelled. (b) Hierarchical representation of bones and their joints in the mouse hind limb. This representation provides the order in which model bones are registered to the sample mesh, which can be modified with ease for experimental purposes.

The topology of the mouse hind limb was represented as a tree (or hierarchy) where nodes and connections correspond to bones and joints, respectively (Figure 1). All nodes have exactly one parent node (except for the root node) with any geometric transformations applied to a parent bone being inherited by its children (i.e. if the 2nd metatarsal is rotated, then so are the 2nd proximal and distal phalanges). This hierarchical model was represented and stored as an eXstensible Markup Language (XML) document, allowing for construction of models with arbitrary hierarchies and traversal sequences.

2.3   Articulated Registration

The articulated registration algorithm follows the scheme outlined in [10], where an initial coarse alignment of a whole mouse atlas with the sample is followed by consecutive registration of individual bones, initialising subsequent registration steps. The method described in this paper differs in several ways to account for the differences in bone anatomy, joint complexity and proximity of parts. In particular (1) there is an additional coarse alignment of model and sample based on their "centres of mass"; (2) rigid (rotation, translation) and affine (rigid + scaling) transformations are carried out in separate ICP registration steps; and (3) motion constraint uses a viewing frustum, to account for the proximity and similarity of neighbouring components. Without incorporating these modifications registration yields unsatisfactory results in the form of misaligned bones. During this process, all transformations are applied to separate instances of the model, leaving individual samples stationary. In order to perform statistical shape analysis, sample bones are segmented (using the registration correspondence) and then inversely transformed into a common coordinate system as shown in Figure 4.

Coarse Alignment. The coarse alignment process globally aligns the model and sample meshes, providing an initialisation for the subsequent articulated registration. The curvature of the model and sample limbs is first approximated by equally subdividing the image volume along the longitudinal axis (the axis about which the specimen is rotated in the micro-CT instrument) and computing the centroid for each subvolume. This gives rise to two corresponding "centre of gravity" curves, from which a rotation matrix can be computed by solving a system of linear equations in a least-squares fashion.

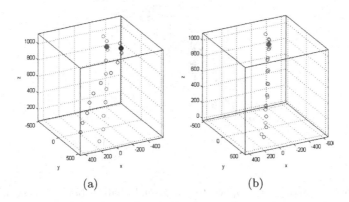

(a)   (b)

Fig. 2. Coarse alignment of model (blue) and sample (red) "centre of gravity curves" shown (a) before coarse alignment, and (b) after coarse alignment. The two larger points shown are the respective centres of mass. The alignment of these points aims to filter out rotational and translational effects associated with mounting the sample in the micro-CT scanner, prior to performing articulated registration.

The rotation matrix serves to align the meshes such that they both face the same direction. This does not however guarantee that the two meshes are aligned along the longitudinal axis. This is achieved by approximating their centres of mass, located near the ankle joint. The whole image volume is first projected onto its xy and yx planes, and the brightest pixels in each projection are then located (corresponding to the thickest regions of the specimen.) Of these pixels the topmost (nearest the leg) is chosen, and the centroid of the slice in which it resides is computed. The difference between the two centres of mass is used to determine the translational offset. The rotation and translation are then applied to the model, aligning it coarsely with the sample mesh. Figure 2 shows the result of applying the two transformations to two example curves.

Motion Constraints. Having coarsely aligned the model and sample mesh, the individual bones are registered by ICP consecutively down the hierarchy, with connected sub-trees inheriting the transformations computed at each step. The bones that comprise the mouse hind limb can be grouped into three shape categories; long bones (metatarsals, phalanges), small bones (tibiale, 1st and 2nd distal tarsal) and irregular bones (talus, calcaneus, 3rd - 5th distal tarsals). Small and irregular bones have limited natural motion, and so the entire search space is made available to the iterative closest point (ICP) algorithm when approximating point correspondence. By contrast, long bones have a greater range of motion which can yield an incorrect registration result if rotation is not constrained. This problem has been solved using a *field of view* approach.

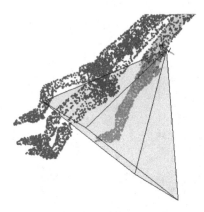

Fig. 3. Motion constraint as applied to a proximal phalanx bone by viewing frustum culling. The set of legal points within the viewing frustum are shown in green, and the set of illegal (culled) points are shown in red.

Having already registered its parent, registration of a child bone begins by finding an initial set of corresponding points by nearest-neighbour criteria. Rather than testing against all of the available sample points, the set is reduced to a set of feasible points that fall within a viewing frustum, parametrised by four angles (up, down, left and right). The viewing frustum is projected from the end of the parent bone along its principal axis, and the vertices that fall outside the frustum are eliminated (Figure 3). Correspondence is then approximated from the remaining points, and the optimal transformation found by ICP. The parametrisation of the viewing frustums for each bone was determined manually, and found to be consistent for all of samples used in the results presented. Having calculated the optimal rigid transformation, the entire search space is opened up once again for an additional ICP step that solves for differences in scaling. The iterative closest point (ICP) algorithm used in this work is a freely available MATLAB implementation[1].

Segmentation and Shape Modelling. The result of registering the articulated model to a set of n training samples is a set of n transformed model instances. The point correspondence that the registration yields is used to segment the individual samples, by propagating labels between model and sample vertices. Each of the meshes is composed of several thousand points, and in all likelihood will not have the same exact amount in each. As a result, not every point will receive a label, and so unlabelled mesh patches are assigned a label based on neighbouring vertices (those that share an edge). Anatomical structures not represented in the model (e.g. claws, small non-articulating bones) are left unlabelled.

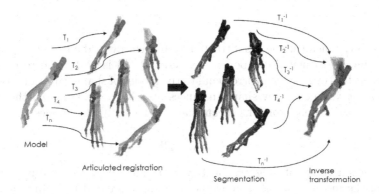

Fig. 4. The registration and segmentation workflow for statistical shape model construction. The process begins with the articulated model being registered onto each of the n samples, which remain stationary. After registration, each sample is segmented according to the learned correspondence, and inversely transformed into the common (model) coordinate system according to the transformations gathered during registration.

The labelled samples are inversely transformed using the learned registration parameters so that the whole training set adopts a common coordinate frame. The coregistered samples can now be integrated into a multi-part statistical model, where shape variation of each individual bone is modelled separately. For each bone, an $n \times 3m$ system matrix is formed (where m is the number of points)

---

[1] Finite Iterative Closest Point: http://www.mathworks.co.uk/matlabcentral/fileexchange/24301-finite-iterative-closest-point)

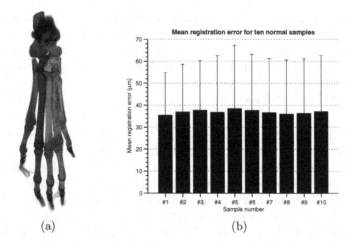

(a)   (b)

Fig. 5. Results of articulated registration of ten samples: (a) the original model overlaid with the registered samples and (b) the mean registration error for the ten samples. The results demonstrate a registration accuracy of less than 40 μm (∼3 voxels) over the whole hind limb (error bars correspond to one standard deviation).

from which the mean shape is subtracted from each row and a covariance matrix P is computed. Principal component analysis (PCA) is performed to compute the eigenvectors of P, which correspond to the modes of shape variation, in order of decreasing variance. New shape instances may be generated from the model as weighted deviations from the mean shape along the first p modes:

$$X = \bar{X} + Pb \tag{1}$$

where b is a vector of weights, constrained to fall within three standard deviations of the mean. Normal bone shapes are approximated by finding a vector b for each bone that minimises the least-squared distance (using the Levenberg-Marquardt algorithm) between the model and sample points. By constraining the deformations to biologically feasible limits, the differences between the model and sample may be attributed to pathological shape changes.

3   Results and Validation

Ten wild-type (normal) mouse hind limb samples (5 females, C57Bl/6, 12 weeks old) were acquired and imaged by micro-CT, and processed according to protocols outlined in Section 2.1. Articulated registration was performed on the ten samples which are shown overlaid with the original model in Figure 5 alongside the mean registration error for each sample. Registration error is defined as the mean Euclidean distance in voxels between model (M) and corresponding sample (S) points:

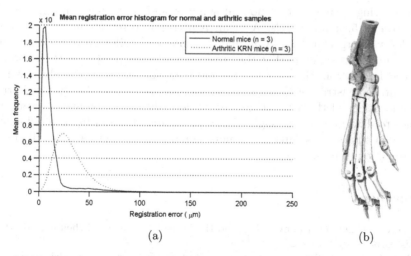

(a)   (b)

Fig. 6. (a) Result of articulated registration with shape model fitting to three unseen normal samples and three unseen arthritic samples. On average, the normal samples are more accurately approximated by the model that the arthritic samples (with mean errors of 5.84 μm and 27.18 μm respectively) indicating the presence of statistically abnormal shape features. (b) An example of a KRN mouse hind limb, with evidence of bone destruction around the metatarsals.

$$E(M, S) = \frac{1}{n} \sum_{i=1}^{n} \sqrt{(M(x_i, y_i, z_i) - S(x_i, y_i, z_i))^2} \tag{2}$$

To test the model's ability to approximate samples from outside the training set, articulated registration and shape model fitting was applied to three normal samples (from outside the training set) and three arthritic samples. The results are shown in Figure 6 as mean error histograms.

4   Conclusion

In this paper, we demonstrated a method for constructing a statistical model of the mouse hind limb. Manual segmentation and labelling of a single sample provides an articulated model which may be used to extract bone shape variation from a set of unlabelled samples. Registration of the model onto a set of ten samples achieved a mean registration error of less than 40 μm ($\sim$ 3 voxels). Whilst some errors are due to natural shape variation, others may attributed to cumulative misregistration of connected parts. The effect of coarse aligment on the final results will therefore be investigated in future work. After registration, labels were transferred onto the samples which were then inversely transformed into a common (model) coordinate system. The co-registered samples were used to build a bone-by-bone statistical model of shape variations via PCA. The ability of the model to represent unseen normal shapes was successfully validated by registering a small set of normal samples and obtaining a mean registration error of 5.84 μm voxels. A mean registration error for unseen abnormal samples was larger, at 27.18 μm, and its mode was shifted towards larger displacements. This suggests that the erosions and spurs present in the abnormal samples depart from the model of normal bone shape. Further analysis will be aimed at demonstrating that the latter results are mainly due to large errors at the locations of the arthritic abnormalities, which may be mapped onto the meshes to determine their height/depth or volume. Computing the differences between an abnormal sample and a normal model at these locations will aid the quantification of pathologies.

References

1. Buckley, C.D.: Science, medicine, and the future: Treatment of rheumatoid arthritis. Brit. Med. J. 315, 236–238 (1997)
2. Asquith, D.L., Miller, A.M., McInnes, I.B., Liew, F.Y.: Animal models of rheumatoid arthritis. Eur. J. Immunol. 39, 2040–2044 (2009)
3. Diarra, D., Stolina, M., Polzer, K., Zwerina, J., et al.: Dickkopf-1 is a master regulator of joint remodeling. Nat. Med. 13, 156–163 (2007)
4. Cootes, T.F., Taylor, C.J., Cooper, D.H., Graham, J., et al.: Active shape models - their training and application. Comput. Vis. Image Und. 6, 38–59 (1995)
5. Yang, Y.: Shape modelling of bones: application to the primate shoulder. Ph.D thesis, Imperial College London, UK (2008)
6. Kainmueller, D., Lamecker, H., Zachow, S., Hege, H.C.: An articulated statistical shape model for accurate hip Joint Segmentation. In: IEEE EMB-M, pp. 6345–6351 (2009)
7. Saha, P.K., Liang, G., Elkins, J.M., Coimbra, A., Duong, L.T., Williams, D.S., Sonka, M.: A New Osteophyte Segmentation Algorithm using Partial Shape Model and its Applications to Rabbit Femur Anterior Cruciate Ligament Transection via Micro-CT Imaging. IEEE T. Bio-Med. Eng. 55, 2212–2227 (2011)
8. Monach, P.A., Mathis, D., Benoist, C.: The K/BxN Arthritis Model. Curr. Protoc. Immunol. 81, 15:22.1–15:22.12 (2008)
9. Garland, M., Heckbert, P.S.: Surface simplification using quadric error metrics. In: SIGGRAPH, pp. 209–216 (1997)
10. Baiker, M., Milles, J., Vossepoel, A.M., Que, I., Kaijzel, E.L., Lowik, C., Reiber, J.H.C., Dijkstra, J., Lelieveldt, B.P.F.: Fully automated whole-body registration in mice using an articulated skeleton atlas. In: IEEE ISBI: From Nano to Macro, pp. 728–731 (2007)

Non-parametric Discrete Registration
with Convex Optimisation

Mattias P. Heinrich[1], Bartlomiej W. Papież[2],
Julia A. Schnabel[2], and Heinz Handels[1]

[1] Institute of Medical Informatics, University of Lübeck, Germany
[2] Institute of Biomedical Engineering,
Department of Engineering, University of Oxford, UK
heinrich@imi.uni-luebeck.de
www.mpheinrich.de

Abstract. Deformable image registration is an important step in
medical image analysis. It enables an automatic labelling of anatomical structures using atlas-based segmentation, motion compensation and
multi-modal fusion. The use of discrete optimisation approaches has recently attracted a lot attention for mainly two reasons. First, they are
able to find an approximate global optimum of the registration cost function and can avoid false local optima. Second, they do not require a
derivative of the similarity metric, which increases their flexibility. However, the necessary quantisation of the deformation space causes a very
large number of degrees of freedom with a high computational complexity. To deal with this, previous work has focussed on parametric transformation models. In this work, we present an efficient non-parametric
discrete registration method using a filter-based similarity cost aggregation and a decomposition of similarity and regularisation term into two
convex optimisation steps. This approach enables non-parametric registration with billions of degrees of freedom with computation times of less
than a minute. We apply our method to two different common medical
image registration tasks, intra-patient 4D-CT lung motion estimation
and inter-subject MRI brain registration for segmentation propagation.
We show improvements on current state-of-the-art performance both in
terms of accuracy and computation time.

1 Introduction and Background

Deformable image registration is an integral part of medical image analysis and
has been the focus of a large amount of research. Most deformable registration algorithms consist of three parts: similarity metric, optimisation strategy
and transformation model, a comprehensive overview of the current literature
is given in [21]. Image registration between an target image I_t and moving image I_m can in general be stated as an energy optimisation problem. The spatial
transformation $\phi = Id + \mathbf{u}$, consisting of identity transform Id and deformation
field $\mathbf{u}$, is sought that minimises the cost function $E(I_t, I_m, \mathbf{u})$.

S. Ourselin and M. Modat (Eds.): WBIR 2014, LNCS 8545, pp. 51–61, 2014.
© Springer International Publishing Switzerland 2014

We define a cost function for deformable registration, which consists of a similarity term $\mathcal{S}$ and a regularisation term $\mathcal{R}$, where α is a positive factor that balances the weighting between both penalties:

$$E(\mathbf{u}) = \mathcal{S}(I_t, I_m, \mathbf{u}) + \alpha \mathcal{R}(\mathbf{u}) \tag{1}$$

Most registration approaches optimise this combined cost function directly. A pointwise similarity term, such as the sum of squared differences, defined for each voxel $\mathbf{x}$: $\mathcal{S}(\mathbf{x}) = (I_t(\mathbf{x}) - I_m(\mathbf{x} + \mathbf{u}))^2$, contains a non-linearity with respect to $\mathbf{u}$. Therefore, it cannot be directly solved using convex optimisation.

Continuous Optimisation: One approach is to linearise the similarity term to obtain an approximate step towards the desired solution. This linearisation is only valid for a small deformation step, the registration thus requires a series of small iterative updates. This results in two disadvantages: large deformations of small anatomical features might be lost, as only a local optimum is found, and many iterations are required to reach convergence. Additionally the linearisation requires the derivative of the similarity to be computed, which restricts the flexibility of continuous optimisation approaches.

MRF-Based Optimisation: In order to overcome the above discussed disadvantages of gradient-based techniques, the use of discrete optimisation has been proposed based on a Markov random field (MRF) formulation [7]. Here, the deformation field $\mathbf{u}$ is not represented by a continuous vector field, but defined as a (dense) set of discrete spatial displacement labels $\mathbf{d} \in \mathcal{L} = \{0, \pm 1, \ldots \pm l_{max}\}^3$. The cost of assigning a certain label $\mathbf{d} \in \mathcal{L}$ to each voxel $\mathbf{x}$ depends on the unary potentials, which correspond to the (pointwise) image similarity and pairwise (or higher-order) interactions (representing the regularisation term). Different optimisation methods can be employed, however, even the simplest inference algorithms (e.g. dynamic programming on a tree [9]) have a high computational complexity. Therefore most previous approaches for discrete optimisation in medical image registration used parametric transformation models[1]. Glocker et al. [7] used a B-spline transformation model and further reduced the complexity by restricting the potential displacements to lie along the three normal axes. In [17] a finite element method is used to parametrise the transformations.

Local Cost Aggregation: Alternatively, local regularisation models have been used for discrete registration (or stereo estimation). In cost aggregation approaches [19], no explicit global regularisation of the deformation field is performed, and the motion is only locally constrained to be smooth by averaging the similarity term over a small window. These techniques work reasonably well and are computationally fast. However, they often require ad-hoc post-processing steps to propagate information into textureless regions.

In this work, we present a different solution, which is based on a dual optimisation technique following the idea of [5]. The non-convex optimisation problem

---

[1] The only exception for 3D registration we know of is [20], where a non-parametric solution is obtained with graph cuts resulting in computation times of 24 hours.

can be split into two convex problems: one for the similarity term and one for the regularisation, by introducing an auxiliary vector field linking both terms. Each term is optimised in alternation, increasing the linking between them until both vector fields converge. This concept has been previously investigated in [2] resulting in the "Pair-And-Smooth, Hybrid Energy based Algorithm" (PASHA), and can be implicitly found in the demons registration approach [24]. However, these approaches are based on gradient-based optimisation of the similarity cost. In contrast, we propose to use a discretised search space to find a better optimum of the similarity term (following the ideas presented in [22] for optical flow estimation) and additionally use a local cost aggregation step.

The remainder of this paper is organised as follows. Sec. 2 introduces our method consisting of local cost aggregation, convex optimisation for global smoothness and minimisation of inverse inconsistencies. The implementation used to efficiently solve the proposed model will be explained in detail. In Sec. 3 we present the employed experiments on two different challenging medical image registration tasks. Sec. 4 discusses the results and gives an outlook on further possible research directives.

2   Methods

Our proposed non-parametric discrete registration method aims to find the deformation field $\mathbf{u}$, which minimises a cost function over the image domain:

$$E(\mathbf{u}) = \sum_{\Omega} \mathcal{S}(I_t, I_m, \mathbf{u}) + \alpha |\nabla \mathbf{u}|^2 \qquad (2)$$

The second term penalises the squared gradient of the displacement field, which forms a diffusive regularisation. The similarity term can be either point-wise or defined over a local neighbourhood (image patch) Ω.

Our method estimates a deformation field in three steps. First, an explicit search is performed over a discrete displacement space only enforcing smoothness by **local cost aggregation** (Sec. 2.1). This yields a prior map of probable displacements based on the similarity term and an initial best displacement for each voxel. Second, **global smoothness** is enforced through alternative updates of the estimated deformations and the similarity distribution using an auxiliary term (Sec. 2.2). Third, **inverse consistency** [6] is achieved by minimising the discrepancy between forward and backward transforms (Sec. 2.3). This can be used to enforce a one-to-one mapping between two images, in order to avoid physically implausible folding of the deformation field.

2.1   Local Cost Aggregation

Following the definition of previous discrete registration approaches, e.g. [9], we restrict the deformations $\mathbf{u}$ to be part a quantised set of 3D displacements $\mathbf{d} \in \mathcal{L}$ for each voxel $\mathbf{x}$:

$$\mathbf{d} \in \mathcal{L} = \{0, \pm q, \pm 2q, \dots, \pm l_{max}\}^3,$$

with a quantisation step q and maximal displacement range of l_{max}. The advantage of this approach compared to a linearisation of the similarity function is that both an iterative solution and a local optimum can be avoided. Analogously, to previous work on local cost aggregation in stereo estimation [12,19], we first construct a six-dimensional displacement space volume (DSV), which extends the image dimensions by three dimensions (for the 3D displacement label space $\mathcal{L}$). Each entry of the DSV represents the point-wise similarity cost of translating a voxel $\mathbf{x}$ with a certain displacement $\mathbf{d}$:

$$DSV(\mathbf{x}, \mathbf{d}) = \mathcal{S}(I_t(\mathbf{x}), I_m(\mathbf{x} + \mathbf{d})) \qquad (3)$$

To enforce constant motion within a small local region, we average the similarity term over a local patch for every voxel. However, a naive implementation of such a windowed cost evaluation would have considerable computational cost. Yet, for uniform or spatially weighted (e.g. B-Spline) patches a cost aggregation with constant complexity regardless of the patch size can be obtained through a spatial convolution (or moving average) filter. The convolution filter K is applied to every 3D subvolume (i.e. in spatial domain) of the DSV with a constant displacement (see [12], Fig. 1 for a visual example of this procedure).

We could stop here and directly obtain a displacement field by selecting the displacement $\mathbf{d}$ with the lowest aggregated cost for each voxel:

$$\mathbf{u} = \underset{\mathbf{d} \in \mathcal{L}}{\operatorname{argmin}}(K \star DSV(\mathbf{d})) \qquad (4)$$

This concept, which is often called winner-takes-all (WTA), already achieves a relatively robust estimation of deformations. An alternative way to obtain a cost aggregation is though iterative diffusion of the similarity images [19], which repeatedly replaces the value of a voxel with a weighted average of its neighbours.

The concept of filter-based local cost aggregation is directly suitable for point-wise similarity metrics. One possible choice is to use the sum of absolute differences (SAD) of self-similarity context (SSC) descriptors as introduced by Heinrich et al. [8]. The descriptors represent the self-similarity of small image patches within a local neighbourhood of each voxel. This yields a twelve-valued vector, which is quantised into a single 64-bit integer. Evaluating the SAD of two vectors $\mathbf{s}_t$ and $\mathbf{s}_m$ with quantised representations S_t and S_m therefore simplifies to calculating their Hamming weight:

$$SSC(\mathbf{x}) = \sum_{i=1}^{12} |s_t(\mathbf{x})^i - s_m(\mathbf{x})^i| = \Xi\{S_t(\mathbf{x}) \oplus S_m(\mathbf{x})\}, \qquad (5)$$

where the function $\Xi\{\cdot\}$ represents the bit-count operation. The advantage of this metric is that it can be evaluated very quickly and has been shown to be robust against local change in contrast and image noise. A local cost aggregation within the DSV follows accordingly to Eqs. 3 and 4.

We can extend the local cost aggregation from point-wise to patch-based similarity metrics. In particular local cross-correlation (LCC) is here of interest, as it has been widely used for medical image registration [1,15]. LCC can be directly calculated over a local window Ω centred around $\mathbf{x}$ by:

$$LCC(\mathbf{x}) = \frac{\sum_\Omega (I_t(\mathbf{x}) - \mu_t)(I_m(\mathbf{x}) - \mu_m)}{\sqrt{\sum_\Omega (I_t(\mathbf{x}) - \mu_t)^2}\sqrt{\sum_\Omega (I_m(\mathbf{x}) - \mu_m)^2}} \tag{6}$$

where μ_m and μ_t define the local intensity mean in moving and target images respectively. These values and the local standard deviations $V_{m,t}(\mathbf{x}) = \sqrt{1/|\Omega| \sum_\Omega (I_{m,t}(\mathbf{x}) - \mu_{m,t})^2}$ do not depend on the translational displacement $\mathbf{d}$ and can therefore be pre-computed once for both images. Following the approach in [14] (similarly presented in [1]), we can efficiently compute LCC for each displacement in constant complexity independent of the patch-size. When expanding the numerator of Eq. 6, we obtain:

$$\frac{1}{|\Omega|} \sum_\Omega I_t(\mathbf{x})I_m(\mathbf{x}) - \mu_t \sum_\Omega I_m(\mathbf{x}) - \mu_m \sum_\Omega I_t(\mathbf{x}) + \mu_t\mu_m.$$

Since $\mu_{t,m} = 1/|\Omega| \sum_\Omega I_{t,m}(\mathbf{x})$, we can simplify this to: $1/|\Omega| \sum_\Omega I_t(\mathbf{x})I_m(\mathbf{x}) - \mu_t\mu_m$. The summation of the first term, can again be more efficiently computed by first taking the point-wise product of the image intensities followed by a constant time averaging filter. Since, the local variances have been pre-computed, evaluating the LCC for each voxel and displacement only requires 10 operations: a huge speed-up compared to the naive approach, especially for large windows.

Using the WTA approach, however, does not enforce any global smoothness and can therefore lead to poor motion estimation for homogenous areas with little texture. For these reasons, most local stereo estimation methods perform post-processing steps to remove false correspondences.

2.2   Global Smoothness with Convex Optimisation

To improve the motion estimation for homogenous areas, we adopt the approach presented by [22], which follows the primal dual approaches for total variation based image processing [5]. An auxiliary second deformation field $\mathbf{v}$ is introduced and the combined cost function $E(\mathbf{v}, \mathbf{u})$ is solved in two alternating steps.

$$E(\mathbf{v}, \mathbf{u}) = DSV(\mathbf{v}) + \frac{1}{2\theta}(\mathbf{v} - \mathbf{u})^2 + \alpha|\nabla\mathbf{u}|^2 \tag{7}$$

The optimal selection of $\mathbf{v}$ with respect to the similarity term, together with the auxiliary middle term can be performed globally optimal, as before, using local cost aggregation and WTA selection (of the DSV plus the coupling term). Note, that the disparity space volume (DSV) has to be computed only once. The regularisation penalty can be solved optimally by a Gaussian smoothing of the deformation field. The parameter α controls the diffusivity of the deformation field and is implicitly set through the variance of the Gaussian kernel σ^2. The update is performed by $\mathbf{u} \leftarrow K_\sigma\mathbf{v}$. The parameter θ models the coupling between similarity and regularisation penalty and is decreased during a number of iterations. In our experiments, we have used five iterations of this dual convex optimisation with $\theta = \theta_0 \cdot \{150, 50, 15, 5, 1.5\}$, where θ_0 is a parameter which should be adapted to the range of a specific similarity metric. For $\theta \to 0$ we reach convergence and $\mathbf{u} = \mathbf{v}$. We have chosen isotropic diffusion regularisation with Gaussian smoothing, which has been widely used for medical image registration, but other regularisation penalties or filters (e.g. bilateral filters [16]) could be easily integrated into this framework.

2.3   Inverse Consistency

Following our above formulation, the registration outcome would be dependent on the choice of target and moving image. To remove this bias and ensure a one-to-one mapping, we use a simple scheme to obtain inverse consistent mappings, given the forward and backward displacement fields $\mathbf{u}_f$ and $\mathbf{u}_b$ respectively (which are independently calculated). We aim to reduce the inverse consistency error (ICE) [6]. This can be achieved according to [8] by iteratively updating the following equations:

$$\mathbf{u}_f^{n+1} = 0.5(\mathbf{u}_f^n - \mathbf{u}_b^n(\mathbf{x} + \mathbf{u}_f^n)) \qquad (8)$$
$$\mathbf{u}_b^{n+1} = 0.5(\mathbf{u}_b^n - \mathbf{u}_f^n(\mathbf{x} + \mathbf{u}_b^n))$$

where the initial (asymmetric) transformation are denoted by a time-point $n = 0$. Empirically, we found that 10 iterations are sufficient to reduce the ICE to insignificantly low values and also ensure the absence negative Jacobian values (and thus singularities) within the deformation fields. Further details on the convergence of this scheme can be found in [10] Ch. 4.4.1.

3   Experiments

In order to show the benefits of our new approach, we compare its performance for two challenging datasets for medical image registration. First, the deformable registration of inter-patient brain MRI scans, and second, intra-patient lung motion estimation of 4D-CT scans. The first experiment employs the Columbia University Medical Center (CUMC) dataset [4], consisting of 1.5 T MRI scans of 12 subjects, which have been manually labeled into 130 anatomical or functional regions. For the second experiment, we use the ten cases of the DIR-lab dataset [3], which has been validated with 300 manual landmarks for both the maximum inspiration and maximum expiration phase of a breathing cycle. The motivation for choosing these two datasets is that both have been widely used to evaluate state-of-the-art deformable registration techniques.

3.1   Parameter Choices

We use a multi-resolution scheme with three levels and downsampling factors of $\{3, 2, 1\}$ for all experiments. We use a **dense displacement sampling (deeds)** [9] with a sampling range of $l_{max} = \{6, 4, 2\}$ voxels for the three resolution levels and a quantisation of $q = 1$ voxel. For the brain and lung dataset, we chose LCC and SSC [8] respectively as similarity metric. To obtain SSC descriptors in a lower resolution, we calculate self-similarity distances in the original image resolution and downsample only the final descriptors. A parameter variation has been performed for a subset of the CUMC12 registration experiment, to examine the influence of the radius r of the box-filter for local cost aggregation (or patch-size of LCC computation respectively), the parameter σ for the diffusive regularisation of deformation fields and θ_0 to scale the range of the similarity metric. The Dice metric $D = 2|A \cap M|/(|A| + |M|)$ between automatic and manual segmentations A and M (calculated separately for each of the 130 label regions) has been chosen to evaluate the quality of registrations. The registration accuracy varies between $D = 50.5 - 50.8\%$ for $0.4 \leq \sigma \leq 1.0$ voxels and $D = 50.4 - 50.8\%$ for $0.25 \leq \theta \leq 4$. Using radii of $\{0, 1, 2, 3, 4\}$ voxels for the LCC metric results in segmentation overlaps of $\{36.0, 50.9, 50.8, 50.3, 49.3\}\%$, indicating a very good robustness except when skipping the cost aggregation entirely. The chosen parameters for all further experiments using the symmetric formulation are: $\sigma = 0.6$, $r = 2$, and $\theta_0 = 1$. The best settings for an asymmetric registration are the same except for $\sigma = 1.2$, which results in $D = 50.8\%$.

3.2 Computation Time

We use an efficient multi-threaded CPU implementation, which is being made available at www.mpheinrich.de/software.html and run experiments on a dual-core processor. When using an asymmetric registration formulation, ≈ 20 sec. (for all resolutions) are spent on calculating the DSV and aggregating its cost locally, and half a minute for the iterative global regularisation, yielding a total time for one 3D brain registration (with a volume size of $256 \times 256 \times 124$) of less than one minute. If a symmetric transformation is required, these computation times double and an additional time of ≈ 40 sec. has to be added for enforcing inverse consistency of the deformation fields. When using the SSC similarity metric, ≈ 10 sec. are spent on calculating the descriptors. These processing times are more then an order of magnitude faster than the top performing algorithms in [13] and further speed-ups could be expected when using a GPU (c.f. [12]).

3.3 Results

The CUMC12 dataset has been used in a comprehensive comparison study of 14 non-linear registration methods in [13]. In those experiments, the Jaccard index $J = (A \cap M)/(A \cup M)$ was used to evaluate the registration accuracy. We are therefore able to directly compare our approach to 14 other algorithms for a total of 132 one-to-one registrations. The same pre-processing of the data as detailed in [13] has been used: in particular removing the skull in the images using the provided brain masks. Our method achieves the highest overlap of all methods, with $J = 36.3\%$, see Fig. 1. The usefulness of the global regularisation step is demonstrated by performing the same experiments as before, but this time only

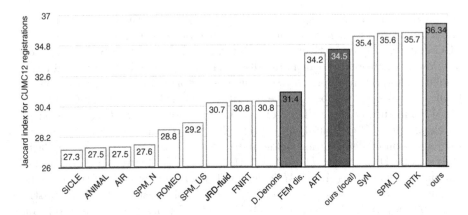

Fig. 1. Jaccard overlap (over 130 regions) for 16 non-linear registration algorithms for CUMC12 dataset. Our approach achieves the highest accuracy with $J = 36.3\%$.

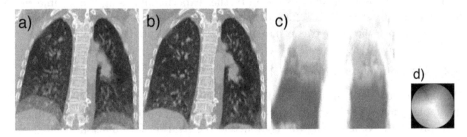

Fig. 2. Coronal view of overlay of inhale and exhale phase of Case # 6 of [3] before (a) and after (b) alignment using our proposed non-parametric discrete registration. The estimated deformation field (c) is represented by HSV colours (d), where the vector orientation is indicated by hue and the deformation length by saturation. The complexity of the deformation field std(Jac) lies between 0.23 and 0.33 for the 10 cases.

use the local cost aggregation (see Eq. 4) followed by one Gaussian smoothing as post-processing. This variant (denoted as "local") achieves only $J = 34.5\%$. We also outperform the FEM based discrete registration approach of, Popuri et al. [17], whose work is the most similar to ours and achieves $J = 31.4\%$. In contrast to us, they use a parametric transformation model, variational smoothing and do not include a global convex optimisation of the regularisation term.

The second experiment is challenging for continuous optimisation approaches, because there is a large discrepancy of the magnitude and direction of the motion inside and outside of the lungs. Currently, most approaches that achieve a high accuracy, e.g. [11] or [18] deal with this problem by segmenting the lungs and masking out the rib-cage and other body parts. In our approach, a discrete sampling of the displacement, with a very large range of possible motion vectors $(6 \times 2 + 1)^3 = 2197$, is used in the lowest resolution to capture large motion of small features. Using the same settings as before (except that we selected

SSC, as we found it works better as similarity metric for this task), we obtain a target registration error of 1.17 mm. This is only marginally higher than the best results, previously achieved for masked registration: 0.99 mm ([11] and [18]). Our approach is so far the most accurate for unmasked registration for this dataset, with an improvement of $\approx$ 0.25 mm to the results of [9] (1.43 mm) and [11] (1.41 mm w/o masks). Figure 2 shows an example registration outcome including the obtained deformation field.

4 Conclusion

We have presented a new framework for discrete medical image registration, which includes both local and global regularisation. The search space of potential deformations is sampled in a dense manner, thus avoiding local minima or the need for an iterative refinement. A local regularisation is integrated by a cost aggregation scheme, which is performed through a spatial filtering of the displacement space volume (DSV). The global diffusive smoothness prior is enforced through an alternating update of the distribution of the locally aggregated image similarity and a global deformation field smoothing through Gaussian convolution. Solving each of the two decoupled functionals separately results in convex optimisation problems that can be solved optimally. After few iterations, this procedure converges to a very good approximation of the optimum of the combined cost function (and a substantial improvement over using only local regularisation). Our approach, which achieves computation times of less than one minute per 3D registration, performs best on the CUMC12 brain dataset in comparison to 15 other state-of-the-art techniques and within 0.2 mm of the best approaches for the DIR-Lab lung dataset. Additional results for the remaining three datasets of the Klein study [13] support the initial findings resulting in Jaccard scores of 56.38% (for LPBA40), 39.54% (for MGH10) and 36.43% (for IBSR18), which each outperform the previously best results.

Further research could improve on the presented results, by integrating additional information, e.g. segmentations or better priors on the deformation field regularity. In the future, we would like to directly compare our approach to global MRF-based optimisation strategies [7,9]. The use of this framework for other challenging medical image registration tasks, including multi-modal registration, is be directly possible. An interesting alternative to the use of identical support regions for each voxel could be the use of multiple potential window sizes to represent simultaneously multiple scales of deformations (c.f. [23]).

Acknowledgements. B.W.P. and J.A.S. would like to acknowledge funding from the CRUK/ EPSRC Cancer Imaging Centre at Oxford.

References

1. Avants, B.B., Tustison, N.J., Song, G., Cook, P.A., Klein, A., Gee, J.C.: A reproducible evaluation of ANTs similarity metric performance in brain image registration. Neuroimage 54(3), 2033–2044 (2011)

2. Cachier, P., Bardinet, E., Dormont, D., Pennec, X., Ayache, N.: Iconic feature based nonrigid registration: The PASHA algorithm. Comput. Vis. Image Underst. 89(2-3), 272–298 (2003)
3. Castillo, R., Castillo, E., Guerra, R., Johnson, V.E., McPhail, T., Garg, A.K., Guerrero, T.: A framework for evaluation of deformable image registration spatial accuracy using large landmark point sets. Phys. Med. Biol. 54(7), 1849 (2009)
4. Caviness Jr., V.S., Meyer, J., Makris, N., Kennedy, D.N.: MRI-based Topographic Parcellation of Human Neocortex: An Anatomically Specified Method with Estimate of Reliability. Journal of Cognitive Neuroscience 8(6), 566–587 (1996)
5. Chambolle, A.: An algorithm for total variation minimization and applications. Journal of Mathematical Imaging and Vision 20(1-2), 89–97 (2004)
6. Christensen, G.E., Johnson, H.J.: Consistent Image Registration. IEEE Trans. Med. Imag. 20(7), 568–582 (2001)
7. Glocker, B., Komodakis, N., Tziritas, G., Navab, N., Paragios, N.: Dense image registration through MRFs and efficient linear programming. Med. Imag. Anal. 12(6), 731–741 (2008)
8. Heinrich, M.P., Jenkinson, M., Papież, B.W., Brady, M., Schnabel, J.A.: Towards Realtime Multimodal Fusion for Image-Guided Interventions Using Self-Similarities. In: Mori, K., Sakuma, I., Sato, Y., Barillot, C., Navab, N. (eds.) MICCAI 2013, Part I. LNCS, vol. 8149, pp. 187–194. Springer, Heidelberg (2013)
9. Heinrich, M.P., Jenkinson, M., Brady, M., Schnabel, J.A.: MRF-based Deformable Registration and Ventilation Estimation of Lung CT. IEEE Trans. Med. Imag. 32(7), 1239–1248 (2013)
10. Heinrich, M.P.: Deformable lung registration for pulmonary image analysis of MRI and CT scans. University of Oxford (2013)
11. Hermann, S., Werner, R.: High Accuracy Optical Flow for 3D Medical Image Registration Using the Census Cost Function. In: Klette, R., Rivera, M., Satoh, S. (eds.) PSIVT 2013. LNCS, vol. 8333, pp. 23–35. Springer, Heidelberg (2014)
12. Hosni, A., Rhemann, C., Bleyer, M., Rother, C., Gelautz, M.: Fast Cost-Volume Filtering for Visual Correspondence and Beyond. IEEE Trans. Pattern Anal. Mach. Intell. 35(2), 504–511 (2013)
13. Klein, A., et al.: Evaluation of 14 nonlinear deformation algorithms applied to human brain MRI registration. Neuroimage 46(3), 786–802 (2008)
14. Lewis, J.P.: Fast normalized cross-correlation. Vision Interface 10(1), 120–123 (1995)
15. Lorenzi, M., Ayache, N., Frisoni, G.B., Pennec, X.: LCC-Demons: a robust and accurate diffeomorphic registration algorithm. NeuroImage 81, 470–483 (2013)
16. Papież, B.W., Heinrich, M.P., Risser, L., Schnabel, J.A.: Complex Lung Motion Estimation via Adaptive Bilateral Filtering of the Deformation Field. In: Mori, K., Sakuma, I., Sato, Y., Barillot, C., Navab, N. (eds.) MICCAI 2013, Part III. LNCS, vol. 8151, pp. 25–32. Springer, Heidelberg (2013)
17. Popuri, K., Cobzas, D., Jägersand, M.: A Variational Formulation for Discrete Registration. In: Mori, K., Sakuma, I., Sato, Y., Barillot, C., Navab, N. (eds.) MICCAI 2013, Part III. LNCS, vol. 8151, pp. 187–194. Springer, Heidelberg (2013)
18. Rühaak, J., Heldmann, S., Kipshagen, T., Fischer, B.: Highly Accurate Fast Lung CT Registration. In: Ourselin, S., Haynor, D.R. (eds.) SPIE Medical Imaging, pp. 1–9 (2013)
19. Scharstein, D., Szeliski, R.: A taxonomy and evaluation of dense two-frame stereo correspondence algorithms. Int. J. Comput. Vision 47(1), 7–42 (2002)

20. So, R.W.K., Tang, T.W.H., Chung, A.C.S.: Non-rigid image registration of brain magnetic resonance images using graph-cuts. Pattern Recognition 44(10-11), 2450–2467 (2011)
21. Sotiras, A., Davatzikos, C., Paragios, N.: Deformable Medical Image Registration: A Survey. IEEE Trans. Med. Imag. 32(7), 1153–1190 (2013)
22. Steinbrücker, F., Pock, T., Cremers, D.: Large displacement optical flow computation without warping. In: ICCV 2009, pp. 1609–1614 (2009)
23. Veksler, O.: Fast Variable Window for Stereo Correspondence using Integral Images. In: CVPR 2003, pp. 1–6 (2003)
24. Vercauteren, T., Pennec, X., Perchant, A., Ayache, N.: Diffeomorphic demons: Efficient non-parametric image registration. NeuroImage 45(1), 61–72 (2009)

Randomly Perturbed Free-Form Deformation for Nonrigid Image Registration

Wei Sun[1], Wiro J. Niessen[1,2], and Stefan Klein[1]

[1] Biomedical Imaging Group Rotterdam,
Departments of Radiology and Medical Informatics,
Erasmus MC, Rotterdam, The Netherlands
{w.sun,w.niessen,s.klein}@erasmusmc.nl
[2] Department of Image Science and Technology,
Faculty of Applied Sciences,
Delft University of Technology, Delft, The Netherlands

Abstract. B-spline based free-form deformation (FFD) is a widely used technique in nonrigid image registration. In general, a third-order B-spline function is used, because of its favorable trade-off between smoothness and computational cost. Compared with the third-order B-splines, a B-spline function with a lower order has shorter support length, which means it is computationally more attractive. However, a lower-order function is seldom used to construct the deformation field for registration since it is less smooth. In this work, we propose a randomly perturbed FFD strategy (RPFFD) which uses a lower-order B-spline FFD with a random perturbation around the original position to approximate a higher-order B-spline FFD in a stochastic fashion. For a given D-dimensional nth-order FFD, its corresponding $(n-1)$th-order RPFFD has $(\frac{n}{n+1})^D$ times lower computational complexity. Experiments on 3D lung and brain data show that, with this lower computational complexity, the proposed RPFFD registration results in even slightly better accuracy and smoothness than the traditional higher-order FFD.

1 Introduction

Nonrigid image registration is widely used in medical image analysis. To model the nonrigid deformation field which is recovered by the registration method, FFD is a popular model and produces competitive results in various registration tasks. In B-spline based FFD registration, B-spline basis functions distributed on a uniformly spaced grid are used to model the transformation [1].

For a given degree of smoothness, B-spline function is a spline function that has minimal support [2]. The B-spline function of order n is obtained by n times convolution of the zeroth-order B-spline. As the n goes to infinity, B-splines converge to the Gaussian function in the limit. Both the support length and the smoothness of B-splines increase with the order n. Compared with the other order B-spline functions, the third-order (cubic) B-spline function is usually regarded as a good trade-off between smoothness and computational cost.

S. Ourselin and M. Modat (Eds.): WBIR 2014, LNCS 8545, pp. 62–71, 2014.
© Springer International Publishing Switzerland 2014

In this research, we propose a random perturbation approach to approximate an nth-order (e.g., cubic) B-spline FFD by an $(n-1)$th-order (e.g., quadratic) B-spline FFD. The technique is inspired by the definition of a B-spline as a convolution of zeroth-order B-splines. In the proposed perturbation process, a uniformly distributed random variable within the range of half a grid spacing is utilized to shift the entire B-spline grid around its original position in each dimension. In RPFFD registration, the perturbation process is combined with a stochastic gradient descent optimizer, which can handle such stochastic fluctuations in the objective function. Through the approximation of nth-order B-spline registration with the randomly perturbed $(n-1)$th-order B-spline registration, the computational cost is inherently reduced in the RPFFD registration thanks to the smaller support region.

2 Method

2.1 Registration Framework

In this work, we focus on parametric intensity-based types of registration methods. Let $F(\mathbf{x}) : \Omega_F \subset \mathbb{R}^D \to \mathbb{R}$ and $M(\mathbf{x}) : \Omega_M \subset \mathbb{R}^D \to \mathbb{R}$ denotes the D-dimensional fixed and moving images where $\mathbf{x} \in \mathbb{R}^D$ represents an image coordinate. Then, the registration problem is formulated as:

$$\hat{\boldsymbol{\mu}} = \arg\min_{\boldsymbol{\mu}} \mathcal{C}(F, M \circ \mathbf{T}_{\boldsymbol{\mu}}), \qquad (1)$$

where $\mathcal{C}$ measures the dissimilarity between the fixed image and the deformed moving image, $\mathbf{T}_{\boldsymbol{\mu}}(\mathbf{x}) : \Omega_F \to \Omega_M$ is a coordinate transformation, and $\boldsymbol{\mu}$ represents the parameter vector of the transformation model. Examples of $\mathcal{C}$ are the sum of squared differences (SSD), normalized correlation coefficient (NCC), and mutual information [3].

In general, an iterative optimization strategy is utilized to determine the optimal set of parameters $\hat{\boldsymbol{\mu}}$,

$$\boldsymbol{\mu}_{k+1} = \boldsymbol{\mu}_k - a_k \boldsymbol{d}_k, \quad k = 1, 2, \dots, K \qquad (2)$$

where $\boldsymbol{d}_k$ is the "optimization direction" at iteration k, and a_k controls the step size along $\boldsymbol{d}_k$.

In gradient-based optimization methods, the definition of $\boldsymbol{d}_k$ is based on the derivative of the cost function with respect to $\boldsymbol{\mu}$, $\partial \mathcal{C}/\partial \boldsymbol{\mu}$. Popular examples of such methods are gradient descent, quasi-Newton, and nonlinear conjugate gradient [4]. It has been shown in [5] that the stochastic gradient descent (SGD) method is a competitive alternative to these deterministic methods. In SGD, $\boldsymbol{d}_k$ is defined as a stochastic approximation of $\partial \mathcal{C}/\partial \boldsymbol{\mu}$,

$$\boldsymbol{\mu}_{k+1} = \boldsymbol{\mu}_k - a_k \tilde{\boldsymbol{g}}(\boldsymbol{\mu}_k), \qquad (3)$$

where $\tilde{\boldsymbol{g}}(\boldsymbol{\mu}_k)$ is the approximate derivative of the cost function evaluated at the current optimization position $\boldsymbol{\mu}_k$. In [5] the stochastic approximation was

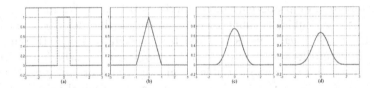

Fig. 1. One-dimensional B-splines with four different orders: (a) $\beta^0(x)$; (b) $\beta^1(x)$; (c) $\beta^2(x)$; (d) $\beta^3(x)$

realized by evaluating the cost function derivative on a small random subset $\widetilde{\Omega}_F \subset \Omega_F$ of image samples, newly selected in each iteration k, thus reducing the computation time per iteration. For example, if we choose SSD as cost function $\mathcal{C}$,

$$\mathcal{C}(F, M \circ \mathbf{T_\mu}) = \frac{1}{|\Omega_F|} \sum_{\mathbf{x}_i \in \Omega_F} (F(\mathbf{x}_i) - M(\mathbf{T_\mu}(\mathbf{x}_i)))^2, \tag{4}$$

then, the stochastic approximation $\tilde{g}(\mu)$ of $\partial \mathcal{C}/\partial \mu$ is calculated as:

$$\tilde{g}(\boldsymbol{\mu}) = \frac{2}{|\widetilde{\Omega}_F|} \sum_{\mathbf{x}_i \in \widetilde{\Omega}_F} \left((F(\mathbf{x}_i) - M(\mathbf{T_\mu}(\mathbf{x}_i))) \left(\frac{\partial \mathbf{T_\mu}}{\partial \boldsymbol{\mu}} \bigg|_{\mathbf{x}_i} \right)^T \left(\frac{\partial M}{\partial \mathbf{y}} \bigg|_{\mathbf{T_\mu}(\mathbf{x}_i)} \right) \right). \tag{5}$$

Convergence in SGD methods can be achieved by letting the step size decay a_k decay according to a pre-defined function. In [6] an adaptive strategy for setting a_k was proposed. This adaptive stochastic gradient descent (ASGD) method is used in our work.

2.2 B-spline Basis Functions

The B-spline function of order n is obtained by n times convolution of the zeroth-order B-spline function [7],

$$\beta^n(x) = \underbrace{\beta^0(x) * \cdots * \beta^0(x)}_{n \text{ times}}, \tag{6}$$

where $\beta^0(x)$ is defined as

$$\beta^0(x) = \begin{cases} 1 : -0.5 \leq x < 0.5 \\ 0 : \text{otherwise} \end{cases}, \tag{7}$$

and the operator '$*$' denotes the convolution operation

$$(f * h)(x) \overset{def}{=} \int_{-\infty}^{+\infty} f(x-t)h(t)dt. \tag{8}$$

Figure 1 shows the shapes of $\beta^0(x)$, $\beta^1(x)$, $\beta^2(x)$, and $\beta^3(x)$. The support length (nonzero domain) of the B-spline function is increased with the spline order.

With increasing spline order, the smoothness improves, but the support region becomes larger.

For a D-dimensional input space, the tensor product of $\beta^n(x)$ is used to span the multidimensional B-spline function $\Phi(\mathbf{x}) : \mathbb{R}^D \to \mathbb{R}$,

$$\Phi_D^n(\mathbf{x}) = \underbrace{\beta^n(x_1) \otimes \cdots \otimes \beta^n(x_D)}_{D \text{ times}}, \tag{9}$$

where '$\otimes$' denotes the tensor product operator.

2.3   B-spline FFD

The traditional FFD transformation model [1] is defined as

$$\mathbf{T}_{\boldsymbol{\mu}}^n(\mathbf{x}) = \mathbf{x} + \sum_{\boldsymbol{\xi} \in \Xi} \mathbf{c}_{\boldsymbol{\xi}} \Phi_D^n(\mathbf{x}/\eta - \boldsymbol{\xi}), \tag{10}$$

where $\Xi \subset \mathbb{Z}^D$ represents a D-dimensional control-point grid, η is the grid spacing, $\mathbf{c}_{\boldsymbol{\xi}}$ is the coefficient vector for a control point $\boldsymbol{\xi}$, and the parameter vector $\boldsymbol{\mu}$ is formed by the elements of all coefficient vectors ($\boldsymbol{\mu} = \{\mathbf{c}_{\boldsymbol{\xi}} \mid \boldsymbol{\xi} \in \Xi\}$). For a given $\boldsymbol{x}$, the summation goes effectively only over all $\boldsymbol{\xi}$ with nonzero $\Phi_D^n(\mathbf{x}/\eta - \boldsymbol{\xi})$ (i.e., over the compact region of support).

As introduced in Section 2.1, a stochastic approximation of the derivative $\partial C / \partial \boldsymbol{\mu}$ is calculated in the SGD based registration, which requires evaluation of $T_{\boldsymbol{\mu}}^n(\mathbf{x})$ and $\partial T_{\boldsymbol{\mu}}^n(\mathbf{x})/\partial \boldsymbol{\mu}$. Calculating these terms dominates the computational costs of nonrigid image registration.

2.4   Randomly Perturbed B-spline FFD

If the nth-order B-spline function is utilized to model the transformation, the number of control points considered in each dimension is $n+1$ inside the support region. Then, the number of control points for a D-dimensional transformation is $(n + 1)^D$. In practical medical image registration tasks, the input images F and M are usually 3D images. Thus, the numbers of control points which need to be considered around one image coordinate are 64 and 27 for $\beta^3(x)$ and $\beta^2(x)$, respectively. As introduced in Section 2.3, the computational cost of nonrigid registration is dominated by evaluating the transformation and its derivative. Therefore, the computational cost could be significantly reduced if the quadratic B-spline function could replace the commonly used cubic B-splines.

As shown in Figure 1 (a), the support region of $\beta^0(x)$ is $[-0.5, 0.5]$ and its value constantly equals to 1 inside this region. From Eqs. (6) and (8), we derive

$$\beta^n(x) = (\beta^{n-1} * \beta^0)(x) = \int_{-\infty}^{+\infty} \beta^{n-1}(x-t)\beta^0(t)dt = \int_{-0.5}^{0.5} \beta^{n-1}(x-t)dt. \tag{11}$$

Inspired by this relation, we propose to treat $t \in [-0.5, 0.5)$ as a random variable with a uniform distribution, and approximate $\beta^n(x)$ by a randomly shifted lower-order B-splines $\beta^{n-1}(x-t)$. This leads to the following definition of the RPFFD transformation model

$$\widetilde{\mathbf{T}}_{\boldsymbol{\mu}}^{n-1}(\mathbf{x}, \mathbf{t}) = \mathbf{x} + \sum_{\boldsymbol{\xi} \in \Xi} \mathbf{c}_{\boldsymbol{\xi}} \Phi_D^{n-1}(\mathbf{x}/\eta - \boldsymbol{\xi} - \mathbf{t}), \tag{12}$$

where $\mathbf{t} = [t_1, t_2, \cdots, t_D]^T$ represent the random shifts in each dimension. Through this way, the entire B-spline control point grid is thus shifted by vector $\mathbf{t}$ but the grid layout is kept.

The proposed RPFFD transformation model fits naturally in the framework of stochastic gradient descent optimization. For the computation of $\partial \mathcal{C}/\partial \boldsymbol{\mu}$, Eq. (5), we use $\widetilde{\mathbf{T}}_{\boldsymbol{\mu}}^{n-1}(\mathbf{x}, \mathbf{t})$ instead of $\mathbf{T}_{\boldsymbol{\mu}}^n(\mathbf{x})$, with a perturbation $\mathbf{t}$ randomly chosen in each iteration k of optimization. We thus obtain a stochastic approximation of the true derivative, at a lower computational cost. It is worth to note that this approximation comes on top of the approximation by randomly subsampling the image as explained in Sec. 2.1. The optimization procedure thus can be written as

$$\boldsymbol{\mu}_{k+1} = \boldsymbol{\mu}_k - a_k \tilde{g}(\boldsymbol{\mu}_k, \mathbf{t}_k), \tag{13}$$

where $\mathbf{t}_k$ is the realization of $\mathbf{t}$ in iteration k. The computationally efficient $(n-1)$th-order B-spline function is utilized only during the optimization process. Once the stochastic gradient descent optimization has finished, the estimated parameters $\hat{\boldsymbol{\mu}}$ are directly plugged into the original nth order B-spline FFD to obtain the final transformation.

Algorithm 1 provides an overview of the proposed RPFFD registration method.

Input: $F \leftarrow$ fixed image, $M \leftarrow$ moving image, $K \leftarrow$ number of iterations, $S \leftarrow$ number of samples $|\widetilde{\Omega}_F|$, and $n \leftarrow$ original B-spline order
Output: Registered moving image $M\left(\mathbf{T}_{\hat{\boldsymbol{\mu}}}^n(\mathbf{x})\right)$
1 Initialize transformation parameters $\boldsymbol{\mu} \leftarrow \mathbf{0}$
2 **for** $k \leftarrow 1$ **to** K **do**
3   Initialize random samples $[\mathbf{x}_1 \ldots \mathbf{x}_S]$, $\tilde{g} = \mathbf{0}$, step size a_k
4   Determine random shift $\mathbf{t}_k$
5   **for** $\mathbf{x} \leftarrow \mathbf{x}_1$ **to** $\mathbf{x}_S$ **do**
6   Evaluate $F(\mathbf{x})$
7         $\mathbf{y} \leftarrow \widetilde{\mathbf{T}}_{\boldsymbol{\mu}}^{n-1}(\mathbf{x}, \mathbf{t}_k)$
8   Interpolate moving image value $M(\mathbf{y})$
9   Calculate gradient $\nabla M(\mathbf{y})$
10   Calculate transformation derivative $\partial \widetilde{\mathbf{T}}_{\boldsymbol{\mu}}^{n-1}(\mathbf{x}, \mathbf{t}_k)/\partial \boldsymbol{\mu}$
11   Calculate contribution to $\tilde{g}$
12   **end**
13   Update transformation parameters $\boldsymbol{\mu} \leftarrow \boldsymbol{\mu} - a_k \tilde{g}$
14 **end**
15 $\hat{\boldsymbol{\mu}} \leftarrow \boldsymbol{\mu}$
16 Instantiate nth-order FFD transformation $\mathbf{T}_{\hat{\boldsymbol{\mu}}}^n(\mathbf{x})$
17 **return** $M\left(\mathbf{T}_{\hat{\boldsymbol{\mu}}}^n(\mathbf{x})\right)$

Algorithm 1. RPFFD registration method

Table 1. Description of compared registration methods

Name	During optimization	Final transformation	Random perturbation
CubicFFD	Cubic	Cubic	Off
QuadraticFFD	Quadratic	Quadratic	Off
QuadraticFFD-M	Quadratic	Cubic	Off
QuadraticRPFFD-M	Quadratic	Quadratic	On
QuadraticRPFFD	Quadratic	Cubic	On

3   Experiments

The performances of the traditional FFD and proposed RPFFD methods were evaluated and compared in terms of registration accuracy, transformation smoothness, and computation time. The experiments were carried on both 3D lung CT and 3D brain MRI scans.

3.1   Registration Methods

In the present work, we focused on B-spline order $n = 3$. We define the standard cubic FFD (CubicFFD) registration method as the reference method. The proposed method using $\widetilde{\mathbf{T}}_{\boldsymbol{\mu}}^{n-1}(\mathbf{x}, \mathbf{t})$ is referred to as QuadraticRPFFD. To gain further insight in the differences between CubicFFD and QuadraticRPFFD, we define three 'intermediate' methods, which are also evaluated. First, we define QuadraticFFD, which is similar to CubicFFD but uses everywhere $n = 2$ (without random perturbation). Second, we define QuadraticFFD-M, which uses $n = 2$ for optimization (without random perturbation), and then plugs the estimated $\hat{\boldsymbol{\mu}}$ into an $n = 3$ FFD to obtain the final transformation. Third, we define QuadraticRPFFD-M, which uses $n = 2$ for optimization with random perturbation, but returns as final transformation $\widetilde{\mathbf{T}}_{\hat{\boldsymbol{\mu}}}^{n-1}(\mathbf{x}, \mathbf{0})$ instead of $\mathbf{T}_{\hat{\boldsymbol{\mu}}}^{n}(\mathbf{x})$.

Table 1 provides an overview of the compared registration methods.

3.2   Experimental Settings

All methods were implemented based on the open source image registration package `elastix` [8]. Similarity measures SSD and NCC were used as dissimilarity terms on lung and brain data, respectively. Trilinear interpolation was used to interpolate the moving image. For the ASGD optimizer, the numbers of random samples S and iterations K were set to 2000 in all experiments. A Gaussian filter using $\{\sigma_1, \ldots, \sigma_4\} = \{4, 2, 1, 0.5\}$ voxels was applied to the input images to create 4 image resolution levels. During the registration, the transformation estimated at a coarser scale was used to initialize the transformation on finer scale. The finest grid spacing η_4 was set to 8mm or 13mm in the experiments on lung data. To avoid too large coarsest grid spacing, we fixed η_1 to be 64mm on the lung data. With η_1 and η_4, the multiresolution grid schedule can be calculated according to $\{\eta_1, \eta_4(\eta_1/\eta_4)^{2/3}, \eta_4(g_1/\eta_4)^{1/3}, \eta_4\}$. Thus, the grid schedules for 8mm and 13mm are $\{\eta_1, \eta_2, \eta_3, \eta_4\} = \{64, 32, 16, 8\}$mm and $\{64, 38, 22, 8\}$mm, respectively. On the brain data, the grid schedule $\{40, 20, 10, 5\}$mm was utilized.

3.3 Experimental Data

We used 10 pairs of DIR-Lab 3D chest CT scans with 300 manually annotated landmarks on the lung structure. The voxel and dimension sizes of lung data are around $1 \times 1 \times 2.5$mm and around $256 \times 256 \times 110$. Lung masks were created to limit the registration to the lung region. The masks were created by thesholding, 3D-6-neighborhood connected component analysis, and morphological closing operation using a spherical kernel with a diameter of nine voxels. For all cases, the exhale phase (moving image) was registered to the inhale phases (fixed image). The mean target registration error (mTRE) which calculates the distance between the transformed and ground truth landmarks was used to measure the registration accuracy. To evaluate the transformation smoothness of registration, the standard deviation of the determinant of spatial Jacobian (D_{SJ}) was used. For a given spatial location $\tilde{x}$ inside the lung mask, D_{SJ} is calculated as

$$D_{SJ} = \left| \frac{\partial \mathbf{T}_\mu}{\partial \boldsymbol{x}}(\tilde{\boldsymbol{x}}) \right|. \tag{14}$$

Because D_{SJ} represents the local volume change of a specific location, the standard deviation of D_{SJ} measures the change of the movement thus giving an indication of the smoothness of a transformation.

The Internet Brain Segmentation Repository (IBSR v2.0), which contains 18 T1-weighted MRI 3D brain scans, was also used to evaluate the registration methods. The volumes of these images are $256 \times 256 \times 128$mm. The voxel sizes are divided into three groups (8: $0.94 \times 0.94 \times 1.5$, 6: $0.84 \times 0.84 \times 1.5$, 4: $1 \times 1 \times 1.5$). Overall mean overlap which measures the overlap between the transformed and ground truth atlases was used to evaluate the registration accuracy. The overall mean overlap is calculated as

$$\text{Overall Mean Overlap} = 2 \frac{\sum_r |M_r \bigcap F_r|}{\sum_r (|M_r| + |F_r|)}, \tag{15}$$

where r represents a certain label, and the overall mean overlap is calculated over all labels. For evaluating smoothness of the transformation, we used the standard deviation of D_{SJ} as defined in Eq. (14), calculated inside a brain mask. The same affine registrations were used to roughly align the data first, and then these initialized results were used as the input data for the nonrigid registration experiments.

4   Results

The results using the finest grid spacings 13mm and 8mm on lung data were pooled and shown as boxplots in Figure 2. Overall, the RPFFD registration has better accuracy and smoothness than the other methods.

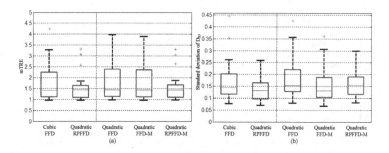

Fig. 2. Results on lung data by different methods: (a) accuracy (mTRE, in mm, lower values are better); (b) smoothness (standard deviation of D_{SJ}, lower values are better)

Figure 3 provides the detailed registration accuracy and smoothness results on the 10 pairs of lung scans, both for finest grid spacings 13mm and 8mm. Figure 3 (a) shows that RPFFD registration (QuadraticRPFFD) produced registration accuracy comparable with or better than the reference method CubicFFD, except for case 8. The smoothness results (Figure 3 (b)) indicate that the QuadraticRPFFD produced the best smoothness over all methods in most cases.

As introduced in Section 2, the quadratic RPFFD has a factor $(\frac{n}{n+1})^D$ lower computational complexity than the cubic FFD. Experimentally, the computation times on subject 1 using an Intel Core i7-2720QM with 8G memory were 139 ± 1 seconds and 86 ± 1 seconds (mean $\pm$ standard deviation over 10 runs) for the CubicFFD and QuadraticRPFFD methods, respectively.

Figure 4 shows the registration results on brain data. Quadratic RPFFD registration generated better registration accuracy than cubic FFD registration, see Figure 4 (a). In terms of smoothness, Figure 4 (b), the proposed QuadraticRPFFD method outperformed all other methods.

The running time of nonrigid registration to register subject 2 to subject 1 on an Intel Core i7-2720QM with 8G memory were 231 ± 1 seconds and 146 ± 1 seconds (mean $\pm$ standard deviation over 10 runs) for the CubicFFD and QuadraticRPFFDmethods, respectively.

5   Discussion

The results indicate that the proposed quadratic RPFFD method outperforms the standard cubic FFD method not only in terms of computation time, as was expected, but also in terms of accuracy and smoothness of the estimated transformation. The 'intermediate' methods, each omitting one or more components of the proposed method, were outperformed by RPFFD as well, suggesting that each element of the algorithm is essential for good performance.

We provide two possible explanations for the improvement in accuracy and smoothness. First, Tustison et al. [9] demonstrated how the conventional B-spline

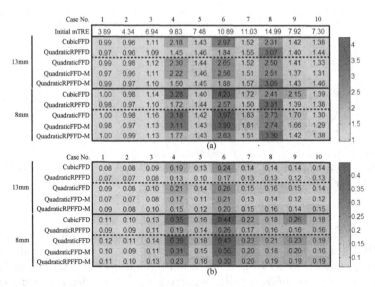

	Case No.	1	2	3	4	5	6	7	8	9	10
	Initial mTRE	3.89	4.34	6.94	9.83	7.48	10.89	11.03	14.99	7.92	7.30
	CubicFFD	0.99	0.96	1.11	2.18	1.43	2.97	1.52	2.31	1.42	1.38
	QuadraticRPFFD	0.97	0.96	1.09	1.45	1.46	1.84	1.55	3.07	1.40	1.44
13mm	QuadraticFFD	0.99	0.98	1.12	2.30	1.44	2.65	1.52	2.50	1.41	1.33
	QuadraticFFD-M	0.97	0.96	1.11	2.22	1.46	2.56	1.51	2.51	1.37	1.31
	QuadraticRPFFD-M	0.99	0.97	1.10	1.50	1.45	1.88	1.57	3.05	1.43	1.46
	CubicFFD	1.00	0.98	1.14	3.28	1.40	4.23	1.72	2.41	2.15	1.39
	QuadraticRPFFD	0.98	0.97	1.10	1.72	1.44	2.57	1.50	3.31	1.39	1.38
8mm	QuadraticFFD	1.00	0.98	1.16	3.18	1.42	3.97	1.83	2.73	1.70	1.30
	QuadraticFFD-M	0.98	0.97	1.13	3.11	1.43	3.90	1.81	2.74	1.66	1.29
	QuadraticRPFFD-M	1.00	0.99	1.13	1.77	1.43	2.63	1.51	3.30	1.42	1.38

(a)

	Case No.	1	2	3	4	5	6	7	8	9	10
	CubicFFD	0.08	0.08	0.09	0.19	0.13	0.24	0.14	0.14	0.14	0.14
	QuadraticRPFFD	0.07	0.07	0.08	0.13	0.10	0.17	0.13	0.13	0.12	0.13
13mm	QuadraticFFD	0.09	0.08	0.10	0.21	0.14	0.26	0.15	0.16	0.15	0.14
	QuadraticFFD-M	0.07	0.07	0.08	0.17	0.11	0.21	0.13	0.14	0.12	0.12
	QuadraticRPFFD-M	0.09	0.08	0.10	0.15	0.12	0.20	0.15	0.16	0.14	0.15
	CubicFFD	0.11	0.10	0.13	0.35	0.16	0.44	0.22	0.18	0.26	0.18
	QuadraticRPFFD	0.09	0.09	0.11	0.19	0.14	0.26	0.17	0.16	0.16	0.16
8mm	QuadraticFFD	0.12	0.11	0.14	0.36	0.18	0.43	0.23	0.21	0.23	0.19
	QuadraticFFD-M	0.10	0.09	0.11	0.31	0.15	0.36	0.20	0.18	0.20	0.16
	QuadraticRPFFD-M	0.11	0.10	0.13	0.23	0.16	0.30	0.20	0.19	0.19	0.19

(b)

Fig. 3. Detailed registration results on lung data by different methods: (a) accuracy (mTRE, in mm, lower values are better); (b) smoothness (standard deviation of D_{SJ}, lower values are better)

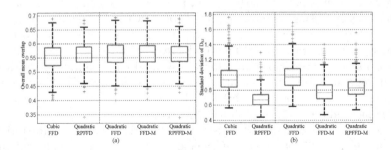

Fig. 4. Results on brain data by different methods: (a) accuracy (overall mean overlap, higher values are better); (b) smoothness (standard deviation of D_{SJ}, lower values are better)

FFD can lead to ill-conditioned optimization spaces, due to the disproportionate B-spline weighting of the control points. To solve the optimization problem caused by FFD registration, a preconditioning strategy was proposed in their work. In our work, by randomly shifting the control point grid, the influences of different control points to the cost function are randomly changed in each iteration. Therefore, the effect of the disproportionate control point weighting might be reduced thanks to the perturbation process in RPFFD. Second, in RPFFD registration, a new stochastic dynamic is introduced to the stochastic gradient descent optimization. The stochastic perturbations in RPFFD may help to avoid the local minima as has been previously reported in the literature on stochastic approximation optimization [10].

In the future, we plan to further investigate these hypotheses, and extend the RPFFD method to different orders of B-splines. The RPFFD method will also be evaluated in combination with different multiresolution strategies [11].

6   Conclusions

In this research, a new randomly perturbed B-splines based FFD (RPFFD) registration method is presented. The new RPFFD method uses a randomly perturbed lower $(n - 1)$th-order B-spline transformation to approximate a higher nth-order B-spline FFD during optimization. Because less control points are involved in RPFFD registration, the method is computationally less expensive than the traditional FFD registration. Besides leading to faster image registration, the RPFFD method also outperforms the traditional FFD method in terms of accuracy and smoothness of the registration results.

References

1. Rueckert, D., Sonoda, L.I., Hayes, C., et al.: Nonrigid registration using free-form deformations: Application to breast MR images. IEEE Transactions on Medical Imaging 18(8), 712–721 (1999)
2. De Boor, C.: A practical guide to splines, vol. 27. Springer, New York (1978)
3. Maintz, J., Viergever, M.A.: A survey of medical image registration. Medical Image Analysis 2(1), 1–36 (1998)
4. Nocedal, J., Wright, S.J.: Numerical optimization. Springer, New York (1999)
5. Klein, S., Staring, M., Pluim, J.P.W.: Evaluation of optimization methods for non-rigid medical image registration using mutual information and B-splines. IEEE Transactions on Image Processing 16(12), 2879–2890 (2007)
6. Klein, S., Pluim, J.P.W., Staring, M., Viergever, M.A.: Adaptive stochastic gradient descent optimisation for image registration. International Journal of Computer Vision 81(3), 227–239 (2009)
7. Unser, M., Aldroubi, A., Eden, M.: Fast B-spline transforms for continuous image representation and interpolation. IEEE Transactions on Pattern Analysis and Machine Intelligence 13(3), 277–285 (1991)
8. Klein, S., Staring, M., Murphy, K., Viergever, M.A., Pluim, J.P.W.: Elastix: a toolbox for intensity-based medical image registration. IEEE Transactions on Medical Imaging 29(1), 196–205 (2010)
9. Tustison, N.J., Avants, B.B., Gee, J.C.: Directly manipulated free-form deformation image registration. IEEE Transactions on Image Processing 18(3), 624–635 (2009)
10. Maryak, J.L., Chin, D.C.: Global random optimization by simultaneous perturbation stochastic approximation. In: Proceedings of the American Control Conference, vol. 2, pp. 756–762. IEEE (2001)
11. Sun, W., Niessen, W.J., van Stralen, M., Klein, S.: Simultaneous multiresolution strategies for nonrigid image registration. IEEE Transactions on Image Processing 22(12), 4905–4917 (2013)

Probabilistic Diffeomorphic Registration: Representing Uncertainty[*]

Demian Wassermann[1,3], Matthew Toews[1],
Marc Niethammer[4], and William Wells III[1,2]

[1] SPL, Brigham and Womens Hospital, Harvard Medical School, Boston, MA, USA
[2] CSAIL, Massachusetts Institute of Technology, Boston, MA, USA
[3] EPI Athena, INRIA Sophia Antipolis-Méditerranée, Sophia Antipolis, France
[4] Department of Computer Science, University of North Carolina, Chapel Hill, NC, USA

Abstract. This paper presents a novel mathematical framework for representing uncertainty in large deformation diffeomorphic image registration. The Bayesian posterior distribution over the deformations aligning a moving and a fixed image is approximated via a variational formulation. A stochastic differential equation (SDE) modeling the deformations as the evolution of a time-varying velocity field leads to a prior density over deformations in the form of a Gaussian process. This permits estimating the full posterior distribution in order to represent uncertainty, in contrast to methods in which the posterior is approximated via Monte Carlo sampling or maximized in maximum a-posteriori (MAP) estimation. The framework is demonstrated in the case of landmark-based image registration, including simulated data and annotated pre and intra-operative 3D images.

1 Introduction

Deformable image registration seeks to identify a deformation field that aligns two images, and is a key component of image analysis applications such as computational anatomy [1,2]. An important body of literature focuses on deformations in the form of diffeomorphisms [3,4,2], one-to-one mappings between image coordinate systems that are smooth and invertible. These properties help in ensuring biologically plausible deformations, and avoiding phenomena such as folding or tearing that may occur in non-diffeomorphic registration approaches [5].

While a good deal of literature has focused on identifying optimal diffeomorphic registration solutions, it would be useful to quantify the inherent uncertainty in these solutions when interpreting the results of registration. Quantification of deformable registration uncertainty, particularly at point locations throughout the image, remains an open problem. The Bayesian approach quantifies probabilistic uncertainty via a posterior distribution over deformations conditioned on image data. Estimating the full posterior in the case of large deformation diffeomorphisms is desirable but computationally challenging, and has typically been avoided. Simpson et al. propose a Bayesian variational framework based on small deformation kinematics [5], however this does not address the general case of large deformations. Markussen proposed a stochastic differential equation (SDE) model for large deformations, however only the computation of

---
[*] This work was supported by grants NIH P41EB015898, R01CA138419 and NSF EECS-1148870.

S. Ourselin and M. Modat (Eds.): WBIR 2014, LNCS 8545, pp. 72–82, 2014.

the maximum a posteriori deformation is provided lacking the estimation of a distribution on the deformations [6]Alternatively, the posterior may be investigated via sampling methods, e.g. Markov chain Monte Carlo (MCMC) [7] or Hamiltonian Monte Carlo [8].

This paper introduces a novel mathematical framework that allows representing and computing of the full Bayesian posterior in the case of large deformation diffeomorphisms. Our framework considers a SDE modeling the deformation field as the evolution of a time-varying velocity field, with additive noise in the form of a Wiener process. A Gaussian process (GP) density results from a locally linear approximation of the SDE and taking the initial deformation field to be Gaussian process distributed. Deformation field uncertainty is quantified by the point-wise covariance of the deformation field throughout the image, and can be summarized, e.g., via the Frobenius norm of the covariance (FC). This can be pictured through the following example: if the FC at a point approaches 0, the marginal density of the transform approaches an impulse function denoting the existence of a single probable solution. On the other hand, when FC is large, the density becomes "broader" denoting a larger set of solutions with high probability at that point. Hence the point-wise FC is a model of uncertainty. Experiments demonstrate our framework in the context of landmark correspondences, where a heteroscedastic model accounts for variable uncertainty in landmark localization. This is particularly useful when estimates of landmark localization variability are available.

2 Methods

2.1 Variational Approximation to Registration

We start by posing the registration problem in a probabilistic framework. Let M and F be moving and fixed objects with domains in Ω_M and Ω_F respectively, and let $\phi : \Omega_M \mapsto \Omega_F$ be a mapping between the two. The registration problem seeks a posterior probability density over mappings ϕ conditioned on data (M, F), which is expressed via Bayes theorem as

$$p(\phi|M, F) = p(\phi)p(M, F|\phi)/p(M, F). \tag{1}$$

In Eq. (1), $p(\phi)$ is a prior density over ϕ embodying geometrical constraints such as smoothness. $p(M, F|\phi)$ is the data attachment factor or likelihood of the map ϕ relating F and M. E.g. the probability that M deformed by ϕ, which we note $\phi \circ M$, is similar to F. Finally, $p(M, F)$ is a normalizing constant.

The direct calculation of the posterior density $p(\phi|M, F)$ is a difficult problem. Hence, we use a variational method to estimate a distribution $q(\phi)$ (abbreviated as q) that is close to $p(\phi|M, F)$ in the sense of the Kullback-Leibler divergence (KL $[\cdot\|\cdot]$). Specifically, we seek q minimizing:

$$\text{KL} \left[q\|p(\phi|M, F)\right] = \text{KL} \left[q\|p(\phi)\right] - \int \log p(M, F|\phi) dq(\phi) + \log p(M, F). \tag{2}$$

In the registration literature the data attachment factor $p(M, F|\phi)$ is typically modeled using a measure of similarity between the registered objects: $m : \Omega_F \times \Omega_F \mapsto \mathbb{R}$

which is minimal when two objects are exactly the same and grows as they become different. Adopting the equality $-\log p(M, F|\phi) = m(\phi \circ M, F)$, Eq. (2) may be rewritten as:

$$\mathrm{KL}\left[q\|p(\phi|M, F)\right] \quad = \quad \mathrm{KL}\left[q\|p(\phi)\right] \; + \; \langle m(\phi \circ M, F)\rangle_q \; + \; \log p(M, F), \quad (3)$$

where $\langle m(\phi \circ M, F)\rangle_q$ is the expected value of m with respect to the density q. There are two main differences of this formulation with respect to common diffeomorphic registration approaches [3,4]. First, instead of seeking a single optimal deformation ϕ, e.g. the maximum a-posteriori (MAP) solution in the Bayesian formulation, we seek to obtain the full distribution $q(\phi)$. In this way, we obtain both the MAP deformation ϕ in addition to the uncertainty at any given point in space, which can be calculated from $q(\phi)$. Second, we obtain $q(\phi)$ by minimizing the data attachment term over a weighted combination of *all possible deformation fields in the family of* ϕ instead of only at a single deformation ϕ.

2.2 Probabilistic Diffeomorphic Deformations

The variational approximation to $p(\phi|M, F)$ described in the previous section requires a parameterization for $q(\phi)$ over which Eq. (3) can be minimized. In this section we derive a novel parameterization in the form of a Gaussian Process (GP). The theoretical basis for our derivation lies in a stochastic interpretation of the work of [1], common to many diffeomorphic registration approaches [2]. Here, we begin by outlining the relevant elements of this work, then we present our derivation in three propositions and their proofs, with our primary contributions being in Propositions 2 and 3.

Following the work of [1], many diffeomorphic deformation formulations seek an optimal registration solution ϕ, e.g. the MAP deformation in Eq. (1), by constraining the map ϕ to be the solution at $t = 1$ of the ordinary differential equation (ODE)

$$\tfrac{d}{dt}\phi_t(x) = v_t(\phi_t(x)), \quad \phi_0(x) = x, \quad t \in [0, 1]. \quad (4)$$

and setting ϕ_1 in Eq. (4) to minimize

$$E(\phi; M, F) = E_v(v) + E_\phi(\phi; M, F), \quad E_v(v) = \frac{1}{2}\int_0^1 \int_{\Omega_m} \|Lv_t(x)\|_2^2 dx dt. \quad (5)$$

From the two terms of E, $E_v(v)$ regularizes the evolution of the time-varying velocity field and $E_\phi(\phi; M, F)$ drives E such that the deformed moving object, $\phi_1 \circ M$, becomes as similar to F as possible. The regularization term $E_v(v)$, is driven by L, a linear differential operator. The key insight here is that given suitable L according to [1], Eq. (5) restricts $\phi_t(x)$ defined as in Eq. (4) to the space of diffeomorphisms [1]. From this, we make the following propositions:

Proposition 1. *Under a probabilistic interpretation, the regularization term $E_v(v)$ in Eq. (5) corresponds to the negative logarithm of the GP prior on the stochastic velocity field* **v**

$$p(\mathbf{v}) = \mathcal{GP}(0, \Sigma_{ts}(x, y)), \quad \Sigma_{ts}(x, y) \in \mathrm{SPD}^d \quad (6)$$

where the covariance function $\Sigma_{ts}(x, y)$, representing the relation between the point x at time t and the point y at time s, is determined by the operator L in Eq. (5).

Proposition 2. *Interpreting the energy $E_v(v)$ in Eq. (5) as the negative logarithm of the density of a stochastic process $\mathbf{v}$ induces a random process ϕ with density $p(\phi)$ on the deformation field of Eq. (4) that is a solution of the stochastic differential equation (SDE)*

$$d\phi_t(x) = v_t(\phi_t(x))dt + \sqrt{\Sigma_t(\phi_t(x))}d\mathbf{W}_t, \tag{7}$$

$$\mathbf{W}_t \sim \mathcal{GP}(0, \Theta_{ts}(x, y)), \quad \Theta_{ts}(x, y) = \min(t, s)\,\mathrm{Id}, \tag{8}$$

where $\sqrt{\Sigma}$ is the square root matrix $\sqrt{\Sigma}\sqrt{\Sigma}^{\mathsf{T}} = \Sigma$; the GP $\mathbf{W}_t \in \mathbb{R}^d$ is called Brownian motion or a Wiener process [9]; $v_t(x) \in \mathbb{R}^d$ is a deterministic velocity field like in Eq. (4); and $\Sigma_t(x) \triangleq \Sigma_{tt}(x, x) \in \mathrm{SPD}^d$ [1], the covariance of the probabilistic prior defined in Prop. 1, is a consequence of Eq. (5).

Proposition 3. *For the stochastic process ϕ with density $p(\phi)$, defined in prop. 2, the mean $\bar{\phi}$ and covariance Λ functions are solutions of the deterministic ODEs*

$$\tfrac{d}{dt}\bar{\phi}_t(x) = \langle v_t\,(\phi_t(x))\rangle_p \tag{9a}$$

$$\Lambda_{ts}(x, y) = \mathrm{cov}_p\left[\phi_t(x), \phi_s(y)\right] = \left\langle \phi_t(x)\phi_s^{\mathsf{T}}(y)\right\rangle_p - \bar{\phi}_t(x)\bar{\phi}_s^{\mathsf{T}}(y) \tag{9b}$$

$$\tfrac{d}{dt}\left\langle \phi_t(x)\phi_s^{\mathsf{T}}(y)\right\rangle_p = \left\langle v_t(\phi_t(x))\phi_s^{\mathsf{T}}(y)\right\rangle_p + \left\langle \phi_t(x)v_s^{\mathsf{T}}(\phi_s(y))\right\rangle_p \tag{9c}$$

$$+ \left\langle \Sigma_{ts}(\phi_t(x), \phi_s(y))\right\rangle_p.$$

Moreover, up to a first order approximation:

$$p(\phi) = \mathcal{GP}(\bar{\phi}_t(x), \Lambda_{ts}(x, y)), \tag{10}$$

The proofs for Propositions 1-3 are as follows:

Proof of Prop. 1 This proposition has been proven by Joshi et. al.[2], here we provide a sketch of the relevant points. We start by relating $E_v(v)$ in Eq. (5) to a probability density on velocity fields as stochastic processes $\mathbf{v}$, $p(\mathbf{v})$:

$$-\log(p(\mathbf{v})) = E_v(v) + const = \frac{1}{2}\int_0^1 \int_{\Omega_M} \|Lv_t(x)\|_2^2 dx dt + const, \tag{11}$$

To show that $p(\mathbf{v})$ is a stochastic process with a particular distribution, we need to prove that any finite sample of the domain $\Omega_M \in \mathbb{R}^d$ has the same parametric distribution [10]. We take N samples $X \in \mathbb{R}^{N\times d}$ in space and $t \in [0, 1]^N$ in time, and let $\mathbf{V}_{ij} = [\mathbf{v}_{t_i}(X_i)]_j \in \mathbb{R}^{N\times d}$. Then we rewrite Eq. (11) as

$$-\log(p(\mathbf{V})) = \tfrac{1}{2}\left(L \,\mathrm{vec}\,\mathbf{V}\right)^{\mathsf{T}} L \,\mathrm{vec}\,\mathbf{V} + const = \tfrac{1}{2}\,\mathrm{vec}\,\mathbf{V}^{\mathsf{T}}L^{\mathsf{T}}L\,\mathrm{vec}\,\mathbf{V} + const, \tag{12}$$

where L is the matrix such that $[L\mathbf{V}_{i\cdot}] = [L\mathbf{v}_{t_i}(X_i)]_j$. Eq. (12) is recognisable as the log probability of a centered multivariate Gaussian with covariance $C = (L^{\mathsf{T}}L)^{-1}$ and, therefore $\mathbf{v}(x)$ is a GP. The covariance function $\Sigma_{ts}(x, y)$ can be calculated as the

---

[1] SPD^d: set of symmetric positive definite matrices of dimension d.

matrix Green's function of the operator L [2]; specifically, if $x, y \in \mathbb{R}^d$, $\Sigma_{ts}(x, y) \in$ SPD^d where $[\Sigma_{ts}(x, y)]_{ij}$ is the covariance between x_i at time t and y_j at time s.

This shows that for a given velocity field $\mathbf{v}(x)$, random perturbations according to the regularization term $E_v(v)$ in Eq. (5) or prior Eq. (11) follow a GP, therefore the velocity fields according to $E_v(v)$ in Eq. (5) have the density specified in Eq. (6) proving Prop. 1.

Proof of Prop. 2 A formal proof of Prop. 2 is beyond the scope of this paper. Instead, using Prop. 1 we argue its validity and provide appropriate references. In Prop. 1 we characterized the density of random perturbations of velocity fields according to Eq. (5). Adding such random perturbations to Eq. (4) leads to Eq. (7).

The second term in Eq. (7) comes from considering the velocity fields v_t of Eq. (4) as a stochastic process according to Prop. 1. We achieve this by perturbing the right hand side of Eq. (4) with noise. The factor $\mathbf{W}_t \in \mathbb{R}^d$ is white noise, which multiplied by $\sqrt{\Sigma_t}$ is a centered Gaussian random variable with covariance Σ_t, a sample drawn from Eq. (6). We noted the *stochastic* velocity field in Eq. (7) $\mathbf{v}$ to distinguish it from the deterministic one v. Eq. (7) ceases to be an ODE as a sample path of $\mathbf{W}_t$ is almost surely not differentiable. Alternatively, using the Itō interpretation of Eq. (7) leads to the SDE in Eq. (7), whose solution is the density on ϕ [9, Chap. 8].

Proof of Prop. 3 The ODE for the mean of the stochastic process ϕ, Eq. (9a), is obtained by calculating the expectation on both sides of Eq. (7). It is a consequence of the linearity of the expected value and the derivative operator and the definition of $\mathbf{W}_t$ as a zero-centered Wiener process in Eq. (8).

To obtain the ODE for the second moment of ϕ, shown in Eq. (9c), we use the Itō product rule [9] to obtain an expression for $d(\phi_t(x)\phi_s^\mathsf{T}(y))$ and substitute it in Eq. (7) obtaining

$$
\begin{aligned}
\left\langle d(\phi_t(x)\phi_s^\mathsf{T}(y)) \right\rangle_p &= d\left\langle \phi_t(x)\phi_s^\mathsf{T}(y) \right\rangle_p = \left\langle v_t(\phi_t(x))dt\phi_s^\mathsf{T}(y) \right\rangle_p + \left\langle \sqrt{\Sigma}_t(\phi_t(x))d\mathbf{W}_t\phi_s^\mathsf{T}(y) \right\rangle_p \\
&+ \left\langle \phi_t(x)(v_s(\phi_s(y)))^\mathsf{T}ds \right\rangle_p + \left\langle \phi_t(x)(\sqrt{\Sigma}_t(\phi_s(y))d\mathbf{W}_s)^\mathsf{T} \right\rangle_p \\
&+ \left\langle \left(v_t(\phi_t(y))dt + \sqrt{\Sigma}_t(\phi_t(y))d\mathbf{W}_t\right)\left(v_s(\phi_s(y))ds + \sqrt{\Sigma}_s(\phi_s(y))d\mathbf{W}_s\right)^\mathsf{T} \right\rangle_p,
\end{aligned}
$$
(13)

which, using the Itō identities for expected values of differentials [9] results in Eq. (9c).

Obtaining a parametric form of the density of ϕ, $p(\phi)$, satisfying the SDE (7) in the general case is an open problem and a wide field of study. However, in the case where the drift v and diffusion coefficient $\sqrt{\Sigma}$ are linear functions on their time and location parameters, and the initial condition $\phi_{t=0}$ is a GP, $\phi_t(x)$ is known to be a GP [9]. With this purpose we define a locally linearized (LL) v and $\sqrt{\Sigma}$ centered at t_0, x_0 [11]:

$$
v_t(x) \approx v_{t_0}(x_0) + \partial_t v_{t_0}(x_0)(t - t_0) + \mathrm{D}^x_{v_{t_0}}(x_0)(x - x_0) \tag{14a}
$$

$$
\sqrt{\Sigma}_t(x) \approx \sqrt{\Sigma}_{t_0}(x_0) + \partial_t \sqrt{\Sigma}_{t_0}(x_0)(t - t_0) + \sum_i \partial_{x_i}\sqrt{\Sigma}_{t_0}(x_0)(x - x_0)_i \tag{14b}
$$

where $\mathrm{D}^x_{v_t}$ is the Jacobian of $v_t(x)$ w.r.t. x and $\partial_t v_t$ its partial derivative w.r.t. t. Considering that L is assumed time-invariant in Prop. 1, the time derivative of $\sqrt{\Sigma}$ in Eq. (14b) is equal to 0. Then, using the LL equations Eqs. (14a) and (14b), we approximate Eq. (7) as

$$d\phi_t(x) \approx (A_t\phi_t(x) + a_t)dt + \left(\sum_i S_t^i\phi_t(x)_i + R_t\right)d\mathbf{W}_t \qquad (15)$$

$$A_t \triangleq \mathsf{D}_{v_{t_0}}^x(x_0) \qquad a_t \triangleq -\mathsf{D}_{v_{t_0}}^x(x_0)x_0 + \partial_t v_{t_0}(x_0)(t - t_0) + v_{t_0}(x_0)$$

$$S_t^i \triangleq \partial_{x_i}\sqrt{\Sigma}_{t_0}(x_0) \quad R_t \triangleq -\sum_i S_t^i \cdot (x_0)_i + \sqrt{\Sigma}_{t_0}(x_0). \qquad (16)$$

The LL approximations in Eqs. (14a) and (15) lead to an approximation of the mean function of ϕ, $\bar{\phi}$, by the solution of the ODE

$$\frac{d\bar{\phi}_t(x)}{dt} \approx v_t(\bar{\phi}_t(x)) \text{ where } v_t(x) \approx (A_t\bar{\phi}_t(x) + a_t), \qquad (17)$$

and its second moment $\left\langle \phi_t(x)\phi_s(y)^\mathsf{T}\right\rangle$ when $t = s$ by

$$\frac{d\left\langle \phi_t(x)\phi_t^\mathsf{T}(y)\right\rangle}{dt} \approx A_t \left\langle \phi_t(x)\phi_t^\mathsf{T}(y)\right\rangle + \left\langle \phi_t(x)\phi_t^\mathsf{T}(y)\right\rangle A_t'^\mathsf{T} + a_t\bar{\phi}_t^\mathsf{T}(y) + \bar{\phi}_t(x)a_t'^\mathsf{T}$$

$$+ \sum_{ij} S_t^i \left\langle \phi_t(x)\phi_t^\mathsf{T}(y)\right\rangle \left(S_t'^j\right)^\mathsf{T} + \left(\sum_i S_t^i\bar{\phi}_t(x)_i\right)R_t'^\mathsf{T} + R_t\left(\sum_i S_t'^i\bar{\phi}_t(y)_i\right)^\mathsf{T} + R_tR_t'^\mathsf{T},$$

$$\qquad (18)$$

where A_t'; a_t'; $S_t'^i$; and R_t' are the same as A_t; a_t; S_t^i; and R_t in Eq. (16) substituting y and y_0 for x and x_0.

As long as the initial condition $\phi_{t=0}$ is a GP, the linear approximation of ϕ_t is a GP uniquely determined by $\bar{\phi}$ and Λ [9]. Then, given a set of stochastic velocity fields $v_0 \ldots v_{t_{M-1}}$ with $t_0 = 0$ and $t_{M-1} = 1$, the parameters of the stochastic process representing the transform ϕ are obtained integrating Eqs. (17) and (18) with the initial conditions $\phi_{t=0} \sim \mathcal{GP}(\bar{\phi}_{t=0}, \Lambda_{t=0})$. Having characterized stochastic transformations representing a diffeomorphic deformation, we are in position to formulate our probabilistic diffeomorphic registration algorithm.

2.3 Probabilistic Diffeomorphic Registration

The stochastic diffeomorphic deformation model of Section 2.2 leads to a GP approximation on deformation fields, whose parameters are determined by v and Σ; we use this model as $q(\phi_1)$, our variational distribution. In this section, we show how to compute the parameters of $q(\phi_1)$ minimizing Eq. (2) for a particular registration problem. Taking the approach of [3], we focus on operators L for the energy Eq. (5) regularizing in space but not in time. Due to the time-independent regularization, the prior on velocity fields of ϕ derived with Prop. 1 is the joint probability of the fields at each time t: $p(\phi_1) = \prod_0^1 p(\mathbf{v}_t)^{dt}$ with $p(\mathbf{v}_t) \sim \mathcal{GP}(0, \Sigma_0)$. Then, we rewrite leftmost term of Eq. (2) as KL $[q\|p(\phi_1)] = \int_0^1$ KL $[q(\mathbf{v}_t)|p(\mathbf{v}_t)]\,dt$. We parameterize each stochastic velocity field $\mathbf{v}_t$ by a N-point set represented as a matrix $X_t \in \mathbb{R}^{N \times d}$ rendering its mean equivalent to a spline model [10]. This sets the distributions of the discretized velocity field prior to $p(\text{vec } \mathbf{v}_t | X_t) = \mathcal{G}(0, S_{t=0} | X_t)$. As in usual LDDMM approaches, we keep the L operator, hence the covariance S, fixed. Hence, the parameterized form of variational approximation to the posterior of the velocity fields becomes $q(\text{vec } \mathbf{v}_t | X_t) = \mathcal{G}(\mu_t, S_{t=0} | X_t)$. Due to GP properties given the mean and covariance functions for the GP, we can characterize the mean and covariance for the discretized velocity field as, $\mu_t(X) = \text{vec } v_t(X)$ and $[S_{t=0}(X)]_{di+k,dj+l} = [\Sigma_{t=0}(X_i, X_j)]_{kl}, i, j = 1 \ldots N, k, l = 0 \ldots d - 1$ [10]. This leads to an objective which we minimize to obtain $q(\phi_1)$ representing the registration problem:

$$\mathcal{E}(q(\phi_1)) = \text{KL}\left[q(\phi_1) \| p(\phi_1)\right] + \langle m(\phi_1 \circ M, F)\rangle_q + \log p(M, F) \tag{19a}$$

$$\text{KL}\left[q(\phi_1) \| p(\phi_1)\right] = \int_0^1 \mu_t^\mathsf{T} S_{t=0}^{-1} \mu_t dt, \text{ s.t. } \tfrac{d\bar{\phi}_t}{dt} \approx \mu_t(\bar{\phi}_t), \bar{\phi}_0 = \text{id}. \tag{19b}$$

Using the ideas of [3], Eq. (19) can be minimized through geodesic shooting [4], i.e. it depends only on M, F and $\mu_{t=0}$. The shooting equations for the proposed probabilistic diffeomorphic registration can be derived using Eq. (19) in combination with the evolution equation based on the most probable velocity field μ. In fact, the problem formulation equations, shown in Eq. (4), stay the same as in [3], only the final condition E_ϕ changes, which is then warped to $t = 0$ for a gradient descent with respect to the initial velocity $\mu_{t=0}$ leading to the objective function of $q(\phi_1)$ parameterized on $\mu_{t=0}$

$$\operatorname*{argmin}_{\mu_{t=0}} \mathcal{E}(q_{\mu_{t=0}}(\phi)) = \tfrac{1}{2}\mu_{t=0}^\mathsf{T} S_{t=0}^{-1} \mu_{t=0}^\mathsf{T} + \langle m(\phi_1 \circ M, F)\rangle_q - \log p(M, F). \tag{20}$$

Up to this point the framework we presented is general for cases where M and F are images or landmarks. Henceforth, we specialize the treatment of the registration problems for the landmark case where M and F are matrices in $\mathbb{R}^{N \times d}$; $m(M, F) = \|M - F\|_2^2$; and the random variable $\boldsymbol{\Phi}_t = \text{vec}(\phi_t \circ M) \triangleq \text{vec } \phi_t(M)$. This allows us to rewrite

$$\langle m(\phi_1 \circ M, F)\rangle_q = \langle m(\boldsymbol{\Phi}_1, F)\rangle_q = \text{tr}\left\langle \boldsymbol{\Phi}_1 \boldsymbol{\Phi}_1^\mathsf{T} \right\rangle_q - 2\bar{\boldsymbol{\Phi}}_1^\mathsf{T} F + \text{tr } F F^\mathsf{T}. \tag{21}$$

Replacing Eq. (21) in Eq. (20) leads to the gradient

$$\nabla_{\mu_{t=0}} \mathcal{E}(q_{\mu_{t=0}}(\phi_1)) = \tfrac{1}{2} S_{t=0}^{-1} \mu_{t=0} - \left(2\bar{\boldsymbol{\Phi}}_1 - 2F\right).$$

Having this gradient, we minimize $\mathcal{E}$ w.r.t. $\mu_{t=0}$ using a gradient descent algorithm.

3   Experiments

We are now in position to perform experiments using our probabilistic diffeomorphic registration algorithm. For all our experiments, we chose the covariance function

$$\Sigma_{ts}(\boldsymbol{x}, \boldsymbol{y})_{ij} = \delta(t - s)\left[\exp\left(-\tfrac{\|\boldsymbol{x}_i - \boldsymbol{y}_j\|_2^2}{2\sigma^2}\right)\right]_{ij} \in \mathbb{R}^{d \times d} \tag{22}$$

where σ^2 is the model parameter. To conclude the specification of the model, we know with certainty that the starting point of the registration algorithm is the identity transform, hence $\phi_0(\boldsymbol{x}) \sim \mathcal{GP}(\boldsymbol{x}, \Sigma_{t=0,s=0}(\boldsymbol{x}, \boldsymbol{y}))$ and $\Sigma_{t=0,s=0}(\boldsymbol{x}, \boldsymbol{y}) = \mathbf{0}$.

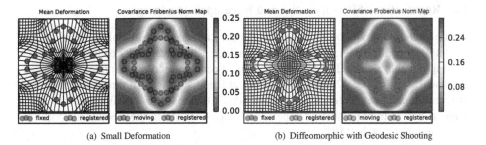

(a) Small Deformation   (b) Diffeomorphic with Geodesic Shooting

Fig. 1 – Comparison between small deformation and diffeomorphic registrations with equal parameter values, the *uncertainty* is represented by the Frobenius norm of the covariance. The small deformation model has a smaller variance in general at the expense of a possibly invalid deformation field away from the landmarks.

3.1 Validity of the Locally Linear Approximation

To test the validity of our GP model for diffeomorphic deformations we compared the GP through the LL method with one of the standard numerical solver for SDEs which does not assume a parametric density on ϕ [9]. We generated two sets of landmarks, as shown in Fig. 1, a circle and one resembling a flower, both of radius $10mm$. Then we generated random initial velocity fields with the covariance function in Eq. (22) with a range of $\sigma \in \{.1, 2, 5\}$. We sampled from the SDE in Eq. (7) using the standard Euler-Maruyama method [9] and then calculated the mean and covariance of the samples at the end time of the simulation. On the other side we calculated the mean and covariance at the same end time using the ODEs in Eqs. (17) and (18). After generating 100 experiments per landmark set and σ value, the mean arrival locations for both methods differed by $.5 \pm .02$ for $\sigma = .1$; $.1 \pm .003$ for $\sigma = 2$ and $.012 \pm .0003$ for $\sigma = 5$ all at least two orders of magnitude smaller than the radius of the datasets; the Frobenius norm of the difference between covariances was 11 ± 1 for $\sigma = .1$; $3 \pm .02$ for $\sigma = 2$; and $.5 \pm .01$ for $\sigma = 5$ which is small in comparison with the original variance of the points 74. This shows good agreement between the LL and the Euler-Maruyama methods.

3.2 Synthetic Registration Experiment

In order to compare our diffeomorphic model with a stochastic short deformation model [5], we implemented our model and then registered the landmarks in the circle shown in green in Fig. 1 to those of the "flower" shown in blue. The results for the short deformation model are illustrated in Fig. 1(a) and those of the diffeomorphic in Fig. 1(b). It is noticeable that in the short deformation model the domain has been warped into a non-invertible deformation which is not possible in the diffeomorphic case [3,1]. We also show the uncertainty in the transform as modeled by the of the deformation field at each point. In Figs. 1(a) and 1(b) it is noticeable how, as expected, the uncertainty is lower close to the landmarks and it grows as we move far away from them. Moreover, in both models the FC values are comparable, showing that the increased complexity of the diffeomorphic model has not increased the uncertainty in the results.

3.3   Registration of Pre-operative and Intra-operative Images

We illustrate the strength of our method in the case of multi-modal registration. We use publicly available images [12] which include 12 clinical cases of brain tumor resection. For these cases T1-MRI images have been acquired pre-surgically, manually annotated with between 20 and 37 anatomical landmarks and a tumor delineation and then intra-operative 3D ultrasound (US) reconstructions were acquired for the same subjects before tumor resection. The same experts annotated the US images with the same landmarks as the MRI.

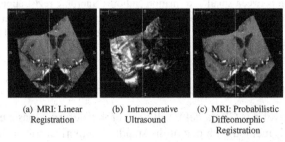

| (a) MRI: Linear Registration | (b) Intraoperative Ultrasound | (c) MRI: Probabilistic Diffeomorphic Registration |

Fig. 2 – Registration of pre-operative and intra-operative images: (a) The pre-operative MRI linearly registered and projected onto the ultrasound space. (b) The intra-operative ultrasound image; and (c) the pre-operative MRI of (a) registered to (b) using our algorithm were we show the warping according to the average registration field. The crosshair indicator shows how correspondence between a-b is not as accurate as the one using deformable registration (c).

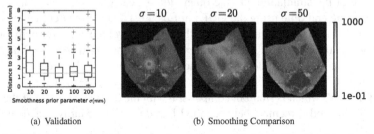

| (a) Validation | (b) Smoothing Comparison |

Fig. 3 – (a): Evaluating registration accuracy against manually labeled landmarks using LOO (see Section 3.3). The green line indicates the average pre-registration distance to the ideal location. The yellow line indicates the median distance to the ideal position of the best configuration, $\sigma = 50mm$. **(b)**: The MRI of Fig. 2 warped according to the mean deformation of the probabilistic diffeomorphic registration using 5 different levels of smoothing. Overlapped on the warped image is the estimated uncertainty. As the smoothness of the prior increases the uncertainty of the warp diminishes spanning from a small neighborhood around the landmark to the rest of the image.

We tested the accuracy of our registration algorithm on areas were there is no explicit information. For this, we used a leave-one-out (LOO) validation. For each subject we took one of the landmarks out, registered all others and then measured the distance of the landmark that we left out with the solution that were obtained by including it in the registration. We show the results in Fig. 3(a). The results are over 12 subjects with between 20 and 37 landmarks per subject. We obtained the best results with

$\sigma = 50mm$. Priors with $\sigma < 50mm$, were not able to move the left-out landmark to the ideal position and had increased variance. Priors, $\sigma > 50mm$, had a closer distance to the ideal location but an increased number of outliers. Finally, we register these subjects using all the available landmarks and, through visual inspection, we are able the see that the deformable registration improves the image matching as shown in Fig. 2. Moreover, we also show how a prior enforcing a stronger smoothness constraint increases the certainty in of the registration in the whole image. We illustrate this in Fig. 3(b) where the increase of the low uncertainty (blue) area of the image correlates with the increase of the smoothness parameter.

4 Discussion and Conclusion

In this paper we presented a probabilistic diffeomorphic registration methodology. By extending the usual diffeomorphic model of [1] from a deterministic ODE formulation to a stochastic one, we were able to include in our model the registration error, or uncertainty. To the best of our knowledge, this is the first algorithm proposing a probabilistic diffeomorphic registration using a parametric density of the diffeomorphic deformations including a numerical method to calculate the parameters. Having presented our model, we devised an algorithm to implement it through a locally linear approximation to a parametric density. We successfully tested this approximation against usual methods for SDEs where a parametric density is not available. Then, we analyzed the performance of our algorithm in synthetic and human data. Our experiments showed that our algorithm produces good results. We measured this quantitatively through a LOO experiment as well as qualitatively by visual assessment of 12 registrations between MRI and US modalities.

References

1. Dupuis, P., Grenander, U.: Variational problems on flows of diffeomorphisms for image matching. Quarterly of Applied Mathematics (1998)
2. Joshi, S.C., Miller, M.: Landmark matching via large deformation diffeomorphisms. TIP (2000)
3. Ashburner, J., Friston, K.J.: Diffeomorphic registration using geodesic shooting and Gauss–Newton optimisation. NImg (2011)
4. Beg, M., Miller, M., Trouvé, A., Younes, L.: Computing large deformation metric mappings via geodesic flows of diffeomorphisms. IJCV (2005)
5. Simpson, I.J.A., Woolrich, M.W., Cardoso, M.J., Cash, D.M., Modat, M., Schnabel, J.A., Ourselin, S.: A Bayesian Approach for Spatially Adaptive Regularisation in Non-rigid Registration. In: Mori, K., Sakuma, I., Sato, Y., Barillot, C., Navab, N. (eds.) MICCAI 2013, Part II. LNCS, vol. 8150, pp. 10–18. Springer, Heidelberg (2013)
6. Markussen, B.: Large deformation diffeomorphisms with application to optic flow. Computer Vision and Image Understanding (2007)
7. Risholm, P., Janoos, F., Norton, I., Golby, A.J., Wells III, W.M.: Bayesian characterization of uncertainty in intra-subject non-rigid registration. Medical Image Analysis (2013)
8. Zhang, M., Singh, N., Fletcher, P.T.: Bayesian estimation of regularization and atlas building in diffeomorphic image registration. In: Gee, J.C., Joshi, S., Pohl, K.M., Wells, W.M., Zöllei, L. (eds.) IPMI 2013. LNCS, vol. 7917, pp. 37–48. Springer, Heidelberg (2013)

9. Kloeden, P.E., Platen, E.: Numerical Solution of Stochastic Differential Equations. Springer (1992)
10. Rasmussen, C.E., Williams, C.K.I.: Gaussian Processes for Machine Learning. The MIT Press (2006)
11. Biscay, R., Jimenez, J.C., Riera, J.J., Valdes, P.A.: Local linearization method for the numerical solution of stochastic differential equations. Ann. Inst. Stat. Math. (1996)
12. Mercier, L., Del Maestro, R.F., Petrecca, K., Araujo, D., Haegelen, C., Collins, D.L.: Online database of clinical MR and ultrasound images of brain tumors. Med. Phys. (2012)

Automated Registration of 3D TEE Datasets of the Descending Aorta for Improved Examination and Quantification of Atheromas Burden

M.C. Carminati[1,2], C. Piazzese[1,3], L. Weinert[4], W. Tsang[5],
G. Tamborini[2], M. Pepi[2], R.M. Lang[4], and E.G. Caiani[1]

[1] Dipartimento di Elettronica, Informazione e Bioingegneria,
Politecnico di Milano, Italy
[2] Centro Cardiologico Monzino IRCSS, Milano, Italy
[3] Università della Svizzera Italiana, Lugano, Switzerland
[4] Noninvasive Cardiac Imaging Laboratories, Department of Cardiology,
University of Chicago, IL, USA
[5] Division of Cardiology, University of Toronto, Canada

Abstract. We propose a robust and efficient approach for the reconstruction of the descending aorta from contiguous 3D transesophageal echocardiographic (TEE) images. It is based on an *ad hoc* protocol, designed to acquire ordered and partially overlapped 3D TEE datasets, followed by automated image registration that relies on this *a priori* knowledge. The method was validated using artificially derived misaligned images, and then applied to 14 consecutive patients. Both qualitative and quantitative results demonstrated the potential feasibility and accuracy of the proposed approach. Its clinical applicability could improve the assessment of aortic total plaque burden from 3D TEE images.

1 Introduction

Rupture of aortic atherosclerotic lesions is a known risk factor for severe complications such as stroke and peripheral embolization, leading to decreased quality of life and excess mortality [1]. Embolic events are more prone to happen when the aortic lesions are classified as severe or complex plaques (or atheromas), namely if they are >4 mm thick or contain ulceration or mobile elements [2]. Neurologic complications may occur in particular after cardiac surgery requiring aortic manipulation and therefore characterization and avoidance of these plaques may help in decreasing embolic risks.

Different modalities, such as contrast angiography and transthoracic echocardiography (TTE) and more recently transesophageal echocardiography (TEE), epiaortic ultrasound, magnetic resonance imaging and computed tomography, have been used to image aortic plaques [2,3,4,5]. Among these, 2D TEE exhibits several advantages, allowing accurate and detailed evaluation of the aorta as well as plaque composition. Nevertheless, visualization and measure is possible only one cross-sectional plane at a time, thus neglecting the evaluation of

S. Ourselin and M. Modat (Eds.): WBIR 2014, LNCS 8545, pp. 83–92, 2014.
© Springer International Publishing Switzerland 2014

true 3D morphology and the extent of atheromas. Recently available 3D TEE technology, both real time and ECG-gated full-volume, potentially allows for a comprehensive evaluation of atheromas in the descending aorta by assessment of their thickness, volume and shape, as lately suggested by [3,6]. However, as the entire aorta cannot fit into a single acquisition, multiple datasets must be acquired and analyzed separately in order to quantify the total amount of plaques and their location at different aortic levels.

Accordingly, our aims were: 1) to develop a novel approach for the reconstruction of the descending aorta from contiguous partially overlapped 3D TEE images, based on an *ad hoc* acquisition protocol and on post-processing image registration, as first step to allow quantification of total plaque burden; 2) to validate it on artificially misaligned images obtained from original 3D TEE datasets; 3) to apply it on clinical data acquired in patients.

2 Methods

2.1 Acquisition Protocol

An *ad hoc* protocol was designed to acquire ordered and partially overlapped 3D TEE datasets of the descending aorta. All the images were acquired using single-beat, narrow-angle acquisition mode (X-7t, Philips, Nederland), at 0° with the TEE probe rotated towards the aorta. The probe was initially placed in the deepest esophageal position, in correspondence with the diaphragm, where the first dataset was acquired. Sequential overlapping segments were obtained by retracting the probe by increments of approximately 1 cm step (z-axis, foot-to-head, Figure 1). This increment was evaluated by monitoring the movement of the TEE tube at the patient's mouth. This process was repeated until reaching the aortic arch. Such procedure ensures spatial correspondence between multiple acquisitions because of the forced path of the TEE probe along the esophagus and large overlap between consecutive volumes due to small gap between contiguous probe positions. No echo parameter was changed during acquisition of images belonging to the same patient. Following this protocol, 14 consecutive patients referred for TEE, were studied and partially overlapped 3D TEE datasets of the descending aorta were acquired. Of the 14 acquired patients, five were characterized by the presence of plaques. A different number of datasets (4 to 11) was acquired for each patient, depending on the presence and extension of atheromas. All datasets were exported in cartesian converted format for further analysis (QLab, Philips, Netherland).

2.2 Registration

For each patient, the registration process aims to reciprocally align all acquired datasets and to bring them in the same reference system. We exploited the *a priori* knowledge about reciprocal position and range of overlap between images to initialize and guide the registration. To this rationale, registration was computed for pairs of contiguous images, as presented in the scheme of Figure 2,

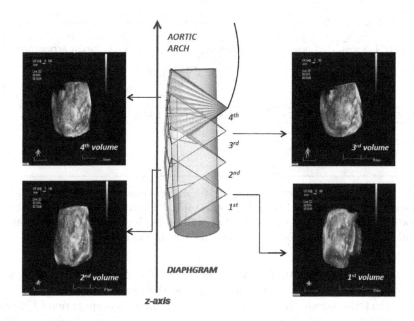

Fig. 1. Schematic describing the acquisition protocol, in which sequential overlapping 3D TEE datasets of the descending aorta were acquired

to take advantage of the information content in the overlapping regions that is maximum in adjacent volumes.

Initialization and Masks Creation. Due to the lack of frame of reference and to the extremely limited presence of anatomical landmarks in aortic TEE datasets, the initial transformation plays a significant role in the success of the registration process.

The initialization procedure was fully automated and relied on the creation of image masks obtained from the original pairs of datasets. First, each volume was thresholded in order to obtain a binary image, with white voxels belonging to the pyramid acquisition. From it, a sub-volume was obtained by setting to black the voxels corresponding to the tip of the pyramid, defined as 1/4 of the total volume of the bounding box including the acquisition pyramid (Figure 3 a)). Finally, voxels belonging to the upper or to the lower sub-volume of the binary image, corresponding to 1/3 of the total volume of the bounding box including the pyramid, were set to zero according to the reciprocal position of the two datasets to be registered. Namely, for the volume in the considered pair obtained in the deepest esophageal position the lower sub-volume was set to zero, and vice versa (Figure 3 b) and c)).

The so-obtained masks highlight the voxels in the original datasets that, in agreement with the acquisition protocol, are expected to be superimposed after registration. Their role was twofold: firstly, by overlying their centers of mass,

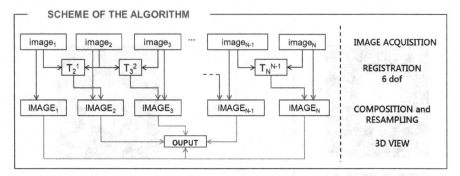

SCHEME OF THE ALGORITHM

Fig. 2. Scheme of the algorithm: starting from the consecutive overlapping images (image$_N$), pairwise registration (T_N^{N-1}) was applied resulting in reciprocally aligned images (IMAGE$_N$). After their composition and resampling into a common reference system, a fusion step is performed to allow 3D view of the output.

it was possible to obtain an adequate and automatic transformation to be used to initialize the registration process. Secondly, they were used in the registration to select the voxels that contributed to the metric computation. This was necessary because TEE aortic datasets are characterized by very limited morphological distinctive features between different datasets, so that, without masking, registration would very likely result in local optima in which pyramidal shapes are overlapping.

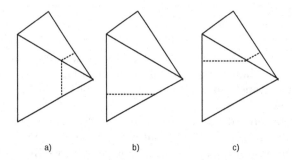

a)   b)   c)

Fig. 3. Masks creation: removal of the tip a), the bottom b) or the top portion c) of the acquisition pyramid to highlight voxels in the dataset that are expected to be superimposed for each pair of dataset after registration

Pairwise Registration and Composition. After initialization, a standard voxel-based multi resolution algorithm was used to register contiguous pair of TEE aortic dataset. A 3D rigid registration approach with three level of multiresolution and gradient descent optimizer was chosen, and normalized cross correlation (NCC) between masked images was set as similarity metric to guide the registration process. The three level multiresolution pyramid was obtained with isotropic downsampling factors of 4, 2 and 1.

To ensure temporal correspondence between datasets belonging to the same patient, the first frame, corresponding to end diastole, was selected for each acquisition and used for the analysis. We assumed that a rigid transformation $(T = \{T_x, T_y, T_z, \theta_x, \theta_y, \theta_z\})$ was adequate to align our datasets, as temporal correspondence was ensured by ECG gating, and acquisition parameters were kept fixed during the entire TEE exam.

After calculating all pairs of registration for each patient, transformations were composed in order to bring all datasets in the same reference system. We considered as the reference image the first volume acquired in the study protocol, i.e. the dataset corresponding to the deepest esophageal position. Then, all transformations were mapped with respect of this first image, according to the following equation:

$$T_1^n = \prod_{i=1}^{n-1} T_i^{i+1} \tag{1}$$

where T_1^n is the transformation of the nth image with respect to position of the first acquired image. The entire algorithm was developed in C++ using the Insight Toolkit [7].

2.3   Validation on Simulated Data

For validation purposes, two datasets were derived from a single 3D TEE dataset with isotropic spatial resolution of 0.17mm, to test the performance of the pairwise registration algorithm. Two sub-volumes (VOI_1 and VOI_2) were obtained by cutting 30% of the upper or lower portion of the original volume along the z axis, respectively, in order to obtain partially overlapped volumes with known ground truth positions. VOI_1 was set as reference image and VOI_2 was artificially misaligned.

Known rototranslations were obtained by randomly sampling a linear distribution of translation values in the range of [-10; +10] mm along the z direction, [-5; +5] mm along x and y direction and of rotation values in the range of [-10°, +10°] along each axis. Translation along z-axis was greater than those along x- and y- axis to simulate misalignment conditions in agreement with the acquisition protocol.

Following this scheme, 30 different transformations were obtained and applied to VOI_2, which was finally resampled along the VOI_1 grid in order to obtain an artificially misaligned dataset. Registration of the datasets was performed as described in Section 2.2, and residual errors after registration were computed. Both multi- and mono-resolution registration approaches were tested and their performance compared in terms of residual errors and computational time.

2.4   Clinical Validation

Several criteria were applied to quantify the pairwise registration accuracy in contiguous datasets in patients. Custom software for semi-automated segmentation of aortic plaques requiring minimal user interaction was used to obtain a 3D mesh from each dataset in which posterior aortic wall and atheromas were identified [6]. The computed geometrical transformation obtained from registration of pairs of contiguous data was then applied to the 3D meshes to allow visual assessment of correspondence between detected plaques (Figure 4). Furthermore, mean surface distance (MSD) and Hausdorff distance (HD) between 3D meshes corresponding to the same plaque, if present, in contiguous datasets were computed. Finally, displacements along z-axis between all consecutive dataset after registration was recorded in order to verify the consistency with the probe displacement defined in the acquisition protocol.

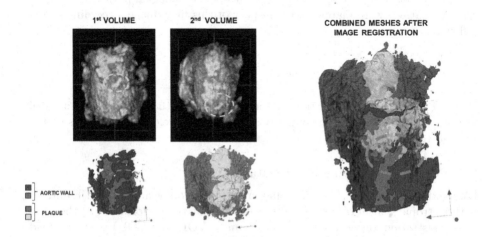

Fig. 4. Example of the clinical validation procedure. Top left: the two contiguous 3D TEE datasets in which a detail of the same plaque was highlighted with a yellow circle. Bottom left: the corresponding result, as 3D mesh, of plaque segmentation obtained with custom software, with a detail of the same plaque highlighted with a blue circle. Right: result of the image registration, defined using the original 3D TEE data, applied to the 3D meshes. The overlap of the two corresponding details of the plaque is highlighted.

3   Results

Residual registration error after simulations on artificially misaligned images, as described in 2.3, are presented in Table 1. Very limited errors were found in both mono and multi resolution approaches. As expected, computational time for multi resolution approach was significantly lower than mono resolution approach: 85s and 161s (median value), respectively, for each pair of registered datasets.

For the 14 consecutive patients, 142 3D TEE datasets were overall acquired and 128 pairwise registrations consequently computed. All registration results were visually checked by an experienced observer as described in Section 2.4 and 90% judged reliable for correspondence of aortic wall and plaques, when present. Values of translations along the z-axis of 6.15 (2.36; 10.09) mm (median

Table 1. Residual registration error in phantom datasets expressed as delta transla-
tions (ΔT_x, ΔT_y, ΔT_z) and rotations ($\Delta \theta_x$, $\Delta \theta_y$, $\Delta \theta_z$). Values are presented as median
(25th; 75th percentile).

	mono resolution	multi resolution
ΔT_x	0.016 (0.01; 0.036) mm	0.012 (0.008; 0.025) mm
ΔT_y	-0.01 (-0.012; -0.006) mm	-0.008 (-0.010; -0.0045) mm
ΔT_z	-0.005 (-0.0142; 0.0004) mm	-0.003 (-0.009; 0.0009) mm
$\Delta \theta_x$	-0.006° (-0.025°; 0.003°)	-0.005°(-0.017°; 0.002°)
$\Delta \theta_y$	0.002° (-0.002°; 0.007°)	0.002° (-0.0005°; 0.0073°)
$\Delta \theta_z$	0.021° (0.018°; 0.026°)	0.018°(0.015°; 0.021°)

and interquartile range) were found, in the range of the probe displacement
defined in the acquisition protocol. In the subset of five patients characterized
by the presence of plaques, 41 3D TEE datasets were overall acquired and 36
pairwise registrations computed. Among these, 18 pairs of volumes presented at
least one corresponding plaque. In these cases, MSD and HD were computed
between pairs of surfaces representing the same plaque in contiguous datasets
resulting in median and interquartile values of 0.9 (0.5; 1.5) mm and 4.7 (3.4; 8)
mm, respectively.

After registration, composition of the transformations with respect with the
first acquired volume allowed for 3D visualization of datasets by means of surface
as well as volume rendering. In the left panel of Figure 5, composed surface
rendering of 9 registered datasets is presented, as resulting segmented mesh, in
which a color code was applied to highlight different plaque thickness. In the

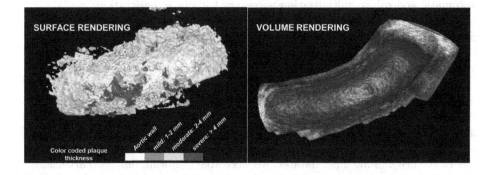

Fig. 5. Example of data composition and fusion: color coded surface rendering of 9
registered datasets (left panel), fused image by means of mean fusion rule, composed
by 10 contiguous dataset (right panel)

right panel, an example of fused image by means of simple mean intensity fusion rule, and composed by 10 contiguous datasets is shown.

4   Discussion

Aortic plaques are not only independent risk factors for stroke and peripheral emboli [8], but their presence was also associated with carotid, coronary and renal artery disease [2,10]. Thus, identification and quantification of aortic atherosclerotic burden in the descending aorta is clinically relevant. TEE is readily available and is routinely performed on patients to identify cardiac source for embolic event as well as during cardiac surgery. Besides, TEE is one of the main imaging modality used to guide percutaneous procedures, where complication rates are increased by peri-procedural plaque embolization. Thus, TEE is a suitable tool for assessing aortic atherosclerosis [9,11].

We proposed a robust and efficient approach for acquiring and composing 3D TEE datasets of the descending aorta. To the best of our knowledge, this is the first time that the registration and composition of 3D TEE contiguous aortic datasets is proposed. This method allows for the 3D morphological reconstruction of the descending aorta from 3D TEE images, by augmenting the field-of-view in respect to the acquisition and analysis from a single position. Thus, it potentially results into precise spatial localization of atherosclerotic plaques and quantification of the total plaque burden for the patient.

Our study is based on a dedicated acquisition protocol, that slightly differs from routine 3D TEE aortic examination, but which complexity is minimal and potentially possible in all patients already undergoing TEE examinations. In [12], Housden et al. rigidly registered 3D TEE cardiac datasets to obtain a compounded image with extended field-of-view and their proposed initialization strategy was based on probe tracking by X-ray imaging. In our study, instead, the acquisition protocol resulted in sequentially ordered and partially overlapped datasets, so that we were able to exploit this *a priori* knowledge to perform automatic and robust initialization necessary for image registration.

The registration step is based on known intensity based multi resolution approach and guided by NCC metric. A similar algorithm was previously adopted by [13], as a first step for multiview fusion of real time 3D TTE images, with the aim of obtaining high quality images of the cardiac chambers. Nevertheless, registration of 3D TEE aortic dataset represents a more difficult task than ventricular images, due to the lack of characteristic structures and anatomical landmarks. As a first step for validation of the pairwise registration, we used two virtually derived artificially misaligned datasets, which results showed very limited residual registration error, proving the robustness of our approach. Due to the limited size of the original 3D TEE dataset, we were able to obtain only two artificially misregistered subvolumes, while up to 11 consecutive volumes were registered and composed for clinical data. However, this first validation was carried out to test the performance of the registration, which in our study was performed for pairs of consecutive volumes. On patients datasets, each registration was first checked by visual inspection and high success rate was reported (90%). In the remaining 10% of cases in which the alignment procedure failed, the ECG gating probably was not able to avoid other deformations, such as pulsatile or breathing motion, and affine or non-rigid registration should be considered. Furthermore, quantitative validation was based on MSD and HD indices, that however was possible only in 5 patients, in which plaques were present. In this limited cohort, we found small MSD values, proving that corresponding plaques in contiguous volumes were correctly overlapped after registration, thus supporting the feasibility and accuracy of the method in the clinical settings. It is worth noting that the reported higher HD values are justified by the fact that maximum distance between surfaces is increased as atheromas located on overlapping areas could also extend to non-overlapping regions. Furthermore, displacement along the z-axis resulting from the registration process between contiguous dataset was studied. This axis is approximately correspondent to the longitudinal axis of the aorta, as the acquisition is forced by the movement of the probe along the esophagus. The relative position of volumes after registration was verified to be consistent with the range allowed in the acquisition protocol. Further validation with gold standard imaging techniques (i.e., CT scans or MRI), in which the entire descending aorta is imaged, is required to provide additional information on the algorithm performance.

In conclusion, 3D TEE contiguous and partially overlapped datasets of the descending aorta can be efficiently registered by an automatic algorithm based on *a priori* knowledge of the acquisition protocol. As such, routine investigation could include systematic 3D data acquisition of the aorta during TEE to improve the information on total aortic plaque burden in the echocardiographic report. This will allow standardization of analysis across echocardiographic laboratories and provide quantification for reporting purposing, which aids in follow-up and use in clinical trials.

References

1. Hogue, C.W., Murphy, S.F., Schechtman, K.B., Dávila-Román, V.G.: Risk factors for early or delayed stroke after cardiac surgery. Circulation 100(6), 642–647 (1999)
2. Kronzon, I., Tunick, P.A.: Aortic atherosclerotic disease and stroke. Circulation 114(1), 63–75 (2006)
3. Bainbridge, D.: 3D imaging for aortic plaque assessment. In: Seminars in Cardiothoracic and Vascular Anesthesia, vol. 9, pp. 163–165. Sage Publications (2005)
4. Kutz, S.M., Lee, V.S., Tunick, P.A., Krinsky, G.A., Kronzon, I.: Atheromas of the thoracic aorta: A comparison of transesophageal echocardiography and breath-hold gadolinium-enhanced 3-dimensional magnetic resonance angiography. Journal of the American Society of Echocardiography 12(10), 853–858 (1999)
5. Harloff, A., Brendecke, S.M., Simon, J., Assefa, D., Wallis, W., Helbing, T., Weber, J., Frydrychowicz, A., Vach, W., Weiller, C., et al.: 3D MRI provides improved visualization and detection of aortic arch plaques compared to transesophageal echocardiography. Journal of Magnetic Resonance Imaging 36(3), 604–611 (2012)

6. Piazzese, C., Tsang, W., Sotaquira, M., Lang, R.M., Caiani, E.G.: Semi-automated detection and quantification of aortic atheromas from three-dimensional transesophageal echocardiography. In: Computing in Cardiology Conference (CinC), pp. 13–16. IEEE (2013)

7. Ibanez, L., Schroeder, W., Ng, L., Cates, J.: The ITK Software Guide, 1st edn. Kitware, Inc. (2003), http://www.itk.org/ItkSoftwareGuide.pdf, ISBN 1-930934-10-6

8. Cohen, A., Tzourio, C., Bertrand, B., Chauvel, C., Bousser, M., Amarenco, P., et al.: Aortic plaque morphology and vascular events a follow-up study in patients with ischemic stroke. Circulation 96(11), 3838–3841 (1997)

9. Vaduganathan, P., Ewton, A., Nagueh, S.F., Weilbaecher, D.G., Safi, H.J., Zoghbi, W.A.: Pathologic correlates of aortic plaques, thrombi and mobile aortic debris imaged in vivo with transesophageal echocardiography. Journal of the American College of Cardiology 30(2), 357–363 (1997)

10. Fazio, G.P., Redberg, R.F., Winslow, T., Schiller, N.B.: Transesophageal echocardiographically detected atherosclerotic aortic plaque is a marker for coronary artery disease. Journal of the American College of Cardiology 21(1), 144–150 (1993)

11. Vegas, A., Meineri, M.: Three-dimensional transesophageal echocardiography is a major advance for intraoperative clinical management of patients undergoing cardiac surgery: a core review. Anesthesia & Analgesia 110(6), 1548–1573 (2010)

12. Housden, R.J., Ma, Y., Arujuna, A., Nijhof, N., Cathier, P., Gijsbers, G., Bullens, R., Gill, J., Rinaldi, C.A., Parish, V., et al.: Extended-field-of-view three-dimensional transesophageal echocardiography using image-based x-ray probe tracking. Ultrasound in Medicine & Biology 39(6), 993–1005 (2013)

13. Rajpoot, K., Grau, V., Noble, J.A., Szmigielski, C., Becher, H.: Multiview fusion 3D echocardiography: improving the information and quality of real-time 3D echocardiography. Ultrasound in Medicine & Biology 37(7), 1056–1072 (2011)

A Hierarchical Coarse-to-Fine Approach for Fundus Image Registration

Kedir M. Adal[1,3], Ronald M. Ensing[1,3], Rosalie Couvert[1,3], Peter van Etten[2],
Jose P. Martinez[2], Koenraad A. Vermeer[1], and L.J. van Vliet[3]

[1] Rotterdam Ophthalmic Institute, Rotterdam, The Netherlands
[2] Rotterdam Eye Hospital, Rotterdam, The Netherlands
[3] Quantitative Imaging Group, Department of Imaging Physics,
Delft University of Technology, Delft, The Netherlands

Abstract. Accurate registration of retinal fundus images is vital in computer aided diagnosis of retinal diseases. This paper presents a robust registration method that makes use of the intensity as well as structural information of the retinal vasculature. In order to correct for illumination variation between images, a normalized-convolution based luminosity and contrast normalization technique is proposed. The normalized images are then aligned based on a vasculature-weighted mean squared difference (MSD) similarity metric. To increase robustness, we designed a multiresolution matching strategy coupled with a hierarchical registration model. The latter employs a deformation model with increasing complexity to estimate the parameters of a global second-order transformation model. The method was applied to combine 400 fundus images from 100 eyes, obtained from an ongoing diabetic retinopathy screening program, into 100 mosaics. Accuracy assessment by experienced clinical experts showed that 89 (out of 100) mosaics were either free of any noticeable misalignment or have a misalignment smaller than the width of the misaligned vessel.

Keywords: Mosaicking, fundus illumination normalization, diabetic retinopathy screening.

1 Introduction

Registration of retinal fundus images plays a crucial role in computer-aided diagnosis and screening of the human eye for various retinal diseases. Depending on the targeted clinical application, fundus image registration can aid retinal examination in three ways. Firstly, mosaicking creates a larger field-of-view by stitching individual images. Such a mosaic facilitates comprehensive retinal examination at a single glance. Secondly, multimodal registration spatially aligns images from different modalities, thereby fusing complementary information into a single image. Thirdly, longitudinal registration aligns a series of fundus images taken over time. This is especially vital in screening or staging of progressive eye diseases such as age-related macular degeneration (AMD) and diabetic retinopathy [1,2].

S. Ourselin and M. Modat (Eds.): WBIR 2014, LNCS 8545, pp. 93–102, 2014.
© Springer International Publishing Switzerland 2014

The success of these clinical applications depends on the accuracy of the registration algorithm. Although several fundus image registration algorithms have been proposed in the past decades [3–9], accurate and robust registration of retinal images still remains a challenge. This is mainly due to the sometimes very small image overlap, severe illumination artifacts near the frame boundaries, and the spatial distortion as a result of mapping the curved retinal surface onto the image plane.

Depending on the image information used for matching, existing algorithms can be grouped into intensity-based and feature-based methods. Intensity based methods make use of the similarity between the intensity or RGB values of raw or pre-processed images [3, 4]. Nicola et al. [3] used mutual information as a similarity criterion to estimate the parameters of a global (rigid) affine model. In [4], the correlation between the binary vasculature masks of segmented fundus image pairs is optimized. These intensity based methods ignore the quadratic and higher order terms of the image distortion.

Feature-based methods [5–9] make use of saliency or landmark points, disregarding most of the structural information embedded in the local correlation of fundus images. In [5], retinal vessel bifurcations and crossover points are used as landmarks in a hierarchical optimization of a quadratic transformation model. Stewart et al. [6] used vessel bifurcations for initialization of a dual-bootstrap iterative closest point (ICP) algorithm to align the vessel centerlines using a quadratic transformation model. Chanwimaluang et al. [7] used the vasculature tree for initialization and the quadratic model parameters are estimated using the vessel bifurcation and crossover points. In [8], a radial distortion correction, estimated using vessel bifurcations, is applied prior to registration in order to correct the distortion caused by the curved to planar surface mapping. Recently, Jian et al. [9] proposed salient feature regions (SFR) as landmark points of fundus images and local features extracted from these points are subsequently matched.

In general, the accuracy and robustness of feature-based methods are highly dependent on the feature detection method, the number of detected features, and their distribution in the image. The latter two conditions are restrictive in registration of fundus images, because vessel branching and crossover points are sparsely and unevenly distributed. Furthermore, this effect gets even worse if the region of overlap between the image pairs becomes smaller.

In this paper, a registration method is proposed that exploits the intensity as well as the structural information of the retinal vasculature. We introduce a novel technique to normalize the green fundus image channel for illumination and contrast variation, thereby improving the visibility of the vasculature and hence the registration accuracy in these regions. The method then aligns retinal vessels based on the normalized images. We designed a multiresolution matching strategy coupled with a hierarchical registration model with a deformation model of increasing complexity for robust optimization of a global second-order transformation model.

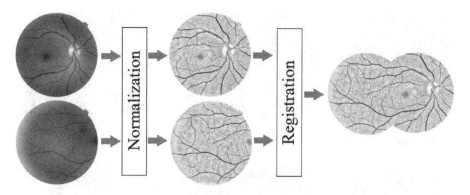

Fig. 1. Overview of the proposed registration framework. First, the green channels of the fundus images are normalized for luminosity and contrast. Then, a hierarchical coarse-to-fine registration method is applied to produce a mosaic.

2   Methods

The proposed method, outlined in figure 1, starts by normalizing the image luminosity and contrast, which vary greatly due to illumination conditions. Then the images are spatially aligned by first estimating the lower order transformation model parameters at a coarse resolution level and propagating the results to the next finer resolution level, where higher order model parameters are introduced. To guide the registration by vasculature regions, more weight was assigned to pixels in these regions.

2.1   Image Normalization

The main limitations of using the raw intensity values of fundus images for registration are the luminosity and contrast variations caused by non-uniform illumination of the retina during image acquisition. In this work, this intra and inter image variation is compensated for by applying an improved version of Foracchia's luminosity and contrast normalization method [10] to the green channel (I_G) of our RGB fundus images. The method relies on the intensity distribution of the retinal background (excluding vessels, optic disc, and lesions) to estimate local luminosity (L) and contrast (C). To compensate for local variations, the normalized image I_N, becomes:

$$I_N = \frac{I_G - L}{C}, \tag{1}$$

where L and C are respectively the sample mean and standard deviation of the background image in the neighborhood of each pixel. However, since the background image is locally masked by retinal features such as blood vessels, a local signal approximation is required to handle this space-variant reliability map in neighborhood operations. In this paper, a higher-order normalized convolution is used to approximate the luminosity map. It takes into account missing or

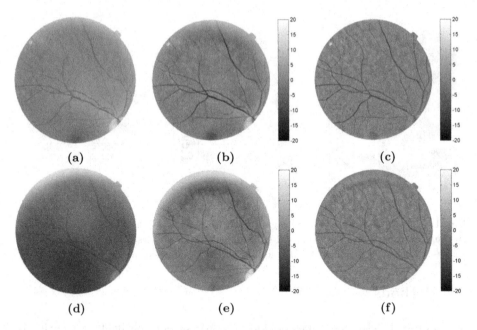

Fig. 2. An example of illumination normalization on a pair of fundus images. (a) and (d) Green channel of fundus images. (b) and (e) Normalized fundus images using the method described in [10]. (c) and (f) Normalized fundus images using the proposed normalized convolution technique.

unreliable data samples and gives a better estimate of linear and quadratic variations in the illumination pattern [11,12]. This is done by projecting each pixel and its neighbors on a set of basis vectors, chosen from the second-order Taylor expansion of the pixel around the neighbors, to create a new representation [12]. The contribution of each neighbor pixel is controlled by a Gaussian applicability function combined with a confidence measure, which encodes the presence or absence of background pixel values.

In figure 2, a typical example of a pair of fundus images from the same eye captured one year apart are shown before and after image normalization. The normalized image pairs (figure 2c and 2f) appear much more similar than the unprocessed image pairs (figure 2a and 2d). Moreover, the normalized convolution approach provides a far better contrast of the fine vasculature compared to the method described in [10] (figure 2b and 2e), especially around the border of the images. This is very crucial in registration of fundus images. As most of the overlap occurs around border regions, the registration accuracy depends on how well the vasculatures in these regions are aligned.

2.2   Registration Initialization

Convergence and robustness of image registration requires a good starting point. In this paper, we propose a robust initialization algorithm using overlap-corrected

cross-correlation, i.e. standard cross-correlation divided by the number of overlapping pixels from which it is computed (see Eq. 2). This allows the cross-
correlation to be invariant to the overlap between images. In order to further
handle rotation between the image pairs (e.g. due to possible head, eye or camera
motion between consecutive image acquisitions), this is done at three rotation
angles, $\alpha = 0°, \pm 5°$, and at a very coarse scale, i.e. by blurring with a Gaussian
filter of $\sigma = 32$ pixels and downsampling by a factor of $s = 16$.

$$I_{\widehat{CC}}(u,v,\alpha) = \frac{\sum\limits_{x=1}^{M}\sum\limits_{y=1}^{N} I_f(x,y)I_m(x',y')}{\sum\limits_{x=1}^{M}\sum\limits_{y=1}^{N} \Omega_f(x,y)\Omega_m(x',y')}, \tag{2}$$

where $I_{\widehat{CC}}$ is the overlap-corrected cross-correlation and I_f and Ω_f (I_m and Ω_m)
are the normalized image and field-of-view mask of the fixed (moving) image of
size $M \times N$, respectively. $(x',y') = (x\cos\alpha - y\sin\alpha + u, x\sin\alpha + y\cos\alpha + v)$
are the rotated and translated pixel coordinates. For each angle, the values of u
and v that maximize $I_{\widehat{CC}}$ are tentatively selected. The optimal angle ($\hat{\alpha}$), and
the corresponding values for u and v, are then selected by minimizing the mean
squared difference (MSD) of $I_f(x,y)$ and $I_m(x',y')$. In our study, since the image
pairs are represented at a very coarse scale, the three angles (five degrees apart)
are enough to find the starting point for the registration.

2.3   Hierarchical Coarse-to-Fine Registration

Since the image pairs are normalized for luminosity and contrast, the MSD can
be used as similarity metric. The registration is further guided by the vasculature regions as they provide the main distinctive structures of fundus images,
thereby restricting the effect of intensity change in the background region due
to factors such as disease progression and artifacts. This is achieved by weighting the contribution of each pixel to the similarity metric using a measure for
vesselness $V(x,y) \in [0,1]$. The vesselness-weighted cost function to minimize is:

$$\varepsilon = \frac{1}{|\Omega|} \sum_{(x,y)\in\Omega} V^2(x,y) \cdot \left[I_f(x,y) - I_m(T(x,y;\Theta))\right]^2, \tag{3}$$

where $T(\cdot)$ is the transformation model parameterized by Θ, I_f and I_m are the
normalized values of the fixed (anchor) and moving (floating) image, respectively,
and Ω is the set of all overlapping pixels in the image pairs. The vesselness maps
of both normalized images were computed from the multi-scale ($\sigma \in [1,9]$ pixels),
second-order local image structure [13]. The pixelwise maximum of the two maps
was then dilated by a disk structuring element of 25 pixels radius and used as a
weight.

As fundus imaging involves mapping the curved retinal surface onto a flat
image plane, a transformation model of at least second-order is required to accurately align images. In this work, a global 12 parameter quadratic transformation
model is used [5]:

Table 1. Transformation model and parameters at each pyramid level of the proposed hierarchical coarse-to-fine registration approach. σ and s are the Gaussian blurring scale and subsampling factor, respectively. The deformation model parameters at each level are optimized using Eqs 3 and 4. Note that $\hat{\alpha}$ is a fixed angle optimized at the initialization stage (section 2.2).

Level	Transformation	Parameters	σ (pixels)	s
1	Translation	$\begin{pmatrix} 0\ 0\ 0\ \cos\hat{\alpha}\ -\sin\hat{\alpha}\ \theta_1 \\ 0\ 0\ 0\ \sin\hat{\alpha}\ \ \cos\hat{\alpha}\ \theta_2 \end{pmatrix}$	16	8
2	Similarity	$\begin{pmatrix} 0\ 0\ 0\ \cos\alpha\ -\sin\alpha\ \theta_1 \\ 0\ 0\ 0\ \sin\alpha\ \ \cos\alpha\ \theta_2 \end{pmatrix}$	8	4
3	Affine	$\begin{pmatrix} 0\ 0\ 0\ \theta_1\ \theta_2\ \theta_3 \\ 0\ 0\ 0\ \theta_4\ \theta_5\ \theta_6 \end{pmatrix}$	4	2
4a	Simplified Quadratic	$\begin{pmatrix} \theta_1\ \theta_1\ 0\ \theta_2\ \theta_3\ \theta_4 \\ \theta_5\ \theta_5\ 0\ \theta_6\ \theta_7\ \theta_8 \end{pmatrix}$	2	2
4b	Quadratic	$\begin{pmatrix} \theta_1\ \theta_2\ \theta_3\ \theta_4\ \theta_5\ \theta_6 \\ \theta_7\ \theta_8\ \theta_9\ \theta_{10}\ \theta_{11}\ \theta_{12} \end{pmatrix}$	1	1

$$T(x, y; \Theta) = \begin{pmatrix} x' \\ y' \end{pmatrix} = \begin{pmatrix} \theta_1\ \theta_2\ \theta_3\ \theta_4\ \theta_5\ \theta_6 \\ \theta_7\ \theta_8\ \theta_9\ \theta_{10}\ \theta_{11}\ \theta_{12} \end{pmatrix} \begin{pmatrix} x^2\ y^2\ xy\ x\ y\ 1 \end{pmatrix}^T, \quad (4)$$

where (x', y') are the transformed pixel coordinates and θ_i is an element of the transformation matrix Θ.

In order to improve the robustness in estimating the parameters of the transformation model, a hierarchical multiresolution method is applied. The method employs a four level coarse-to-fine Gaussian pyramid, in which the complexity of the deformation model increases with every step downwards in the pyramid: first translation-only at the top level, second translation and rotation, third an affine transform followed by a simplified quadratic model (4a) and finally a full quadratic model (4b). The simplified quadratic model assumes an isotropic second-order deformation along both x and y dimensions. Each level of the Gaussian pyramid is formed by blurring and downsampling. Table 1 summarizes the transformation models, the blurring scale, and subsampling factors.

At each level of the pyramid, the model parameters which minimize the cost function ε, are optimized using Levenberg-Marquardt. In order to take into account the difference of the magnitude of each parameter's search space, a scaling technique is employed. In addition, the parameters are orthogonalized with respect to each other so as to mitigate intra-parameter correlation. Since the optimization of each level is initialized by the results of the previous level, the risk of getting stuck into a local minimum is greatly reduced. Moreover, the hierarchical coarse-to-fine approach speeds up the convergence of the Levenberg-Marquardt algorithm by providing an appropriate initial estimate of parameters at successive pyramid levels.

3   Experiments and Results

3.1   Data Description

Data for this study was obtained from an ongoing diabetic retinopathy screening program at the Rotterdam Eye Hospital. 70 diabetes patients who visited the hospital in two consecutive years for diabetic retinopathy screening were included. During each visit, four images of macula-centered, optic nerve-centered, superior, and temporal regions of the retina were acquired from each eye. 400 images from 100 eyes, selected randomly from the first or the second year, were combined into 100 mosaics. At least one eye of each patient was included in this study.

3.2   Data Processing

For each eye, the image having the largest overlap with the remaining three images was selected as the fixed image. Then, starting with the fixed image as intermediate result, each of the three images were registered sequentially to the intermediate result in order of decreasing overlap area with the fixed image. The overlap between image pairs was as low as 14%, with an average of 48%. In total, 300 registrations were accomplished to create the 100 mosaics.

After registration, instead of averaging the overlapping area, each mosaic was constructed by overlaying the four individual images on top of each other. This is particularly important to assess the registration accuracy of fine vasculatures as combining by averaging conceals any misalignment or yields spurious blurring in the overlap regions. By changing the order of overlay, each image appeared in the top layer once, resulting in four mosaics. These mosaics were put together to form a mosaic video which was then used for grading.

3.3   Fundus Mosaic Grading

Unlike the conventional approach where the centerline error between the aligned vessels is used to quantify the accuracy of alignment, we let clinical experts do the evaluation. Two experienced graders, which are involved in the diabetic retinopathy screening program, independently assessed the accuracy of the normalized mosaic images. Each of the graders evaluated the accuracy of the overall

Table 2. Evaluation results of 100 mosaics from both graders. Each grader evaluated half of all the data.

Grade	No. of mosaics		
	Grader 1	Grader 2	Total
Off	1	2	3
Not Acceptable	8	0	8
Acceptable	35	10	45
Perfect	6	38	44

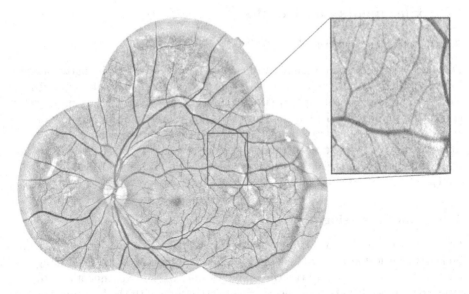

Fig. 3. A fundus mosaic which was graded as 'perfect'. The zoomed in and overlaid image patch shows part of the mosaic in which three images overlapped.

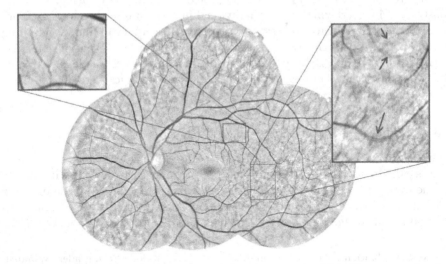

Fig. 4. A fundus mosaic which was graded as 'not acceptable'. The arrows in the zoomed in and overlaid image patch mark the misaligned micro-vessels, resulting in a blurred or double appearance of the vessels. The image patch on the left shows accurately aligned fine vasculatures.

mosaic by assessing how well the vasculatures in the overlap region were aligned and assigned a grade to it. Mosaics were graded based on the region with the worst alignment. The possible grades were:

- **Off:** an image is placed at an incorrect location.
- **Not Acceptable:** a misalignment larger than the width of a misaligned vessel.
- **Acceptable:** a misalignment smaller than the width of a misaligned vessel.
- **Perfect:** no noticeable misalignment.

It should also be noted that in our evaluation a mosaic is considered as 'not acceptable' even if the misalignment occurs in a very small fraction of the overlap region between two images.

3.4   Results

The evaluation results from both graders are summarized in table 2. Figure 3 shows a mosaic image which was graded as 'perfect'. A mosaic which was graded as 'not acceptable' is shown in figure 4. The overlap regions in the mosaics of figure 3 and 4 are constructed by averaging.

4   Discussion and Conclusion

In this paper, we present a robust hierarchical coarse-to-fine registration method for fundus images. The intensity as well as the structural information of the retinal vasculature are exploited to spatially align the four images. The method registers retinal images after normalization for luminosity and contrast variation within and between images. The alignment is done based on the vasculature-weighted MSD of the normalized images, solving the inherent limitation of feature-based algorithms of being dependent on the number and distribution of features. The robustness benefited greatly from the multiresolution matching strategy. We coupled a hierarchical coarse-to-fine registration with a deformation model of increasing complexity to estimate the parameters of a global second-order spatial transformation model. Careful initialization of each step with the results of the previous scale reduced the risk of getting trapped in a local minimum during the optimization.

Among the 100 mosaics created by the proposed method, 44 mosaics were free of any noticeable misalignment ('perfect' grade) and 45 mosaics received an 'acceptable' grade. Three mosaics were graded as 'off', all due to a failure in the first initialization stage. One of these failures could be attributed to a very poor image quality. Note that none of the 400 images were used to develop the method.

In the remaining eight mosaics, even though the accuracy of the alignment was good in most of the overlap area, a small misalignment of one or two micro-vessels resulted in a 'not acceptable' grade. The misalignments in these mosaics occurred mostly in fine vasculature regions (see figure 4). Here, the low signal-to-noise ratio resulted in a weak second-order local structure and, therefore, a low vesselness weight. In these cases, the registration was mainly guided by larger vasculature in regions around it.

In future work, we plan to evaluate a larger data set and include inter-observer agreement in our evaluation. The accuracy of the algorithm will also be evaluated for registering images from inter-visit retinal examinations. Finally, we have plans to compare the performance of our approach with other retinal image registration methods.

References

1. Abràmoff, M.D., Garvin, M., Sonka, M.: Retinal imaging and image analysis. IEEE Reviews in Biomedical Engineering 3, 169–208 (2010)
2. Zhou, L., Rzeszotarski, M.S., Singerman, L.J., Chokreff, J.M.: The detection and quantification of retinopathy using digital angiograms. IEEE Transactions on Medical Imaging 13(4), 619–626 (1994)
3. Ritter, N., Owens, R., Cooper, J., Eikelboom, R.H., Van Saarloos, P.P.: Registration of stereo and temporal images of the retina. IEEE Transactions on Medical Imaging 18(5), 404–418 (1999)
4. Matsopoulos, G.K., Mouravliansky, N.A., Delibasis, K.K., Nikita, K.S.: Automatic retinal image registration scheme using global optimization techniques. IEEE Transactions on Information Technology in Biomedicine 3(1), 47–60 (1999)
5. Can, A., Stewart, C.V., Roysam, B., Tanenbaum, H.L.: A feature-based, robust, hierarchical algorithm for registering pairs of images of the curved human retina. IEEE Transactions on Pattern Analysis and Machine Intelligence 24(3), 347–364 (2002)
6. Stewart, C.V., Tsai, C.L., Roysam, B.: The dual-bootstrap iterative closest point algorithm with application to retinal image registration. IEEE Transactions on Medical Imaging 22(11), 1379–1394 (2003)
7. Chanwimaluang, T., Fan, G., Fransen, S.R.: Hybrid retinal image registration. IEEE Transactions on Information Technology in Biomedicine 10(1), 129–142 (2006)
8. Lee, S., Abràmoff, M.D., Reinhardt, J.M.: Feature-based pairwise retinal image registration by radial distortion correction. In: Medical Imaging, p. 651220. International Society for Optics and Photonics (2007)
9. Zheng, J., Tian, J., Deng, K., Dai, X., Zhang, X., Xu, M.: Salient feature region: a new method for retinal image registration. IEEE Transactions on Information Technology in Biomedicine 15(2), 221–232 (2011)
10. Foracchia, M., Grisan, E., Ruggeri, A.: Luminosity and contrast normalization in retinal images. Medical Image Analysis 9(3), 179–190 (2005)
11. Knutsson, H., Westin, C.F.: Normalized and differential convolution. In: Proceedings of the 1993 IEEE Computer Society Conference on Computer Vision and Pattern Recognition, CVPR 1993, pp. 515–523 (1993)
12. van Wijk, C., Truyen, R., van Gelder, R.E., van Vliet, L.J., Vos, F.M.: On normalized convolution to measure curvature features for automatic polyp detection. In: Barillot, C., Haynor, D.R., Hellier, P. (eds.) MICCAI 2004. LNCS, vol. 3216, pp. 200–208. Springer, Heidelberg (2004)
13. Frangi, A.F., Niessen, W.J., Vincken, K.L., Viergever, M.A.: Multiscale vessel enhancement filtering. In: Wells, W.M., Colchester, A.C.F., Delp, S.L. (eds.) MICCAI 1998. LNCS, vol. 1496, pp. 130–137. Springer, Heidelberg (1998)

Combining Image Registration, Respiratory Motion Modelling, and Motion Compensated Image Reconstruction

Jamie R. McClelland, Benjamin A.S. Champion, and David J. Hawkes

Centre for Medical Image Computing, University College London, London, UK

Abstract. Respiratory motion models relate the motion of the internal anatomy, which can be difficult to directly measure during image guided interventions or image acquisitions, to easily acquired respiratory surrogate signal(s), such as the motion of the skin surface. The motion models are usually built in two steps: 1) determine the motion from some prior imaging data, e.g. using image registration, 2) fit a correspondence model relating the motion to the surrogate signal(s). In this paper we present a generalized framework for combining the image registration and correspondence model fitting steps into a single optimization. Not only does this give a more theoretically efficient and robust approach to building the motion model, but it also enables the use of 'partial' imaging data such as individual MR slices or CBCT projections, where it is not possible to determine the full 3D motion from a single image. The framework can also incorporate motion compensated image reconstruction by iterating between model fitting and image reconstruction. This means it is possible to estimate both the motion and the motion compensated reconstruction just from the partial imaging data and a respiratory surrogate signal.

We have used a simple 2D 'lung-like' software phantom to demonstrate a proof of principle of our framework, for both simulated 'thick-slice' data and projection data, representing MR and CBCT data respectively. We have implemented the framework using a simple demons like registration algorithm and a linear correspondence model relating the motion to two surrogate signals.

1 Introduction

Respiratory motion is often a problem when acquiring images or planning and guiding interventions (e.g. surgery, radiotherapy) in the abdomen and thorax. It can cause artefacts in reconstructed images, limiting their utility, and can cause misalignment between the planned intervention and the moving anatomy, limiting the accuracy of the guidance and leading to uncertainties in the delivered treatment. One solution to the problem of respiratory motion, which has been proposed for a wide range of different applications, is the use of respiratory motion models [1].

There are three elements to these motion models: the motion of the organ/anatomy of interest, respiratory surrogate data, and a correspondence model. If the motion of interest is known during the procedure (the image acquisition or the image guided intervention) then it can be corrected for, e.g. by performing a motion compensated

S. Ourselin and M. Modat (Eds.): WBIR 2014, LNCS 8545, pp. 103–113, 2014.

image reconstruction [2,3], or by 'animating' the treatment/intervention plan to follow the motion [4]. However, it is usually very difficult or impossible to directly measure the full motion of interest during the procedure due to limitations of the imaging equipment and/or impositions made by the intervention. In contrast, the respiratory surrogate data should be easy to acquire during the procedure, but cannot be used directly to compensate for the motion. The respiratory surrogate data is usually one or more simple 1D signals, such as the displacement of the skin surface or diaphragm, or the tidal volume measured with spirometry. The correspondence model relates the surrogate signal(s) to the motion of interest, and is fitted to some prior data before the start of the procedure (Fig 1). During the procedure the model is then used to estimate the motion of interest from measurements of the surrogate signal(s).

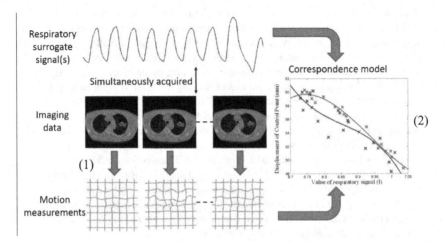

Fig. 1. An illustration of how a respiratory motion model is typically built. Respiratory surrogate data is simultaneously acquired with imaging data. Image registration is then used to determine the motion from the imaging data (1). Once the motion has been determined a correspondence model is fitted which relates the motion to the surrogate data (2).

The prior data used to fit the correspondence models consists of simultaneously acquired surrogate signal(s) and imaging data. The motion models are usually constructed in two distinct steps: 1) determine the respiratory motion from the imaging data using image registration, and 2) fit the correspondence model relating the surrogate signal(s) to the motion determined in step 1 (Fig 1). In this paper we propose a new generalized framework that combines the image registration and the model fitting into a single optimization. Not only does this give a more theoretically efficient and robust approach to determining and modelling the motion, but it also enables the use of 'partial' imaging data such as CBCT projections, or individual MR slices, where it is not possible to determine the full 3D motion from a single image. Additionally, it is straightforward to incorporate motion compensated image reconstruction into this framework using an iterative scheme.

This means the framework is particularly well suited to motion compensated image reconstruction applications, as the motion model can be fitted to the 'unreconstructed' partial imaging data, rather than requiring some previously reconstructed imaging data for fitting the motion model. E.g., some authors have proposed building a motion model from 4DCT data, and using this motion model to motion compensate a CBCT scan acquired at a later time [2]. This can lead to problems when there are differences in the motion and/or anatomy between the 4DCT data and the CBCT scan (as is often seen during the course of radiotherapy). Using the framework proposed here it is possible to build the motion model directly from the CBCT projection data, and then use the model to motion compensate the CBCT reconstruction [5]. No prior 4DCT data is required.

It should be noted that a few publications that could be said to already fit into the framework proposed here, e.g. [5,6]. However, these publications have all been focused on a particular application, registration algorithm, and motion model, whereas the framework presented here is a generalized framework that can be applied to a wide range of applications, registration algorithms, and motion models.

2   Theory and Methodology

2.1   Respiratory Motion Models

To build a respiratory motion model imaging data must be simultaneously acquired with one or more respiratory surrogate signals. The imaging data consists of N_t distinct images, $I_1 \cdots I_{N_t}$, each acquired at a different time-point and representing a different respiratory state. These should cover at least one breath cycle, although sometimes several breath cycles will be imaged so that inter-cycle variations can be observed and modelled. A reference-state image, I_0, is also required. This could be one of the images already acquired or it could be some other image, e.g. a high quality breath-hold image.

The typical approach to building respiratory motion models is to first determine the motion from the image data using image registration, and to then fit a correspondence model that relates the motion to the surrogate signals using a methods such as linear least squares [1]. To determine the respiratory motion image registration is performed between I_0 and each of the other images, I_n, where $n = 1...N_t$. Each registration is usually performed independently. The motion at time-point n can then be represented by the motion parameters, M_n, which describe the spatial transformation resulting from the registration to image I_n.

A respiratory correspondence model is parameterized by a set of model parameters, R, and relates M_n to the surrogate signals, $S_n = s_{1,n} \cdots s_{N_s,n}$, where N_s is the number of surrogate signals measured at each time-point, n, i.e. M_n is a function of S_n and R:

$$M_n = f(S_n, R)$$

E.g. a linear correspondence model relating the motion to two surrogate signals can be parameterized by 3 model parameters (for each motion parameter):

$$M_n = R_1 s_{1,n} + R_2 s_{2,n} + R_3$$

Many correspondence models have been proposed in the literature, as detailed in [1]. Any of these models, including linear, polynomial, and B-spline models, can be used within the framework presented below.

2.2   Combining Image Registration and Respiratory Motion Modelling

The framework presented in this paper does not follow the typical approach described above. Instead, it directly optimizes the correspondence model parameters on all the image data simultaneously, such that the motion estimated by the correspondence model can be used to transform the reference-state image to best match the image data.

Most image registration algorithms attempt to optimize the value of a cost function which expresses how good the registration is:

$$C(\mathbf{I}_1, \mathbf{I}_2, \mathbf{M})$$

This is a function of the motion parameters, $\mathbf{M}$, and two images, $\mathbf{I}_1$ and $\mathbf{I}_2$, where $\mathbf{I}_2$ is usually the result of transforming another image according to the motion parameters:

$$\mathbf{I}_2 = T(\mathbf{I}_0, \mathbf{M})$$

T is the function that applies the transformation parameterized by $\mathbf{M}$ to the image $\mathbf{I}_0$. Note, in this work $\mathbf{I}_0$ is the moving image, as this is more convenient when using partial imaging data. The cost function, C, usually consists of one or more similarity terms and zero or more constraint terms. A common approach is to calculate the gradient of C with respect to the motion parameters:

$$\frac{\partial C}{\partial \mathbf{M}}$$

and then use an optimization method such as gradient descent or conjugate gradient to find the optimal values of $\mathbf{M}$ that give the best value of C.

From the respiratory correspondence model it is possible to calculate the gradient of the motion parameters, $\mathbf{M}$, with respect to the model parameters, $\mathbf{R}$, e.g. for the linear correspondence model above:

$$\frac{\partial \mathbf{M}}{\partial \mathbf{R}_1} = s_1, \qquad \frac{\partial \mathbf{M}}{\partial \mathbf{R}_2} = s_2, \qquad \frac{\partial \mathbf{M}}{\partial \mathbf{R}_3} = 1$$

The chain rule can be used to find the gradient of the cost function with respect to the correspondence model parameters, i.e.:

$$\frac{\partial C}{\partial \mathbf{R}} = \frac{\partial C}{\partial \mathbf{M}} \frac{\partial \mathbf{M}}{\partial \mathbf{R}}$$

and this can be used to directly optimize the model parameters to give the best value of the cost function on the image data.

The model parameters should be optimized on all the image data simultaneously, so the total cost function over all images needs to be calculated:

$$C_{total} = \sum_{n=1}^{N_t} C_n$$

where $C_n = C(I_n, I_{T_n}, M_n)$, $I_{T_n} = T(I_0, M_n)$, $M_n = f(S_n, R)$

S_n is the values of the surrogate signals at time n, and R is the current model parameters. Likewise, the gradient of the total cost function over all images needs to be calculated:

$$\frac{\partial C_{total}}{\partial R} = \sum_{n=1}^{N_t} \frac{\partial C_n}{\partial R}$$

where $\frac{\partial C_n}{\partial R}$ is the gradient of the cost function with respect to the model parameters calculated using image, I_n, and surrogate signals, S_n. The gradient of the total cost function can then be used to find the optimal values of R using the same optimization method as used for standard image registration between two images, e.g. gradient descent.

2.3   Using Partial Imaging Data

With the framework described above it is possible to use 'partial' imaging data, such as single slices or projections, instead of full images, providing the total partial image data still sufficiently samples the motion over the region of interest. When using partial imaging data it is necessary to model the image acquisition/reconstruction process:

$$P_n = A_n(I_n) + \varepsilon_n$$

where P_n is the partial imaging data at time n, I_n is the full image at time n, ε_n is the imaging noise, and A_n is the function which simulates the image acquisition at time n. E.g. for projection data A_n would be the forward-projection operator and for slice data A_n would be the slice selection profile. Using A_n the cost function can be calculated for each partial image, P_n:

$$C_n = C(P_n, A_n(I_{T_n}), M_n)$$

To calculate $\frac{\partial C}{\partial M}$ the difference image between the two input images is often required. When using partial imaging data it is necessary to transform the difference image from the space of the partial images, P_n, into the space of the full images, I_n, as the spatial transform parameterized by M_n is defined is the space of the full images. This is done using the adjoint of the function A_n, written as A_n^*, e.g. the adjoint of the forward projection operator is the back projection operator.

For example, if using Sum of Squared Differences (SSD) as the cost function and the linear correspondence model with two surrogate signals from the previous examples, then:

$$C_n = \left\| \mathbf{P}_n - A_n(\mathbf{I}_{T_n}) \right\|_2^2$$

$$\frac{\partial C_n}{\partial \mathbf{R}_1} = \left(-2A_n^* \left(\mathbf{P}_n - A_n(\mathbf{I}_{T_n}) \right) \nabla \mathbf{I}_{T_n} \right) s_1$$

$$\frac{\partial C_n}{\partial \mathbf{R}_2} = \left(-2A_n^* \left(\mathbf{P}_n - A_n(\mathbf{I}_{T_n}) \right) \nabla \mathbf{I}_{T_n} \right) s_2$$

$$\frac{\partial C_n}{\partial \mathbf{R}_3} = -2A_n^* \left(\mathbf{P}_n - A_n(\mathbf{I}_{T_n}) \right) \nabla \mathbf{I}_{T_n}$$

2.4   Incorporating Motion Compensated Image Reconstruction

The framework as described above assumes we have a full reference-state image, $\mathbf{I}_0$, available. However, the framework can easily be combined with motion compensated image reconstruction in an iterative approach, meaning a prior reference-state image is not required.

A number of publications have described how motion compensated image reconstructions can be performed for different imaging modalities, providing the motion is known [2,3]. The motion compensated image reconstruction can be combined into the framework described above by iterating between the image reconstruction and model fitting [5]. Firstly, a standard (non-motion compensated) reconstruction is performed from the partial imaging data. The result will contain blurring and other artefacts caused by motion, but can be used as an initial estimate of $\mathbf{I}_0$. This is used to fit the model parameters, $\mathbf{R}$, as described above. The fitted motion model is then used to perform a motion compensated reconstruction and obtain a better estimate of $\mathbf{I}_0$. The process then continues to iterate between fitting $\mathbf{R}$ using the most recent $\mathbf{I}_0$, and performing a motion compensated image reconstruction of $\mathbf{I}_0$ using the most recent values of $\mathbf{R}$.

As the model fitting framework described above is itself iterative, and will likely be performed using a multi-resolution scheme (as such schemes are commonly employed in image registration algorithms), there are different options for how often to perform the motion compensated image reconstruction: 1) every time $\frac{\partial C}{\partial \mathbf{R}}$ is recalculated, 2) after fitting the model parameters at the current resolution level, 3) after fully fitting the model parameters at all resolution levels.

3   Phantom Experiments

In order to demonstrate our framework we have performed a number of experiments using a simple 2D 'lung-like' software phantom of size 128 x 128 pixels (Fig 2a). To 'animate' the phantom we used a linear correspondence model with two surrogate signals. The first signal, s_1, was the displacement of the skin surface measured from a real patient, and the second signal, s_2, was the temporal gradient of the first signal (Fig 2b), i.e. the 2nd signal is a derived surrogate signal [1]. The motion parameters, **M**, represented a deformation field with a 2D vector at each pixel. As the reference-state image corresponded to surrogate values of 0, the 'offset' model parameter, $\mathbf{R}_3$, was not required, so there were 4 model parameters for each pixel (the x and y components of $\mathbf{R}_1$ and $\mathbf{R}_2$). We manually defined the true correspondence models parameters, $\mathbf{R}^{true}$, so that they were smoothly varying over the phantom (Fig 2c) and produced plausible looking respiratory motion that includes non-linear deformation and both intra- and inter-cycle variation (the motion is different during inhalation and exhalation and during different breath cycles).

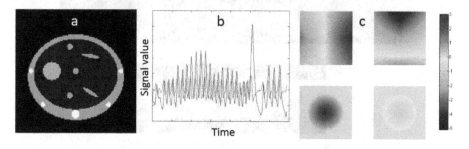

Fig. 2. a) 2D 'lung-like' software phantom. b) surrogate signals used to animate the phantom, s_1 is plotted in blue and s_2 is plotted in red. c) top-left: x component of $\mathbf{R}_1^{true}$, top-right: y component of $\mathbf{R}_1^{true}$, bottom-left: x component of $\mathbf{R}_2^{true}$, bottom-right: y component of $\mathbf{R}_2^{true}$.

We then simulated the acquisition of 3 different types of imaging data (Fig 3):

1. Full 2D images representing 4DCT like data. 13 images were simulated, covering one complete breath cycle. 5% Gaussian noise was added to the images. Fig 3a.
2. 1D slices representing MR like data. The slices were 5 pixels wide and a Gaussian slice profile was used. The slice spacing was 1 pixel (i.e. overlapping slices), and slices were acquired from each location in both the x and y directions. Each slices was acquired 3 times, giving a total of 768 slices. 5% Gaussian noise was added to the slices. Fig 3b.
3. 1D projections representing CBCT projection like data. Projections were acquired with an angular spacing of 1° and a total of 360 projections. 1% Gaussian noise was added to the projection data. Fig 3 c.

To fit the correspondence model parameters, $\mathbf{R}^{fit}$, to the imaging data we implemented a simple 'demons-like' registration algorithm. No constraint term was used but $\frac{\partial C}{\partial \mathbf{R}}$ was smoothed with a Gaussian filter (standard deviation = 5 pixels) prior to updating the model parameters. SSD was used as the similarity measure. The optimization was done using gradient descent and a multi-resolution scheme with 3 resolution levels, and stopped when the cost function improved by less than 0.1%. For the slice and projection data the model fitting was performed both using the original reference-state image used to simulate the image acquisition, and using motion compensated image reconstruction from the partial data. The motion compensated reconstruction was updated after fitting the model parameters at the each resolution level (option 2 in section 2.4).

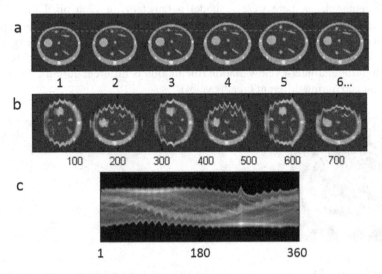

Fig. 3. Simulated imaging data. a) full 2D image (6 of 13 images shown), b) 1D slices, c) 1D projections. Image number is plotted on the x axis.

4   Results

Table 1 gives the mean, standard deviation, and maximum of the absolute difference between R^{true} and R^{fit} for each of the fitted models, as well as the absolute values of R^{true} for comparison. The summary statistics are calculated over all 4 model parameters for all pixels inside the phantom. To assess how well the original motion can be reproduced by the fitted models we also calculated the Euclidean distance between M^{true} and M^{fit} (the pixel displacements generated by R^{true} and R^{fit} respectively). Table 2 gives the mean, standard deviation, and maximum values calculated over all pixels inside the phantom and all time-points used in the simulated image acquisitions. The values for M^{true} are also given to indicate how much motion occurred (these values are from the slice acquisition as this had the most time-points, but the values for the other acquisitions are similar).

It can be seen from Tables 1 and 2 that when using the full images the models can be fitted very well and the motion can be reproduced very accurately. The results are worse for the partial imaging data, as may be expected, but the models are still fitted well and the majority of the motion is reproduced accurately. The mean values are lower for the slice data, but the maximum values are lower for the projection data. The results are worse when performing motion compensated reconstructions than when using the original reference-state image, as would be expected. However, the model parameters and the motion can still be recovered reasonably well, even when the reference-state image is not available.

Table 1. Summary statistics for the absolute differences between $\mathbf{R}^{true}$ and $\mathbf{R}^{fit}$ for each of the fitted models, and for absolute values of $\mathbf{R}^{true}$. F: full 2D images, S: 1D slices, S-MCR: 1D slices using motion compensated image reconstruction, P: 1D projections, P-MCR: 1D projections using motion compensated image reconstruction.

	$\mathbf{R}^{true}$	$\mathbf{R}^{true}$ - $\mathbf{R}^{fit}$ for model fitted to:				
		F	S	S-MCR	P	P-MCR
Mean	0.89	0.07	0.17	0.23	0.22	0.33
Std. Dev.	0.80	0.10	0.24	0.31	0.26	0.30
Max.	3.87	0.69	1.53	1.98	1.37	1.56

Table 2. Summary statistics for the Euclidean distance between $\mathbf{M}^{true}$ and $\mathbf{M}^{fit}$ for each of the fitted models, and the Euclidean distance of $\mathbf{M}^{true}$. F: full 2D images, S: 1D slices, S-MCR: 1D slices using motion compensated image reconstruction, P: 1D projections, P-MCR: 1D projections using motion compensated image reconstruction. All values are in pixels.

	$\|\mathbf{M}^{true}\|_2$	$\|\mathbf{M}^{true} - \mathbf{M}^{fit}\|_2$ for model fitted to:				
		F	S	S-MCR	P	P-MCR
Mean	1.65	0.10	0.22	0.30	0.33	0.49
Std. Dev.	1.60	0.10	0.23	0.28	0.38	0.43
Max.	19.90	0.78	9.75	10.50	6.69	6.49

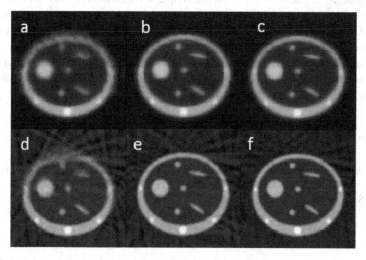

Fig. 4. Motion compensated reconstructions from slice data (top) and projection data (bottom) using (a, d) no motion compensation, (b, e) $\mathbf{M}^{fit}$, and (c, f) $\mathbf{M}^{true}$

Figure 4 shows the motion compensated reconstructions from the slice and projection data using no motion (i.e. a standard reconstruction), $\mathbf{M}^{fit}$, and $\mathbf{M}^{true}$. It can be seen that the motion compensated reconstructions are clearly superior to the non-motion compensated reconstructions. The reconstructions using $\mathbf{M}^{fit}$ are very similar to those using $\mathbf{M}^{true}$, indicating the fitted models can adequately reproduce the motion for the purpose of performing motion compensated image reconstructions.

5   Conclusions

In this paper we presented a general framework that can be used to combine image registration, respiratory motion modelling, and motion compensated image reconstruction. This framework can be used with any registration algorithm that uses the gradient of the cost function to optimize the registration and any respiratory correspondence model where the gradient of the motion with respect to the model parameters can be calculated. This includes most registration algorithms that are commonly used, and all correspondence models that we are aware of in the literature.

To demonstrate this framework we implemented it using a 'demons-like' registration algorithm and a linear correspondence model using two surrogate signals. We used a simple 2D software phantom to simulate the acquisition of full images, slice image data, and projection image data. For all types of image data the framework was able to fit the model directly to the image data and to give a good estimate of the true motion. We also showed that motion compensated image reconstruction can be included in the framework using an iterative approach, and that we were able to reconstruct images that were very similar to those obtained when the true motion was used.

On-going work includes implementing the framework with an efficient open-source registration package based on the B-spline registration algorithm (NiftyReg[1]), and thoroughly validating the framework using a variety of real clinical data, including MR, CBCT projections, and 4DCT. The framework can then be applied to a wide range of medical imaging applications that are affected by respiratory motion. In each of these applications it will be necessary to investigate the ideal combination of image data, registration algorithm (and settings), respiratory surrogate signals and correspondence model, and image reconstruction algorithm (if required).

References

1. McClelland, J.R., Hawkes, D.J., Schaeffter, T., King, A.P.: Respiratory motion models: A review. Medical Image Analysis 17, 19–42 (2013)
2. Rit, S., Wolthaus, J.W.H., van Herk, M., Sonke, J.-J.: On-the-fly motion-compensated cone-beam CT using an a priori model of the respiratory motion. Medical Physics 36, 2283–2296 (2009)

---

[1] http://sourceforge.net/projects/niftyreg/

3. Batchelor, P.G., Atkinson, D., Irarrazaval, P., Hill, D.L.G., Hajnal, J., Larkman, D.: Matrix description of general motion correction applied to multishot images. Magnetic Resonance in Medicine 54, 1273–1280 (2005)
4. Schweikard, A., Glosser, G., Bodduluri, M., Murphy, M.J., Adler, J.R.: Robotic motion compensation for respiratory movement during radiosurgery. Computer Aided Surgery 5, 263–277 (2000)
5. Martin, J., McClelland, J., Yip, C., Thomas, C., Hartill, C., Ahmad, S., O'Brien, R., Meir, I., Landau, D., Hawkes, D.: Building motion models of lung tumours from cone-bean CT for radiotherapy applications. Physics in Medicine and Biology 58, 1809–1822 (2013)
6. Hinkle, J., Szegedi, M., Wang, B., Salter, B., Joshi, S.: 4D CT image reconstruction with diffeomorphic motion model. Medical Image Analysis 16, 1307–1316 (2012)

Fluorescence-Based Enhanced Reality
for Colorectal Endoscopic Surgery

F. Selka[1,2], V. Agnus[1], S. Nicolau[1], A. Bessaid[2],
L. Soler[1,3], J. Marescaux[1,3], and M. Diana[3]

[1] IRCAD 1 Place de l'Hopital, Strasbourg, France
[2] Biomedical Engineering Laboratory, Abou Bekr Belkaid University, Algeria
[3] IHU 1 Place de l'Hopital, Strasbourg, France
selka.faical@gmail.com

Abstract. Minimally Invasive Surgery (MIS) application using computer vision algorithms, helps surgeons to increase intervention safety. With the availability of the fluorescence camera in MIS surgery, the anastomosis procedure becomes safer to avoid ischemia.We propose an Augmented Reality (AR) software that non-rigidly registers the ischemic map based on fluorescence signal on the live endoscopic sequence. The efficiency of the proposed system relies on robust feature tracking and accurate image registration using image deformation. Experimental results on *in-vivo* data have shown that the proposed system satisfies the clinical requirements.

Keywords: feature tracking, augmented reality, non-rigid registration.

1 Introduction

Colorectal cancer is the third cancer in the world with more than 1.3 million new cases diagnosed every year [1]. The standard surgical treatment is an anastomosis: the surgeon removes the segment of the colon containing the tumors and sews the healthy remaining parts of the colon together. To perform the resection, the surgeon needs to clamp vessels irrigating the segment containing the tumors. Once clamped, vessel color begins to get bluer due to ischemia (shortage of oxygen damaging the cells) giving a rough idea of the sites where resection must be performed. In case of the resection and suture site are not properly selected and undergo an ischemia, the anastomosis will not cure and leakages will occur. When such an anastomosis is performed, the surgeon must revise his surgery (in 2% of cases) to remove anastomosis leakages due to ischemia. For this postoperative complication the death rate is 32% [2]. Therefore, an accurate identification of the frontier between ischemic sites and safe ones is a critical task.

As already mentioned, it is currently detected by bluish discoloration of tissues (cyanosis) compared to normal ones, but this approach requires ischemia to have occurred at least one hour before. Moreover this diagnosis method is very subjective and surgeon experience dependent. Among recent research to quantitatively

S. Ourselin and M. Modat (Eds.): WBIR 2014, LNCS 8545, pp. 114–123, 2014.

evaluate ischemia [3], a very promising one can reduce by 60% revision of anastomosis thanks to the fluorescence properties of Indocyanine Green (ICG) when injected intravenously [4]. Nowadays, fluorescence cameras have been miniaturized and are already available for minimally invasive surgery (MIS). Typically, we use a D-light P Camera (Karl Storz) which allows, thanks to specific filters, to switch between normal view and fluorescence view (switching delay of 1s). We have recently shown [5] how we can compute a probability map of ischemia using ICG and its fluorescence signal, which allows to define accurate frontiers of ischemic sites.

This map (Fig.1.c) is generated from the temporal evolution of fluorescence signal (Fig.1.a-b) of each pixel in the video (a slow evolution of fluorescence means a higher risk of ischemia). We highlight that the fluorescence signal reaches the same intensity in the whole video after 50 seconds. Therefore, after this delay, switching to the endoscopic fluorescence mode to visually assess ischemia locations is useless.

In the current software (gray part of Fig.1), this map is then superimposed on the endoscopic reference image (captured just before fluorescence video) and displayed on a second screen to the surgeon when he performs the resection (Fig.1.d). Obviously, the system would be much more efficient if we could superimpose the map on the live endoscopic view. This would ease the surgeons task who must perform a mental registration of the static image that contains reference view and computed ischemia map. Indeed breathing, the peristaltic movement of the colon and instrument interactions with tissues continuously modify the surgical scene.

In this paper, we propose a method to non rigidly register this map in real-time (Fig.1.e-g) and show that our method is accurate despite colon deformation and camera motion. The contribution of our paper is mainly related to the application since it is based upon existing techniques. We firstly propose a methodology adapted to our context to register in real time the ischemic map. Secondly,we evaluate on clinical relevant data the accuracy of our approach.

The paper is organized as follows. We describe in Sec.2 how the ischemic map is updated using feature tracking. Sec.3 is dedicated to the validation protocol, where we show that the accuracy of our non-rigid registration on clinical data is promising for further tests.

2   Feature-Based Non-rigid Registration of Ischemic Map

The method used in this paper to register the ischemic map is divided in two parts. Firstly, we explain our method to estimate the motion of selected features on the structure of interest. Secondly, we explain how we compute a dense deformation map from these sparse features and thus non rigidly register the ischemic map.

2.1   Feature Tracking and Robust Matching

Feature Detection and Descriptor. To reach our purpose, we need to track the colon motion in the image despite occlusions due to instruments and without any assumption about the chronological order of frames to be processed. To meet these needs, feature tracking based on feature matching techniques seems to be the most appropriate. In general, feature matching algorithms find a set of potential matches between two sets of features extracted from two images by exploiting their similar appearance. The features are extracted using a feature detector. The appearance is determined by the feature representation, which includes colors, corners, scale, intensity, which is usually computed using a feature descriptor. This information must be distinctive for each feature to guarantee a high correspondence in matching features.

We choose to use the SURF [6] detector to detect features based on our tracking performance evaluation [7] on pig colon tissues, which shows that the SURF detector has the best performance in terms of feature distribution. We choose BRISK [8] to calculate the descriptor of detected features: it creates binary descriptors that work with Hamming distance instead of Euclidean, which allows for very fast matching computation necessary for our application.

Feature Detection and Descriptor. However, initial matches based on appearance only may contain a large number of mismatches (outliers): this is due to appearance similarity of features in pig colon images. Outliers are obviously problematic to compute a consistent image deformation (inaccurate registration, artefacts: see Fig.2).

There are a number of filters (physical proximity, scale similarity, orientation, descriptor distance ratio...) that have been proposed to improve robustness of selected feature matching [9][10]. In our context, we cannot rely on smooth temporal transition between two frames because we compare the live image to a reference one acquired several minutes before with a different camera position and a different colon shape due to peristaltic motion and instrument interaction. Therefore, we discard the physical proximity, scale and orientation filters and we propose the following strategy.

Let S_R be the set of features detected in the reference image and S_L the set of features detected in the live image. For each feature of S_R, we find the two best matches in the live image using Hamming distance between descriptors, and for each feature in S_L, their two best matches in the reference image. We get respectively two sets of matches $M_{R \to L}, M_{L \to R}$, where each feature is matched on two candidates. The next step consists in filtering these matches. For this purpose we propose two steps.

Firstly, for each set $(M_{R \to L}, M_{L \to R})$ we reject both candidate matches if their associated Hamming distance is too close. If the measured distance is very low for the first candidate match and much greater for the second one, we accept the first match as a good one. We selected a ratio of 0.65 from experimental results. Secondly, from the remaining matches of the two sets $(M_{R \to L}, M_{L \to R})$ we extract the matches that are in agreement with both sets. This means that, for a match to be accepted, both points must be the best matching feature of the other.

Using this approach we propose a highly restricting filter, which can discard possible good matches. However, our application cannot afford any outlier and it is thus crucial to guarantee robust feature matching. We will see in Sec.3 that this conservative choice allows a sufficient number of good matches for our application.

2.2   Image Deformation

The method we use is based on 2D registration and not 3D which is sufficient for our application. In fact, during the surgical procedure (from the beginning of the fluorescence to the definition of resection sites) we expect little perspective motion of the scene, since camera motion remains limited by the trocart. In this paper, we use the method described in [11] to estimate image deformation from a set of sparse matched features and register the ischemic map. The image deformation is based on Moving Least Squares (MLS) using various classes of linear functions including affine, similarity and rigid transformations. The choice of MLS methods is motivated by the fact that they are easy to implement and provide a very fast computation of deformations.

Let P be a set of features in the reference image (Fig.1.a) and Q the set of corresponding features in the live image (Fig.1.e). Given a point v in the reference image, they compute the best transformation $I_v(x) : \mathbb{R}^2 \to \mathbb{R}^2$ that minimizes

$$\sum_{p_i \in P, q_i \in Q} w_i |I_v(p_i) - q_i|^2 \tag{1}$$

Where w_i are weights expressed as $w_i = \frac{1}{|p_i - v|^{2\alpha}}$. Therefore, they obtain a different transformation $I_v(x)$ for each transformation class (affine, similarity, rigid). Finally they obtain a dense motion field that we use to deform and register the ischemic map (Fig.1.f). We loop this registration procedure during the definition of resection sites by the surgeon.

3   Experiments and Evaluation

The performance of our proposed method using soft-tissue tracking was evaluated on *in-vivo* datasets of pig colon. We use 5 video sequences with a resolution of 768×576 and $25 fps$ corresponding to 5 different pigs. We use the OpenCV implementation of SURF detector and BRISK descriptor for feature tracking. The MLS deformation method was written without neither parallelization nor optimisation of the code. For all the videos in this paper, we used grids with (144×115) vertices in order to apply the deformation instead of applying deformation for each pixel to reduce computation time. We then use a bilinear interpolation to fill the resulting quads as in the seminal paper [11]. Computing the deformation field for each pixel increases the accuracy on average by

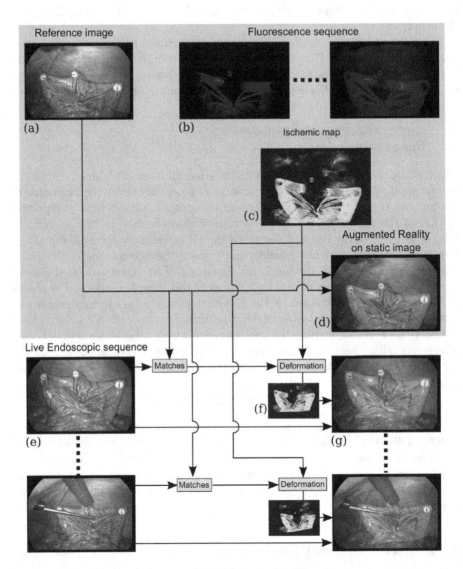

Fig. 1. Diagram of the Fluorescence-based Enhanced Reality, showing the reference image (a), the fluorescence sequence (b) and the ischemic map (c) generated from the temporal evolution of fluorescence signal. Previous approach (in gray square): the ischemic map (c) is superimposed on the reference image (a) providing a static augmented reality view (d). New approach: we perform feature matching between the reference image (a) and the live image (e). From the matched features, we deform the ischemic map (c) to obtain an updated ischemic map (f). We then superimpose the updated ischemic map (f) on the live sequence (e) providing a dynamic augmented reality view (g).

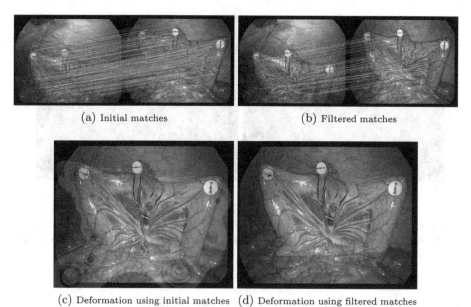

(a) Initial matches   (b) Filtered matches

(c) Deformation using initial matches   (d) Deformation using filtered matches

Fig. 2. The influence of feature matching outlier on image deformation quality

2% but dramatically increases computational time and thus do not satisfy our requirement.

We firstly describe in Sec.3.1 how we obtain ground truth data to evaluate our registration method and present the accuracy results. Secondly, we discuss in Sec.3.2 the computational performance of each MLS method with respect to our real-time constraint.

3.1 Accuracy Registration Performance

Our video set contains varying conditions such as image transformation, tissue change (peristaltic movements, interaction of surgical tools), illumination changes and occlusions. The ground truth data for our evaluation is obtained manually by annotating 10 points on the colon (tissue of interest) that are

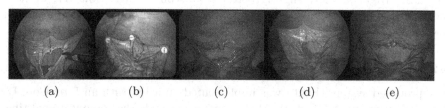

(a)   (b)   (c)   (d)   (e)

Fig. 3. Example of MIS images sequences of the 5 different pigs used in our experiments

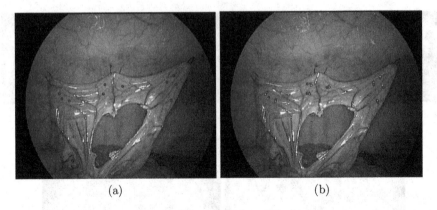

(a)   (b)

Fig. 4. Evaluation of image registration. (a) before deformation, (b) after deformation. Green points: the ground truth, yellow points: the estimated points using MLS Rigid, green line: the ground truth displacement.

tracked on 10 distant frames which shows large deformation and camera motion. We make sure that the clicked points are relatively not too close (minimum distance of 20 pixels) to the matched features in the process.

This allows us to quantitatively evaluate the non-rigid registration provided by our method and to show its interest for the colon. Fig.4 shows an example of ground truth points (green) tracked on two different frames and the estimated points using image deformation field. We highlight that 6 pixels correspond approximately to 1 mm, which is the thickness of colon vessels measured using a ruler during the surgical procedure. In Tab.1 we provide the result of registration error using three different methods: MLS Affine, Rigid and Similarity for an example video sequence (Fig.3b). For each annotated point we give the average error and the average point displacement over the 10 frames. We notice that for this example sequence the MLS Rigid gives the best registration result, which remains under 1 mm.

In Tab.2 we provide the average error registration over the 10 points and the 10 frames of the three different methods for the different video sequences. The error tolerance for the surgeon for this kind of intervention being about 5 mm [12] and thus our first *in-vivo* evaluation clearly shows that our approach has the potential to fulfil clinical requirements of this application. Although, we note that MLS Rigid provides slightly better results on average. However, we need more data to clearly understand in which case one method outperform another one.

3.2   Computational Performance

The proposed system (Fig.6) was implemented on a PC with an Intel Core I7-3.4 GHz processor, 8 GB of RAM. In Fig.5 we provide the computational time for MLS methods for a different number of matched features used to register the

Table 1. The average error registration and its standard deviation of the MLS Affine, Rigid and Similarity (Simil) methods for an example sequence (Fig.3b)

Points	pt 0	pt 1	pt 2	pt 3	pt 4	pt 5	pt 6	pt 7	pt 8	pt 9
Displacement (pixels)	47.3 ±40.3	46.5 ±40.4	47.2 ±41.6	46.9 ±41.1	51.1 ±43.2	52.8 ±44.7	47.8 ±40.7	48.5 ±41.6	47.4 ±40.5	48.2 ±41.1
Method	MLS Affine									
Error (pixels)	2.6 ± 2.2	4.5 ± 3.7	2.9 ± 1	4.5 ± 3.9	2.8 ± 2.2	6.1 ± 6.5	4.1 ± 2.2	3.1 ± 2.4	2.4 ± 1.6	4.5 ± 3.7
Method	MLS Rigid									
Error (pixels)	1.6 ± 1.2	1.2 ± 1.7	1.1 ± 0.4	1.4 ± 1.8	2.6 ±0.6	4.7 ± 1.9	1.6 ± 1.2	1.1 ± 0.5	2.7 ± 2.7	3.6 ± 4.8
Method	MLS Simil									
Error (pixels)	1.5 ± 1.6	4.3 ± 3.4	2.4 ± 0.7	4.3 ± 4.1	2.5 ± 2.1	6.1 ±6.6	3.2 ± 2.3	3.1 ± 2.6	2.4 ± 1.6	4.1 ± 4

Table 2. The average error registration in pixels and its standard deviation for the MLS Affine, Rigid and Similarity method for each video sequences

Videos	Fig.3a	Fig.3b	Fig.3c	Fig.3d	Fig.3e	Average
Affine	3.7 ± 0.9	3.7± 1.4	3.4 ± 1.1	6.2 ± 1.3	1.7 ± 0.6	3.7± 0.6
Rigid	3.9 ± 0.4	2.1± 1.6	3.4 ± 0.7	6.1 ± 1.1	1.9 ± 0.6	3.4± 0.4
Simil	3.6 ± 0.7	3.3 ± 1.5	3.1 ± 1.1	6.3 ± 1.2	1.6 ± 0.5	3.5 ± 0.5

image. We can clearly see that the deformation time is linear with the number of points used to calculate deformation. We also notice that the MLS Affine transformation provides the best result in terms of computation time (about $0.18s$ for about 200 features). However the computational time can be reduced with better code optimization. We highlight that on average, the number of matched features used for our experiment is about 240 points where the proposed feature tracking algorithm takes $0.07s$, which includes feature detection, descriptor and

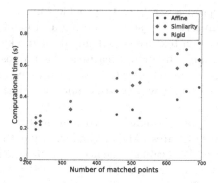

Fig. 5. Computational time depending on the number of matched points used to calculate the registration using image deformation based on MLS (Affine, Similarity and Rigid)

matching computation. Computation time is thus mainly due to the deformation computation. The software provides a registration of 5 frames per second, which satisfy surgeon needs. However it would be preferable to optimise this computation time by optimising and parallelising the code.

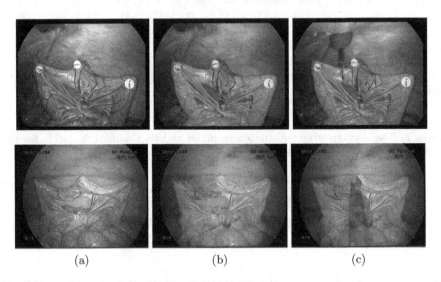

(a)	(b)	(c)

Fig. 6. Illustration of the augmented view provided by our system on several live images, which underwent large deformation and occlusions. a. Reference image, b. superimposition of ischemic map on reference image, c. non-rigid registration of the ischemic map.

4   Conclusion

In this paper, we propose a strategy to provide an AR system which helps surgeons localize ischemia risk, by superimposing a probability map onto a live endoscopic video. The colon texture is well suited for tracking thanks to vessels bifurcations providing highly distinctive features. The proposed AR system relies on this feature tracking and matching which is robust for complete and prolonged occlusion so we are able to recover the ischemic map during the definition of resection sites.

Our method relies on feature tracking to non-rigidly register a probability map using Moving Least Squares (Affine, Similarity and Rigid) transformation on a live endoscopic view. We evaluate the accuracy and the computational time of the proposed methods and we show that the results greatly satisfy surgeons needs. Future research will focus on evaluating our proposed method on human data and extending our application to more surgical procedures, such as stomach bypass using visual guidance based on fluorescence imaging.

References

1. Ferlay, J., et al.: GLOBOCAN 2012 v1.0 Cancer Incidence and Mortality Worldwide: IARC CancerBase No. 11 (2013)
2. Choi, H.K., Law, W.L., Ho, J.W.C.: Leakage after resection and intraperitoneal anastomosis for colorectal malignancy: analysis of risk factors. Diseases of the Colon and Rectum 49, 1719–1725 (2006)
3. Urbanavičius, L., et al.: How to assess intestinal viability during surgery: A review of techniques. World Journal of Gastrointestinal Surgery 3, 59–69 (2011)
4. Kudszus, S., et al.: Intraoperative laser fluorescence angiography in colorectal surgery: a noninvasive analysis to reduce the rate of anastomotic leakage. Langenbeck's Archives of Surgery 395, 1025–1030 (2010)
5. Diana, M., et al.: Enhanced-reality video fluorescence: A real-time assessment of intestinal viability. Annals of Surgery 259(4), 700–707 (2014)
6. Bay, H., Tuytelaars, T., Van Gool, L.: SURF: Speeded up robust features. In: Leonardis, A., Bischof, H., Pinz, A. (eds.) ECCV 2006, Part I. LNCS, vol. 3951, pp. 404–417. Springer, Heidelberg (2006)
7. Selka, F., Nicolau, S.A., Agnus, V., Bessaid, A., Marescaux, J., Soler, L.: Evaluation of endoscopic image enhancement for feature tracking: A new validation framework. In: Liao, H., Linte, C.A., Masamune, K., Peters, T.M., Zheng, G. (eds.) MIAR/AE-CAI 2013. LNCS, vol. 8090, pp. 75–85. Springer, Heidelberg (2013)
8. Leutenegger, S., et al.: BRISK: Binary Robust invariant scalable keypoints. In: 2011 International Conference on Computer Vision, pp. 2548–2555 (November 2011)
9. Yip, M., et al.: Tissue Tracking and Registration for Image-Guided Surgery. IEEE Transactions on Medical Imaging 31, 2169–2182 (2012)
10. Puerto-Souza, G., Mariottini, G.: A Fast and Accurate Feature-Matching Algorithm for Minimally-Invasive Endoscopic Images. IEEE Transactions on Medical Imaging (January 2013)
11. Schaefer, S., McPhail, T., Warren, J.: Image deformation using moving least squares. ACM Transactions on Graphics, TOG (2006)
12. Diana, M., et al.: Probe-based confocal laser endomicroscopy (cellvizio) and enhanced-reality for real-time assessment of intestinal microcirculation at the future anastomotic site. Accepted to SAGES (2014)

Fast and Robust 3D to 2D Image Registration by Backprojection of Gradient Covariances

Žiga Špiclin, Boštjan Likar, and Franjo Pernuš

Faculty of Electrical Engineering, Laboratory of Imaging Technologies,
University of Ljubljana, Tržaška 25, 1000 Ljubljana, Slovenia
{ziga.spiclin,bostjan.likar,franjo.pernus}@fe.uni-lj.si

Abstract. Visualization and analysis of intra-operative images in image-guided radiotherapy and surgery are mainly limited to 2D X-ray imaging, which could be beneficially fused with information-rich pre-operative 3D image information by means of 3D-2D image registration. To keep the radiation dose delivered by the X-ray system low, the intra-operative imaging is usually limited to a single projection view. Registration of 3D to a single 2D image is a very challenging registration task for most of current state-of-the-art 3D-2D image registration methods. We propose a novel 3D-2D rigid registration method based on evaluation of similarity between corresponding 3D and 2D gradient covariances, which are mapped into the same space using backprojection. Normalized scalar product of covariances is computed as similarity measure. Performance of the proposed and state-of-the-art 3D-2D image registration methods was evaluated on two publicly available image datasets, one of cerebral angiograms and the other of a spine cadaver, using standardized evaluation methodology. Results showed that the proposed method outperformed the current state-of-the-art methods and achieved registration accuracy of 0.5 mm, capture range of 9 mm and success rate >80%. Considering also that GPU-enabled execution times ranged from 0.5–2.0 seconds, the proposed method has the potential to enhance with 3D information the visualization and analysis of intra-operative 2D images.

Keywords: Image-guided surgery, 3D-2D image registration, gradient backprojection, covariance, similarity measure, quantitative evaluation.

1 Introduction

Image registration is an indispensable tool for the visualization and analysis of pre- and post-operative images, planning of interventions and in clinical imaging studies. However, it is yet to play a more proactive role in the visualization and analysis of intra-operative images, for example in image-guided radiotherapy (IGRT) and image-guided surgery (IGS). Imaging systems used in IGRT and IGS are required to be of high spatial and high temporal resolution, which leaves X-ray imaging as the only technology currently feasible for use in the operating room. As patient dose is the main concern with X-rays, imaging is limited to 2D. Bringing the information-rich 3D pre-operative images and treatment plans into

S. Ourselin and M. Modat (Eds.): WBIR 2014, LNCS 8545, pp. 124–133, 2014.

the operating room, and to enable intra-operative 3D visualization and analysis, requires accurate, robust and fast 3D-2D image registration methods.

Due to dimensional inconsistence, the 3D-2D image registration is an ill-posed problem, which is often regularized by simultaneously considering at least two 2D images from different projection views [4]. Some IGS systems achieve this by using a biplane X-ray imaging system; however, the biplane X-ray is used only in complex treatment procedures, in which twice higher radiation dose delivered to the patient is an acceptable trade-off. Since radiation dose presents a hazardous risk for patient health, it is desirable to perform IGS procedures using a single 2D view. Performing 3D-2D image registration using a single 2D view, however, presents a challenging task for most of current state-of-the-art methods.

According to a recent survey [4], 3D-2D registration methods are categorized as calibration-based and intrinsic (intensity-, feature- and gradient-based or hybrid) or extrinsic image-based methods. While the calibration-based methods [9] cannot compensate for patient movement, the extrinsic image-based methods [12] are impractical as they require that known artificial objects be introduced into the imaged scene; therefore, only the intrinsic image-based methods are considered for IGRT and IGS. Furthermore, the feature-based methods can be applied only if a reliable and straightforward segmentation can be used to determine the edges and surfaces of structures of interest. Intensity-based methods[1] recast the 3D-2D to 2D-2D registration by aligning the 2D modality to simulated 2D images, called digitally reconstructed radiographs (DRRs). DRRs are obtained by casting virtual rays through a pre-operative 3D image. For DRR to 2D modality registration a robust similarity measures (SMs) such as mutual information (MI), gradient difference and pattern intensity can be used [1]. Gradient-based methods are promising since they encode structural information, and are very efficiently projected from 3D to 2D [3,5] or backprojected from 2D to 3D [11], making them far less computationally demanding than DRR-generation needed in the intensity based methods. The main drawback, however, is that gradient-based method are more sensitive image noise and small 3D image transformations; thus, they usually have a higher chance of registration failure. To overcome this, Mitrović et al. [5] proposed a neighborhood-based gradient-matching process, but which was dedicated for registration of tubular structures like vessels. Even though several state-of-the-art 3D-2D registration methods exist, few or even none have been proved accurate, robust and fast enough for 3D to single 2D view image registration [4].

In this paper, we propose a novel 3D-2D registration method based on measuring similarity between gradient covariances in 3D and 2D images. Gradient covariances capture the distribution of gradients in the 3D or 2D neighborhoods and thus, compared to intensity gradients alone, seem more robust as registration features. 3D and 2D gradient covariances are mapped into the same space using backprojection [11] (Fig. 1) and their similarity, measured by normalized scalar product of covariances, is maximized to obtain register 3D and 2D images. Performance of the proposed and state-of-the-art 3D-2D image registration methods was evaluated on two publicly available image datasets, first of cerebral angiograms [5] and the second of a spine cadaver [10], using standardized evaluation methodology [2]. Results demonstrate that the proposed method outperformed the current state-of-the-art methods and achieved registration accuracy of 0.5 mm, capture range of 9 mm, success rate >80% and execution times from 0.5–2.0 seconds.

2   Image Registration Methodology

3D-2D registration is concerned with positioning the coordinate system of a pre-operative 3D image (S_v) in a world coordinate system S_w so as to align corresponding anatomical structures on 2D and projected 3D image. The pose of the 2D image S_p (in the detector plane $\mathcal{P}$) is known a priori based on a calibration of the imaging system, e.g. C-arm. The degree-of-freedom of spatial transformation $\mathbf{T}$, which is applied to the 3D image, should be selected based on the physical properties and the expected nature of motion of the imaged anatomy. Since we will test our method on images of cerebral angiograms and lumbar vertebrae, we consider here a rigid-body transformation. To best align the 3D to 2D image, one needs to find an optimal transformation $\mathbf{T} = \mathbf{T}(p)$ defined by six rigid-body parameters $p = [t_x\, t_y\, t_z\, \alpha_x\, \alpha_y\, \alpha_z]^{\mathrm{T}}$. Fig. 1 shows the geometrical setup of the 3D to 2D registration problem and the idea behind the gradient covariance based 3D-2D registration method, which is proposed in the next subsections. First, the methodology of gradient backprojection proposed by Tomaževič [11] is briefly explained, followed by derivation of covariance backprojection and the covariance based measure of 3D and 2D image similarity.

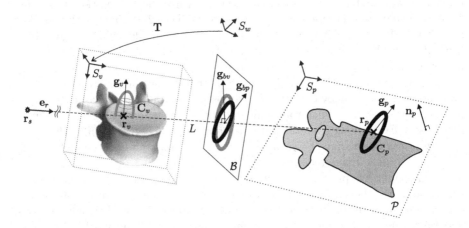

Fig. 1. Geometrical setup of 3D to 2D image registration and illustration of the proposed backprojection of gradient covariance (cf. text below for details)

2.1   Gradient Backprojection

Let the X-ray source $\mathbf{r}_s$ be at the origin of a coordinate system S and let the detector plane $\mathcal{P}$ perpendicular to z axis of S (Fig. 1). 2D intensity image P can be written in spherical coordinates (ρ, Θ, φ) as $P(\mathbf{r}_p) = P(\Theta, \varphi)$. The relationship between the 3D image intensity $V(\mathbf{r})$ and attenuation coefficient $\mu(\rho)$ can be expressed by a linear attenuation model $V(\mathbf{r}) = \int_L \mu(\rho)d\rho$. Then, the 3D intensity gradient corresponds to the gradient of attenuation coefficient $\mu(\mathbf{r})$ in point $\mathbf{r}$, which for spherical coordinates $\mathbf{r} = (\rho, \Theta, \varphi)$ is expressed as

$$\nabla V(\mathbf{r}) = \nabla_\rho \mu(\rho, \Theta, \varphi) + \nabla_t \mu(\rho, \Theta, \varphi). \tag{1}$$

where $\nabla_\rho \mu(\mathbf{r})$ and $\nabla_t \mu(\mathbf{r})$ are radial and tangential, respectively, to the projection beam L. The second term corresponds to 2D intensity gradient

$$\nabla P(\mathbf{r}_p) = \frac{1}{\rho} \int_{\rho_1}^{\rho_2} \tilde{\rho} \nabla_t \mu(\tilde{\rho}, \Theta, \varphi) \, d\tilde{\rho}. \tag{2}$$

The intensity gradient $\mathbf{g}_{bv}$ in plane $\mathcal{B}$ is tangential to vector $\mathbf{e}_r$ on L and equals $\nabla_t V(\mathbf{r}_v)$. Let $\hat{\mathbf{g}}_{bp} \sim \nabla V_t(\mathbf{r}_v)$, then the intensity gradient in the detector plane $\mathcal{P}$ is obtained by orthogonal projection

$$\mathbf{g}_p = (\mathbf{n} \times \hat{\mathbf{g}}_{bp}) \times \mathbf{n}_p). \tag{3}$$

The inverse mapping from $\mathcal{P}$ to $\mathcal{B}$ is an oblique (back)projection expressed as [11]

$$\hat{\mathbf{g}}_{bp} = \frac{(\mathbf{n}_p \times \mathbf{g}_p) \times \mathbf{e}_r}{\mathbf{n}_p \circ \mathbf{e}_r}. \tag{4}$$

According to (1) the 2D intensity gradient $\mathbf{g}_{bp}$ is composed of radial (ρ) and tangential components (t) of the 3D intensity gradient, however, using (2) only the tangential component is projected to 2D plane $\mathcal{P}$ as

$$\mathbf{g}_p = \frac{1}{\|\mathbf{r}_p - \mathbf{r}_s\|} \int_L \|\mathbf{r}_v - \mathbf{r}_s\| \nabla V(\mathbf{r}_v) \, d\rho. \tag{5}$$

Hence, the backprojected gradient must be scaled according to its distance from the X-ray source $\mathbf{r}_s$, i.e.

$$\mathbf{g}_{bp} = \frac{\|\mathbf{r}_p - \mathbf{r}_s\|}{\|\mathbf{r}_v - \mathbf{r}_s\|} \cdot \frac{(\mathbf{n}_p \times \mathbf{g}_p) \times \mathbf{e}_r}{\mathbf{n}_p \circ \mathbf{e}_r}. \tag{6}$$

2.2   Gradient Covariance Backprojection

Gradient covariances encode the shape of intensity gradient distribution in some neighborhood and can be efficiently mapped between 3D and 2D spaces using the gradient backprojection methodology and projection operators. Operator $\Gamma_\mathcal{B} = \mathbf{I}_3 - \mathbf{e}_r \mathbf{e}_r^{\mathrm{T}}$ is an orthogonal projection from $\mathbf{r}$ to plane $\mathcal{B}$ such that

$$\mathbf{g}_{bv}(\mathbf{r}) = \Gamma_\mathcal{B}(\mathbf{r}) \mathbf{g}_v. \tag{7}$$

Similarly, backprojection of the 2D intensity gradient is obtained by (6) and is written in matrix form as

$$\mathbf{g}_{bp}(\mathbf{r}) = c(\mathbf{r})\,\Gamma_{\mathcal{B}^{-1}}(\mathbf{r})\,\mathbf{g}_p\,, \tag{8}$$

where $c(\mathbf{r}) = \|\mathbf{r}_p - \mathbf{r}_s\|/\|\mathbf{r} - \mathbf{r}_s\|$ and $\Gamma_{\mathcal{B}^{-1}} = -(\mathbf{e}_r \circ \mathbf{n}_p)^{-1}[\mathbf{e}_r]_\times[\mathbf{n}_p]_\times$. Symbol $[\mathbf{a}]_\times$ denotes a skew-symmetric matrix of a 3-element vector $\mathbf{a}$

$$[\mathbf{a}]_\times = \begin{bmatrix} 0 & -a_3 & a_2 \\ a_3 & 0 & -a_1 \\ -a_2 & a_1 & 0 \end{bmatrix}. \tag{9}$$

Based on (7) and (8) the covariance matrix originating from neighborhood Ω_v in 3D is computed as

$$\mathbf{C}_v(\mathbf{r}) = \int_{\Omega_v} \mathbf{g}_{bv}(\mathbf{r})\,\mathbf{g}_{bv}(\mathbf{r})^{\mathrm{T}} \approx \Gamma_{\mathcal{B}}\left[\int_{\Omega_v} \mathbf{g}_v\,\mathbf{g}_v^{\mathrm{T}}\right]\Gamma_{\mathcal{B}}^{\mathrm{T}}\,, \tag{10}$$

while covariance matrix originating from neighborhood Ω_p in 2D as

$$\mathbf{C}_p(\mathbf{r}) = \int_{\Omega_p} \mathbf{g}_{bp}(\mathbf{r})\,\mathbf{g}_{bp}(\mathbf{r})^{\mathrm{T}} \approx c^2\,\Gamma_{\mathcal{B}^{-1}}\left[\int_{\Omega_p} \mathbf{g}_p\,\mathbf{g}_p^{\mathrm{T}}\right]\Gamma_{\mathcal{B}^{-1}}^{\mathrm{T}}\,. \tag{11}$$

Expressions in square brackets of Eqs. (10) and (11) are the respective 3D and 2D gradient covariances, computed in neighborhoods $\Omega_v = \Omega_v(\mathbf{r}_v, h)$ and $\Omega_p = \Omega_p(\mathbf{r}_p, c \cdot h)$ around corresponding 3D and 2D points $\mathbf{r}_v$ and $\mathbf{r}_p$. Parameter h represents window size of the neighborhood. In (10) and (11) we assume that the projection operators $\Gamma_{\mathcal{B}}$ and $\Gamma_{\mathcal{B}^{-1}}$ and factor c are invariant to $\mathbf{r}$ within neighborhoods Ω_v and Ω_p, respectively, given that h is sufficiently small. Corresponding covariance matrices $\mathbf{C}_v(\mathbf{r})$ and $\mathbf{C}_p(\mathbf{r})$ are used to define similarity measure between 3D and 2D images.

2.3   Similarity Measure

Covariance matrices in (10) and (11) are positive semi-definite symmetric matrices, the similarity or dissimilarity of which can be measured by various similarity measures [6]. Here, we will use tensor scalar product (TSP) given as

$$s_{TSP}(\mathbf{C}_v, \mathbf{C}_p) = \mathbf{C}_v : \mathbf{C}_p = \mathrm{Trace}(\mathbf{C}_v\mathbf{C}_p) = \sum_{i=1}^{n}\sum_{j=1}^{n} \lambda_{v,i}\lambda_{p,j}(\mathbf{e}_{v,i} \circ \mathbf{e}_{p,j})^2\,, \tag{12}$$

where n is the dimensionality of tensors, $\lambda_{\star,k}$ is the k-th eigenvalue of $\mathbf{C}_\star$ and $\mathbf{e}_{\star,k}$ is the corresponding eigenvector. Note that (12) is analog to the sine weighting function of the SM used to compare 3D to backprojected 2D gradients in [11]. Since TSP is sensitive to relative size of covariance matrix elements, we use normalized TSP (NTSP)

$$s_{NTSP}(\mathbf{C}_v, \mathbf{C}_p) = \frac{\mathbf{C}_v : \mathbf{C}_p}{\|\lambda(\mathbf{C}_v)\|\,\|\lambda(\mathbf{C}_p)\|} = \frac{s_{TSP}(\mathbf{C}_v, \mathbf{C}_p)}{\mathrm{Trace}(\mathbf{C}_v)\mathrm{Trace}(\mathbf{C}_p)}\,. \tag{13}$$

The final similarity measure is computed for points $\mathbf{r}_v$ with K strongest intensity gradients $\|\mathbf{g}_{bf}(\mathbf{r}_v)\|$ as

$$\text{SM} = \sum_{i=1}^{K} s_{NTSP}(\mathbf{C}_v, \mathbf{C}_p).$$ (14)

The parameters p of the rigid-body 3D-2D registration are obtained by maximizing the SM. The proposed backprojection gradient covariance 3D-2D registration method will be referred to as BGC in the experiments.

3 Image Registration Experiments

Performance of the proposed and state-of-the-art 3D-2D image registration methods was evaluated on two publicly available image datasets, first of cerebral angiograms[5] and the second of a spine cadaver[10]. For 3D and 2D image pairs in these two datasets, rigid registration has been established by aligning fiducial markers attached to patient or imaged anatomy, thus the reference or gold standard registrations are highly accurate and known. By using the gold standard registrations and the standardized evaluation methodology[2] we performed an objective and quantitative evaluation of 3D-2D registration methods.

3.1 Evaluation Criteria

Criteria for evaluation of 3D-2D registration methods were based on measuring the initial and final alignment of 3D targets, which were already defined on the anatomy of interest in each of the datasets[5,10], with respect to (w.r.t.) their goldstandard position. Initial positions of 3D images were defined in terms of mean target registration error (mTRE), generated in the range 0–20 mm mTRE w.r.t. the gold standard position by randomly sampling rigid body transformations. After executing 3D-2D registration, accuracy of alignment was measured by mean reprojection distance (mRPD) as it is less sensitive to small deviations of the out-of-plane translation[2], which is ill-defined for registration of 3D to single 2D image. mRPD is the mean of minimal distances between the 3D target points in the goldstandard position and lines connecting the X-ray source and the 3D target points in the registered position. Registration was considered successful if mRPD < 2 mm. Overall accuracy of the 3D-2D registration was defined as MEAN±STD of mRPD of all successful registrations. Overall success rate (SR) was defined as the percentage of successful registrations, while capture range (CR) was defined as the mTRE distance to the first 1 mm subinterval with less than 95% of successful registrations. Execution times were also measured.

3.2 Experiment Description

On the dataset of cerebral angiograms, 3D-2D registration methods were tested on ten pairs of 3D digitally subtracted angiograms (3D-DSAs) and 2D-DSA images, acquired in the lateral (LAT) projection. As in [5], the 3D and 2D images were smoothed and resampled to 0.75 mm and 0.3 mm isotropic resolution, respectively. The initial positions of for each 3D-DSA image were defined by Mitrović *et al.* [5] and ranged from 0–20 mm mTRE, with 20 position per each 1 mm subinterval of mTRE. For all ten pairs, there were a total of 4000 initial positions. The benefit of using the given initial positions is that the obtained registration results can be directly compared to the ones reported in [5]. Additionally, we tested a method based on gradient projection [3] referred to as GPR. The proposed BGC method was tested with window size h set to 2 mm. To be able to compare our results to [5], we used Powell's directional set method with Brent's line search [7] to find the rigid-body parameters with both the GPR and the proposed BGC method (PB-BGC). BGC was also tested with the more recent BOBYQA derivative-free optimization [8] (QA-BGC).

Registrations on the spine cadaver dataset[10] involved five 3D CT images of L1–5 lumbar vertebrae and 18 2D X-ray views, which were acquired in the range $0 - 170°$ around the axis of the spine cadaver. As the initial positions were not a priori defined, they were generated by randomly selecting four 2D X-ray views per each 3D CT image, which formed 20 3D-2D image pairs. For each image pair, 20 rigid body transformations were generated by randomly sampling translations and rotations from the range of 0–20 mm and 0–10°, such that the obtained transformations, relative to the goldstandard position, presented mTRE in the range of 0–20 mm with one initial position per each 1 mm subinterval of mTRE. This resulted in 400 different initial positions across all the image pairs. Prior to registration the 3D and 2D images were smoothed and resampled to 0.75 mm isotropic resolution. Four methods were tested, i.e. DRR-based registration using mutual information metric, gradient-based GPR[3] and BGB[11] methods and the proposed BGC. BGC was executed with window size h set either to 0.1 or 1 mm, and by first executing with $h = 1$ mm and improving the obtained registration by executing with $h = 0.1$ mm. Methods were executed on NVidia 450GTS GPU using BOBYQA derivative-free optimization [8].

3.3   Results

Evaluation results of 3D-2D registration on datasets of cerebral angiograms and of spine cadaver are reported in Tables 1 and 2, respectively. When registering cerebral angiograms, the proposed BGC method achieved slighly higher accuracy with QA as compared to PB optimization method, while SR, CR and execution times were similar. The proposed BGC methods improved the SR and CR compared to the state-of-the-art methods, most notably extending the CR by 3 mm over the MGP+BGB method. Even though MGP+BGB was more accurate than BGC (0.28 vs. 0.42 mm), the registration accuracy of BGC was in subpixel regime (< 0.75 mm).

On the spine cadaver datasets, BGC also achieved subpixel accuracy (0.56 mm) for small window size h. In general, by decreasing the window size h the registration accuracy of the BGC method improved. Conversely, by increasing h the SR and CR improved as more registration trials converged from the farther

Table 1. MEAN±STD of mRPD of successful registrations, success rates (SR), capture ranges (CR) and execution times for computed for registrations of ten 3D-DSA and lateral (LAT) 2D-DSA image pairs for cerebral angiograms [5]. The best result for each evaluation criteria is marked in **bold**.

Method	MEAN ± STD [mm]	SR [%]	CR [mm]	Time [s]
MIP-MI	0.30 ± 0.29	77.4	5	84.3
GPR	0.61 ± 0.23	61.2	2	45.7
BGB*	0.40 ± 0.37	52.4	3	11.6
MGP*	0.61 ± 0.37	73.2	5	**0.5**
MGP*+BGB*	**0.28 ± 0.21**	79.5	6	15.3
PB-BGC$_{h=2}$	0.51 ± 0.29	**82.2**	**9**	1.8
QA-BGC$_{h=2}$	0.42 ± 0.25	78.2	8	2.0

*Not computed on GPU.

Table 2. MEAN±STD of mRPD of successful registrations, success rates (SR), capture ranges (CR) and execution times computed for registrations of 20 3D CT and X-ray image pairs of lumbar vertebrae [10]. The best result for each evaluation criteria is marked in **bold**.

Method	MEAN ± STD [mm]	SR [%]	CR [mm]	Time [s]
DRR-MI	0.60 ± 0.25	39.3	2	9.4
GPR	0.55 ± 0.30	36.5	2	5.1
BGB	**0.31 ± 0.18**	61.3	4	**0.5**
BGC$_{h=0.1}$	0.57 ± 0.35	58.8	5	**0.5**
BGC$_{h=1}$	0.93 ± 0.37	80.5	9	**0.5**
BGC$_{h=1+0.1}$	0.56 ± 0.28	**80.8**	**9**	0.8

initial positions. This is an interesting feature of the proposed BGC method, which was exploited in multi-scale registration BGC$_{h=1+0.1}$ so as to improve, in overall, the registration accuracy, SR and CR. BGC method achieved CR of 9 mm, thus more than doubling the CR of state-of-the-art methods, while SR was higher by 20%. The execution times reported in Tables 1 and 2 show that even with GPU-enabled DRR/MIP generation the projection-based methods (DRR-MI, MIP-MI and GPR) were an order of magnitude slower than GPU-enabled hybrid MGP or gradient-based BGB and BGC methods.

Fig. 2 shows cumulative SRs w.r.t. the initial mTRE for all of the tested methods. In terms of SR, the proposed BGC methods consistently outperformed the tested methods on both datasets.

4 Discussion

In this paper, we proposed a novel 3D-2D registration method based on measuring similarity between 3D and 2D gradient covariances. The 2D covariances

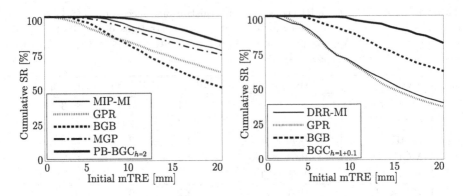

Fig. 2. Cumulative success rates (SR) w.r.t. initial mTRE for the tested methods on the cerebral angiogram (*left*) and spine cadaver (*right*) datasets

were mapped into the same space as the 3D gradient covariances by using the proposed covariance backprojection methodology. The proposed 3D-2D registration method maximized normalized scalar product between 3D and 2D covariances. Performance of the proposed and state-of-the-art 3D-2D image registration methods was evaluated on two publicly available image datasets, one of cerebral angiograms and the other of a spine cadaver, using standardized evaluation methodology. Results showed that the proposed method outperformed the current state-of-the-art methods and achieved registration accuracy of 0.5 mm, capture range of 9 mm and success rate >80%.

The key advantage of the proposed method is a much higher success rate (SR) and capture range (CR) compared to state-of-the-art methods. High SR of 3D-2D registration method is very important factor during image-guided surgery, during which each registration failure will significantly interrupt the treatment process, requiring manual intervention. The proposed method achieved SRs of more than 80% on two image datasets of different anatomies, while the SRs of state-of-the-art methods varied from 40%–80%. Secondly, high CR is important as the initial guess of the position of 3D image prior to registration need not be very precise. I.e. given a rough initial position that is within the CR of the method, the 3D-2D registration method will, with high confidence, be able to accurately align the 3D with the 2D image. The proposed method had CR that was up to twice as high as the CR of state-of-the-art methods, both on the datasets of cerebral angiograms and the datasets of spine cadaver. Considering also that GPU-enabled execution times were from 0.5–2.0 seconds, the proposed method has a high potential for implementation as part of an image-guided system in surgery or radiotherapy, enabling one to enhance with 3D information the visualization and analysis of intra-operative 2D images.

Acknowledgments. This research was supported by the Ministry of Education, Science and Sport, Slovenia, under grants J2-5473, L2-5472, and L2-4072.

References

1. Hipwell, J., Penney, G., McLaughlin, R., Rhode, K., Summers, P., Cox, T., Byrne, J., Noble, J., Hawkes, D.: Intensity-based 2-D-3-D registration of cerebral angiograms. IEEE Transactions on Medical Imaging 22(11), 1417–1426 (2003)
2. van de Kraats, E., Penney, G., Tomaževič, D., van Walsum, T., Niessen, W.: Standardized evaluation methodology for 2-D-3-D registration. IEEE Transactions on Medical Imaging 24(9), 1177–1189 (2005)
3. Livyatan, H., Yaniv, Z., Joskowicz, L.: Gradient-based 2-D/3-D rigid registration of fluoroscopic X-ray to CT. IEEE Transactions on Medical Imaging 22(11), 1395–1406 (2003), PMID: 14606673
4. Markelj, P., Tomaževič, D., Likar, B., Pernuš, F.: A review of 3D/2D registration methods for image-guided interventions. Medical Image Analysis 16(3), 642–661 (2012)
5. Mitrović, U., Špiclin, Z., Likar, B., Pernuš, F.: 3D-2D registration of cerebral angiograms: a method and evaluation on clinical images. IEEE Transactions on Medical Imaging 32(8), 1550–1563 (2013)
6. Peeters, T., Rodrigues, P.R., Vilanova, A., ter Haar Romeny, B.M.: Analysis of distance/similarity measures for diffusion tensor imaging. In: Visualization and Processing of Tensor Fields, pp. 113–136. Springer (2009)
7. Powell, M.J.D.: An efficient method for finding the minimum of a function of several variables without calculating derivatives. The Computer Journal 7(2), 155–162 (1964)
8. Powell, M.J.D.: The BOBYQA algorithm for bound constrained optimization without derivatives. Department of Applied Mathematics and Theoretical Physics, Cambridge, England, technical report NA2009/06 (2009)
9. Ruijters, D., Homan, R., Mielekamp, P., van de Haar, P., Babic, D.: Validation of 3D multimodality roadmapping in interventional neuroradiology. Physics in Medicine and Biology 56(16), 5335–5354 (2011)
10. Tomaževič, D., Likar, B., Pernuš, F.: Gold standard data for evaluation and comparison of 3D/2D registration methods. Computer Aided Surgery 9(4), 137–144 (2004)
11. Tomaževič, D., Likar, B., Slivnik, T., Pernuš, F.: 3-D/2-D registration of CT and MR to X-ray images. IEEE Transactions on Medical Imaging 22(11), 1407–1416 (2003)
12. Truong, M., Aslam, A., Ginks, M., Rinaldi, C., Rezavi, R., Penney, G., Rhode, K.: 2D-3D registration of cardiac images using catheter constraints. Computers in Cardiology, 605–608 (2009)

Combined PET-MR Brain Registration to Discriminate between Alzheimer's Disease and Healthy Controls

Liam Cattell[1,*], Julia A. Schnabel[1], Jerome Declerck[2], and Chloe Hutton[2]

[1] Institute of Biomedical Engineering, Department of Engineering Science,
University of Oxford, UK
[2] Siemens Molecular Imaging, Oxford, UK

Abstract. Previous amyloid positron emission tomography (PET) imaging studies have shown that Alzheimer's disease (AD) patients exhibit higher standardised uptake value ratios (SUVRs) than healthy controls. Automatic methods for SUVR calculation in brain images are typically based on registration of PET brain data to a template, followed by computation of the mean uptake ratio in a set of regions in the template space. Resulting SUVRs will therefore have some dependence on the registration method. It is widely accepted that registration based on anatomical information provides optimal results. However, in clinical practice, good quality anatomical data may not be available and registration is often based on PET data alone. We investigate the effect of using functional and structural image information during the registration of PET volumes to a template, by comparing six registration methods: affine registration, non-linear registration using PET-driven demons, non-linear registration using magnetic resonance (MR) driven demons, and our novel joint PET-MR registration technique with three different combination weightings. Our registration method jointly registers PET-MR brain volume pairs, by combining the incremental updates computed in single-modality local correlation coefficient demons registrations. All six registration methods resulted in significantly higher mean SUVRs for diseased subjects compared to healthy subjects. Furthermore, the combined PET-MR registration method resulted in a small, but significant, increase in the mean Dice overlaps between cortical regions in the MR brain volumes and the MR template, compared with the single-modality registration methods. These results suggest that a non-linear, combined PET-MR registration method can perform at least as well as the single-modality registration methods in terms of the separation between SUVRs and Dice overlaps, and may be well suited to discriminate between populations of AD patients and healthy controls.

1 Introduction

Alzheimer's Disease (AD) affects more than 25 million people worldwide [1], and is significantly more prevalent in the older population. Although the exact

---

* This work is funded by an Industrial CASE award grant from the EPSRC (11440394) with sponsorship from Siemens Molecular Imaging.

S. Ourselin and M. Modat (Eds.): WBIR 2014, LNCS 8545, pp. 134–143, 2014.

cause of AD is unknown, the presence of fibrillar amyloid-β (Aβ) is central to the pathogenesis of the disease.

Positron emission tomography (PET) imaging is increasingly used to assess the Aβ burden in patients with dementia, and the standardised uptake value ratio (SUVR) has become a common measure for PET radiotracers in brain studies [2]. Studies have shown that AD patients exhibit higher ^{18}F-florbetapir SUVRs than cognitively normal controls [3]. The SUVR is calculated by computing the mean uptake of tracer in a region of interest, divided by uptake in a normalisation region (where the uptake is non-specific). Typically, prior to SUVR calculation, the PET volume is registered to a template space in which the regions of interest are defined. Current methods for quantitative analysis of amyloid imaging use affine or non-linear registration methods to achieve alignment to the PET template [4]. Consequently, SUVRs can be somewhat dependent on the quality of the registration.

Although widely accepted that using anatomical images to drive the registration of functional images improves their diagnostic value, it has not been clearly investigated and reported in the literature. Using joint PET and magnetic resonance (MR) image information would exploit all the available data, and could potentially capture changes present in both modalities. In turn, this could lead to more precise SUVRs. Furthermore, in a clinical setting, optimal quality MR and/or PET images may not be available. In this situation, a registration approach which is capable of using a weighted combination of the two modalities could be useful.

The purpose of this work is to investigate the effect of using joint modality image information during registration of PET volumes to a template. To achieve this we propose a novel approach to combined non-linear PET-MR brain registration. We extend the diffeomorphic demons registration framework [5], by combining the individual update steps in simultaneous single-modality demons registrations. Unlike existing multi-channel demons methods [6,7], which only use anatomical images, we combine functional and anatomical information at each iteration. Furthermore, to account for any non-uniform bias distribution in the images, we employ a local correlation coefficient (LCC) image similarity metric [8,9], rather than the standard sum of squared differences (SSD).

We compared SUVRs following affine registration and five PET-MR LCC-demons registrations, each with a different weighted combination of PET and MR updates. For this study, 38 subjects (19 AD, 19 healthy controls) were pre-selected from the Alzheimer's Disease Neuroimaging Initiative (ADNI) database[1]. The templates were constructed using the images from ten randomly selected subjects (5 AD, 5 healthy controls). Registrations were then conducted on the remaining 28 subjects. Cortex-to-cerebellum SUVRs were calculated in six cortical regions, as described in [3].

The remainder of this paper is structured as follows: In Section 2, we outline our registration algorithm. Section 3 introduces the PET-MR dataset, and the steps involved in creating the MR and PET templates. Section 4 describes

---

[1] http://adni.loni.ucla.edu/

the experiments and results. Finally, Section 5 discusses the advantages and limitations of our combined non-linear PET-MR registration compared with alternative methods, and concludes this work.

2   Methods

2.1   Diffeomorphic Demons

The diffeomorphic demons registration algorithm, introduced by Vercauteren et al. [5], estimates the diffeomorphic transformation s between a fixed image F and a moving image M. Finding the displacement field s involves the optimisation of an energy function:

$$E(s) = \frac{1}{\sigma_i^2}\text{Sim}(F, M \circ s) + \frac{1}{\sigma_x^2}\text{Dist}(s, c) + \frac{1}{\sigma_T^2}\text{Reg}(s) \qquad (1)$$

where $\text{Sim}(F, M \circ s)$ is an image similarity measure and $\text{Reg}(s)$ is a regularisation term. To allow for some errors in s, Cachier et al. [8] introduced the $\text{Dist}(s, c)$ term. This forces the displacement field s to be close to the exact correspondences c.

To ensure that the registration is invertible, an update step is found on the Lie group through the exponential mapping from a velocity vector field $\mathbf{u}$ to diffeomorphisms. Thus, the diffeomorphic demons algorithm can be described by:

Algorithm 1. Diffeomorphic Demons

- Given the current deformation field s, compute an update field $\mathbf{u}$
- $c \leftarrow s \circ \exp(\mathbf{u})$
- Regularise c by convolving with a Gaussian filter, such that $s \leftarrow G * c$

2.2   Local Correlation Coefficient

In the classical form, the choice of single-modality similarity measure is the sum of squared differences (SSD) between the image intensities at each voxel. Despite its simple implementation, SSD is a global criterion and assumes a linear relationship between the image intensities. This makes it extremely sensitive to the locally varying intensity biases often found in medical images.

By assuming that the bias distribution is locally uniform, Cachier et al. [8] proposed a local implementation of the correlation coefficient (LCC). The LCC similarity ρ implicitly estimates the locally affine relationship between the image intensities, thus accounting for additive and multiplicative bias:

$$\rho(F, M) = \int_\sigma \frac{\overline{FM}}{\sqrt{\overline{F^2} \cdot \overline{M^2}}} \qquad (2)$$

where $\overline{F} = \mathbf{G}_\sigma * F(x)$ is the local mean image defined by convolution with a Gaussian $\mathbf{G}_\sigma$ of kernel size σ.

Unlike SSD, the LCC criterion has a parameter which needs to be chosen based on the application (i.e. the kernel size σ of the Gaussian filter). However, LCC optimisation fits neatly into the demons registration framework, in contrast to mutual information [10], which requires the estimation of the global joint intensity histogram of the images. If $\mathrm{Sim}(F, M \circ s)$ is replaced by $\rho^2(F, M \circ s)$ in (1), the correspondence energy can be written as:

$$E(F, M) = \frac{1}{\sigma_i^2}\rho^2(F, M) + \frac{1}{\sigma_x^2}\|\mathbf{u}\|^2 \tag{3}$$

The resulting update velocity field is computed using:

$$\mathbf{u} = -\frac{2\Lambda}{\|\Lambda\|^2 - \frac{4}{\rho^2}\frac{\sigma_i^2}{\sigma_x^2}} \tag{4}$$

where

$$\Lambda = \left(\frac{\mathbf{G}_\sigma * (F\nabla M^T - M\nabla F^T)}{\mathbf{G}_\sigma * (FM)} + \frac{\mathbf{G}_\sigma * (F\nabla F^T)}{\mathbf{G}_\sigma * (F^2)} - \frac{\mathbf{G}_\sigma * (M\nabla M^T)}{\mathbf{G}_\sigma * (M^2)} \right) \tag{5}$$

The derivation of the optimisation of (3) with respect to a symmetric update is presented in [9], and we refer the reader to that work for more details.

2.3 Extending Diffeomorphic LCC-Demons by Combining Multiple Update Fields

In our proposed combined PET-MR registration algorithm, we first assume that the pairs of PET and MR volumes for each subject are rigidly registered. The non-linear registration of the PET-MR image pairs is then performed using PET to PET and MR to MR registration (as described in Sections 2.1 and 2.2), but combining the individual update fields at each iteration as follows:

$$\mathbf{u} = \alpha\mathbf{u}_{\mathrm{MR}} + (1 - \alpha)\mathbf{u}_{\mathrm{PET}}, \quad 0 \le \alpha \le 1 \tag{6}$$

where the relative contribution of each modality can be controlled by varying the weighting α. Hence, the diffeomorphic demons algorithm is modified as described in Algorithm 2:

Algorithm 2. Combined PET-MR Diffeomorphic LCC-Demons Registration

- Use (4) to compute an update field $\mathbf{u}_{\mathrm{MR}}$ for the two MR images, and an update field $\mathbf{u}_{\mathrm{PET}}$ for the two PET images.
- Use (6) to compute the combined update velocity field $\mathbf{u}$
- $c \leftarrow s \circ \exp(\mathbf{u})$
- Regularise c by convolving with a Gaussian filter, such that $s \leftarrow G * c$
- Apply s to the moving MR image and the moving PET image

3   Materials

3.1   ADNI Data and Initialisation

In this study, 38 subjects (19 AD, 19 cognitively normal controls) were selected from the Alzheimer's Disease Neuroimaging Initiative (ADNI) online database. Each subject had a pair of ^{18}F-florbetapir Aβ PET and T1-weighted MR volumes, acquired no more than 12 months apart.

Prior to the non-linear registrations, the PET volumes were rigidly registered to their corresponding MR volumes using FLIRT [11,12]. The brains were then extracted from the whole-head MR and PET images, by constructing a mask from the tissue segmentations of the MR images (obtained using SPM8 [13]). Finally, again using FLIRT, the MR brain volumes were affinely registered to a template in MNI space. The non-linear MNI152 brain template used by FSL[2] was chosen as the template. The resulting transformations were also applied to the PET brain volumes. During this process, all images were resampled to a resolution of $1 \times 1 \times 1$ mm/voxel.

3.2   Template Construction

In an attempt to reduce the bias associated with selecting an exemplar subject as the template, an MR template was created iteratively from 10 of the 38 subjects (5 AD, 5 healthy) using the method proposed by Guimond et al. in [14]. In brief, the method involves non-linearly registering the subjects to an initial reference image. The new reference image is constructed by averaging the intensities of the registered images, and deforming this image by the mean inverse transformation from all the subjects to the reference. This entire process is repeated until the estimated template no longer changes between iterations.

A PET template could be constructed in a similar fashion, however, to ensure an unbiased starting point for the combined PET-MR registration, the MR and PET templates need to be perfectly registered. Therefore, a pseudo-PET template was synthesised from the MR template. This was achieved by combining its tissue segmentations with different weighting factors to resemble an amyloid PET image.

Figure 1 shows an axial slice from the MR and synthetic PET templates.

4   Experiments and Results

4.1   Affine Registration

The MR volumes of the 28 subjects excluded from the template creation were affinely registered to the MR template using FLIRT [11,12]. The resulting transformations were then applied to the corresponding PET volumes.

---

[2] http://fsl.fmrib.ox.ac.uk/

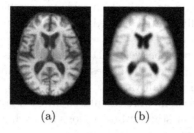

(a)   (b)

Fig. 1. Example axial slice of (a) the iterative MR template, and (b) the synthetic PET template

4.2   Non-linear Registration

Starting with the affinely registered images, five separate PET-MR LCC-demons registrations were conducted for each of the 28 subjects: $\alpha = 0$ (i.e. PET to PET registration), $\alpha = 1$ (i.e. MR to MR registration), and $\alpha = \{0.25, 0.5, 0.75\}$ for the proposed combined PET-MR registration (with increasing influence of the MR volumes).

The registration parameters for the LCC-demons were taken from [9]: $\sigma_{LCC} = 2$ and $\sigma_i/\sigma_x = 0.05$, with a multi-resolution, multi-scale scheme of $30 \times 99 \times 10$ iterations (coarse to fine).

4.3   Dice Overlap

To evaluate the performance of the different registration methods, the Dice overlap was calculated for each subject's MR after registration, with respect to the MR template [15].

The subject cortical region atlases were created automatically using an independent and established registration method. To achieve this, SPM8 was used to perform non-linear registration of each whole-head MR volume (in native subject space) to MNI space [13]. The resulting inverse deformation fields were used to resample the Automatic Anatomic Labelling (AAL) atlas regions [16] to native subject space. Following this procedure, any transformations applied to the MR brain volumes (e.g. those described in Sections 3.1, 4.1 and 4.2) were also applied to the corresponding atlas.

The MR template atlas was constructed by taking the deformed atlases of the subjects comprising the template, and combining them using a majority vote rule at each voxel [17].

Paired t-tests on the mean Dice overlap were conducted between each registration method and every other.

4.4   Standardised Uptake Value Ratio

Following registration, SUVRs were calculated from the mean ^{18}F-florbetapir uptake in six cortical regions of interest (medial orbital frontal, parietal, temporal, precuneus, posterior cingulate and anterior cingulate), with reference to the cerebellum. The target and normalisation regions were based on the AAL atlas regions [16], and manually dilated/eroded so they were visually similar to those presented in [3,4].

In order to best distinguish between AD patients and healthy individuals using SUVRs, the registration method should result in a large difference in mean SUVR between the groups, and a small variance for each group. Therefore, the SUVR means and standard deviations were calculated for each group, and a two-sample t-test, allowing for different standard deviations for each group, was used to test whether the population means were different.

4.5   Results

Figure 2 shows an example registered PET image from both groups, for all six registration methods. To aid visual assessment of the registrations, the bottom row of Fig. 2 shows a close up of the ventricles, with the outline of the PET template ventricle superimposed in red.

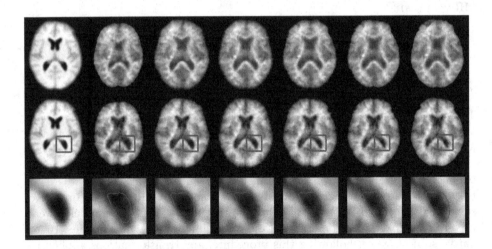

Fig. 2. Example PET registration results for a subject with Alzheimer's disease (top), and a healthy control (middle). The bottom row shows a close-up of the region highlighted in the middle row, with the outline of the PET template ventricle superimposed in red. The left-most column shows the pseudo-PET template. The remaining columns (left to right) represent each registration method: affine, PET to PET ($\alpha = 0$), proposed combined PET-MR ($\alpha = \{0.25, 0.5, 0.75\}$), and MR to MR ($\alpha = 1$). All non-linear registration methods show improved registration over the affine method.

Table 1 presents the mean (standard deviation) Dice overlap (by registration method) of labels in the registered MR volumes and the MR template. The paired t-tests between all of the registration methods show that the non-linear methods demonstrate significantly higher overlap than the affine registration method ($p < 0.05$, corrected for 15 comparisons). Moreover, the combined PET-MR registration methods ($\alpha = \{0.25, 0.5, 0.75\}$) have significantly higher mean Dice values than the non-linear, single-modality methods ($\alpha = \{0, 1\}$).

The mean SUVR of each group (AD or cognitively normal controls) for each registration method, as well as the corresponding t-values, are also presented in Table 1. Across all six registration methods, the AD group has a significantly higher mean SUVR than the control group ($p < 0.01$).

Table 1. Mean (standard deviation) Dice overlap, mean (standard deviation) SUVR, and t-value by registration method: affine, PET to PET ($\alpha = 0$), proposed combined PET-MR ($\alpha = \{0.25, 0.5, 0.75\}$), and MR to MR ($\alpha = 1$). The best results are highlighted in bold.

	Affine	$\alpha = 0$	$\alpha = 0.25$	$\alpha = 0.5$	$\alpha = 0.75$	$\alpha = 1$
Dice overlap	0.65	0.69	**0.73**	**0.73**	**0.73**	0.72
	(0.04)	(0.03)	**(0.02)**	**(0.02)**	**(0.02)**	**(0.02)**
SUVR AD	1.46	1.45	1.45	1.45	1.45	1.46
	(0.28)	**(0.25)**	**(0.25)**	**(0.25)**	**(0.25)**	(0.26)
SUVR Controls	1.12	1.12	1.11	1.11	1.11	1.11
	(0.25)	(0.23)	(0.22)	**(0.21)**	**(0.21)**	**(0.21)**
t-value	3.42	3.67	3.75	3.84	**3.91**	3.88

5   Discussion and Conclusion

The results displayed in Fig. 2 show improved registration for the non-linear methods compared with the affine method. This is especially apparent in the close-up of the ventricles. The mean Dice values in Table 1 further support this visual assessment, since the non-linear registration methods demonstrate a significantly higher overlap between cortical regions in the registered MR images and the MR template than the affine registration method.

Unsurprisingly, applying the deformation field from the PET to PET ($\alpha = 0$) registration to the MR volume offered only a small, though statistically significant, improvement in mean Dice overlap compared to the affine method. This is likely due to the lack of distinct edges in the PET brain volumes, resulting in a smoother deformation field than MR to MR registration. The results also show that the combined PET-MR registration methods ($\alpha = \{0.25, 0.5, 0.75\}$) had significantly higher mean Dice values (same standard deviations) than the MR to MR ($\alpha = 1$) method. This may be due to the functional information acting as a spatially varying regulariser on the LCC-demons updates.

In this work, the cortical region atlases used to compute Dice overlaps were created using an independent registration method (SPM8). Although systematic differences may exist between the SPM8 and LCC-demons registration methods, these should have minimal effect on the Dice overlaps, which are compared between LCC-demons methods only.

Due to the large variation in elderly brains, and differences in the progression of AD, a range of SUVRs is expected in both groups. Nevertheless, the mean SUVRs (and standard deviations) in this study fall within the range reported in [3]. Furthermore, the five non-linear registration methods exhibited smaller standard deviations than the affine registration method, suggesting more precise SUVRs. In addition, Table 1 suggests that the combined PET-MR LCC-demons registration method using $\alpha = 0.75$, which exhibits the largest t-value in our experiments, is well suited to discriminate between two populations of cognitively healthy individuals and AD patients.

In this paper we have proposed a combined PET-MR registration method, using a novel weighting between single-modality updates within the LCC-demons framework. Our method exploits all of the available data, and our results suggest that this method can perform at least as well as the single-modality registration methods with regards to the Dice overlaps and separation between SUVRs. In the future, we will further assess the choice of the weighting parameter α, including a spatially varying weighting of the update combination, on a larger validation data set. We will also investigate the effectiveness of this method on images of sub-optimal quality.

References

1. Wimo, A., Winblad, B., Aguero-Torres, H., Von Strauss, E.: The magnitude of dementia occurrence in the world. Alzheimer Disease and Associated Disorders 17(2), 63–67 (2003)
2. Raniga, P., Bourgeat, P., Fripp, J., Acosta, A., Villemagne, V., Rowe, C., Masters, C., Jones, G., O'Keefe, G., Salvado, O., Ourselin, S.: Automated ^{11}C-PiB standardised uptake value ratio. Academic Radiology 15(11), 1376–1389 (2008)
3. Fleisher, A., Chen, K., Liu, X., Roontiva, A., Thiyyagura, P., Ayutyanont, N., Joshi, A., Clark, C., Mintun, M., Pontecorvo, M., Doraiswamy, P., Johnson, K., Skovronsky, D., Reiman, E.: Using positron emission tomography and florbetapir f 18 to image cortical amyloid in patients with mild cognitive impairment or dementia due to Alzheimer disease. Archives of Neurology 68(11), 1404–1411 (2011)
4. Hutton, C., Declerck, J., Mintun, M., Pontecorvo, M., Joshi, A.: Quantification of florbetapir f18 pet: Comparison of two methods. In: Annual Congress of the European Association of Nuclear Medicine (2013)
5. Vercauteren, T., Pennec, X., Perchant, A., Ayache, N.: Diffeomorphic demons: Efficient non-parametric image registration. NeuroImage 45(1), S61–S72 (2009)
6. Peyrat, J., Delingette, H., Sermesant, M., Xu, C., Ayache, N.: Registration of 4D cardiac CT sequences under trajectory constraints with multichannel diffeomorphic demons. IEEE Transactions on Medical Imaging 29(7), 1351–1368 (2010)
7. Forsberg, D., Rathi, Y., Bouix, S., Wassermann, D., Knutsson, H., Westin, C.-F.: Improving registration using multi-channel diffeomorphic demons combined with certainty maps. In: Liu, T., Shen, D., Ibanez, L., Tao, X. (eds.) MBIA 2011. LNCS, vol. 7012, pp. 19–26. Springer, Heidelberg (2011)
8. Cachier, P., Bardinet, E., Dormont, D., Pennec, X., Ayache, N.: Iconic feature based nonrigid registration: the PASHA algorithm. Computer Vision and Image Understanding 89, 272–298 (2003)

9. Lorenzi, M., Ayache, N., Frisoni, G., Pennec, X.: LCC-Demons: A robust and accurate symmetric diffeomorphic registration algorithm. NeuroImage 81, 470–483 (2013)
10. Studholme, C., Hill, D., Hawkes, D.: Automated 3-d registration of MR and CT images of the head. Medical Image Analyis 1, 163–175 (1996)
11. Jenkinson, M., Smith, S.: A global optimisation method for robust affine registration of brain images. Medical Image Analysis 5(2), 143–156 (2001)
12. Jenkinson, M., Bannister, P., Brady, J., Smith, S.: Improved optimisation for the robust an accurate linear registration an motion correction of brain images. NeuroImage 17(2), 825–841 (2002)
13. Ashburner, J., Friston, K.: Unified segmentation. NeuroImage 26, 839–851 (2005)
14. Guimond, A., Meunier, J., Thirion, J.P.: Average brain models: A convergence study. Computer Vision and Image Understanding 77(2), 192–210 (2000)
15. Zijdenbos, A., Dawant, B., Margolin, R., Palmer, A.: Morphometric analysis of white matter lesions in mr images: method and validation. IEEE Transactions on Medical Imaging 13(4), 716–724 (1994)
16. Tzourio-Mazoyer, N., Landeau, B., Papathanassiou, D., Crivello, F., Etard, O., Delcroix, N., Mazoyer, B., Joliot, M.: Automated anatomical labelling of activations in SPM using a macroscopic anatomical parcellation of the MNI MRI single subject brain. NeuroImage 15(1), 273–289 (2002)
17. Heckemann, R., Hajnal, J., Aljabar, P., Rueckert, D., Hammers, A.: Automatic anatomical brain MRI segmentation combining label propagation and decision fusion. NeuroImage 33, 115–126 (2006)

Deformable Registration of Multi-modal Microscopic Images Using a Pyramidal Interactive Registration-Learning Methodology

Tingying Peng[1], Mehmet Yigitsoy[1], Abouzar Eslami[1],
Christine Bayer[2], and Nassir Navab[1]

[1] Computer Aided Medical Procedures (CAMP), Technical University of Munich, Germany
[2] Department of Radiation Oncology, Technical University of Munich, Germany
tingying.peng@tum.de

Abstract. Co-registration of multi-modal microscopic images can integrate benefits of each modality, yet major challenges come from inherent difference between staining, distortions of specimens and various artefacts. In this paper, we propose a new interactive registration-learning method to register functional fluorescence (IF) and structural histology (HE) images in a pyramidal fashion. We synthesize HE image from the multi-channel IF image using a supervised machine learning technique and hence reduce the multi-modality registration problem into a mono-modality one, in which case the normalised cross correlation is used as the similarity measure. Unlike conventional applications of supervised learning, our classifier is not trained by 'ground-truth' (perfectly-registered) training dataset, as they are not available. Instead, we use a relatively noisy training dataset (affinely-registered) as an initialization and rely on the robustness of machine learning to the outliers and label updates via pyramidal deformable registration to gain better learning and predictions. In this sense, the proposed methodology has potential to be adapted in other learning problems as the manual labelling is usually imprecise and very difficult in the case of heterogeneous tissues.

Keywords: Microscopy, multimodality, deformable registration, noisy robust supervised learning.

1   Introduction

The fast development of multi-modality microscopes and other molecular and cellular techniques allows simultaneous or consecutive biological image acquisition on a single specimen, using multiple techniques [1]. For example, in the preclinical cancer research, fluorescence image (IF) is widely used in studying the tumour function using targeted biomarkers. On the other hand, the Haematoxylin and Eosin (H&E) stain (the most common histological stain) colours cell nuclei and identifies necrotic region in tumours. Accurate co-registration of these datasets can combine the structural and functional properties of tissue to allow a more complete picture of tumour microenvironment and hence the benefits of using each modality can be maximised. However,

S. Ourselin and M. Modat (Eds.): WBIR 2014, LNCS 8545, pp. 144–153, 2014.

multi-modality image registration is nontrivial in general and particular challenges arise for multimodal microscopic images in the following aspects (as shown in Figure 1): 1) dissimilar appearance due to generic difference between functional image (IF) and morphological image (HE); 2) non-rigid distortions such as holes, folding and tears during the histological sectioning and staining; 3) common artefacts such as uneven illumination, dust and air bubbles and staining variations.

So far, the most popular approach in the multi-modal image registration is to maximize the mutual information (MI) of the images based on their joint intensity histogram [2], which favours similar or correlated statistical properties of the two modalities. Although MI works relatively well for rigid alignments [3], it becomes particularly challenging when dealing with non-rigid registration, as the number of false local optima increases [4]. Other approaches extract a modality-independent structure representation from both images and use a L1 or L2 distance measure to assess their similarity [5, 6]. However, the assumption of common structure is not valid for registering functional and structure images.

Another attempt that explores registration between different modalities is to simulate one modality from another, based on modelling the physics of image acquisition [7], or using a image retrieval approach [8]. The strength of this approach is that the simulation provides visual representation of the second modality, which itself can be of clinical interest when the image of that modality is not available or severely distorted.

In this paper, we also simulate one modality from another to reduce the multi-modality registration problem into an intra-modality registration. Since it is very difficult to quantify the relationship between multiple biomarkers imaged by separate modalities using explicit mathematical equations, a learning approach is used here to explore the implicit relationship between modalities. Though a supervised learning is used during registration, our method does not require the use of perfectly registered image pairs as training datasets, as they are not always available for biological images. In fact, confirmation of 'perfectly-registered' multi-modal biological images is not generally a trivial task. Alternatively, our method uses only 'roughly-registered' image data (affine registered in our case) as the first learning base and relies on the ability of learning algorithm to reject label noise and the interaction of subsequent deformable registration and machine learning to improve the learning and registration simultaneously. Though other previous unsupervised learning-based registration that do not require 'perfectly-registered' image data have been proposed [9, 10], our work differ from them in that a supervised learning technique is used for feature selection and therefore an elaborate search of matching labels is avoided.

2   Registration Framework

The general approach of the registration between the IF and HE images introduced here is a pyramidal interactive registration-learning method (PIRLM). After creating Gaussian pyramids of the actual and the simulated HE images, the deformable transformation parameters obtained from the previous coarser pyramid level are used to align the IF and HE images at the next level (Fig. 2). The aligned images serve as training data for the robust boosting model and for the model predictions. The updated simulation of HE image is used to further guide the subsequent deformable registration. At the coarsest scale, the inputs are the initial affinely aligned IF and HE images. In contrast to previous iterative classification and registration approach proposed in [11], we updates our labels by registration whereas in [11] features were updated instead.

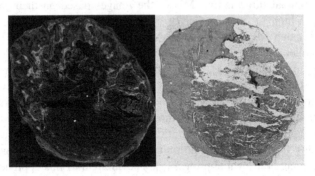

Fig. 1. Example of a fluorescence image (IF) (left) and an HE stain image (right) of the same histological specimen. The slice represents one whole tumour cross-section. The three colour channels in IF represent three fluorescence stains (red: microvessels, green: hypoxia, blue: perfusion). In this example, the deformation of the HE image was caused by rupture during removal of the cover slip between stainings.

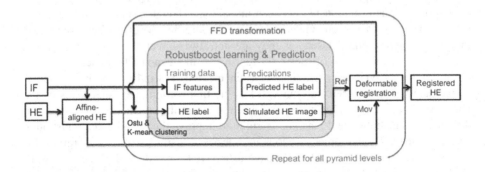

Fig. 2. Schematics of the pyramid interactive registration-learning method (PIRLM) to align the IF and HE images. The deformation model used is cubic B-splines based free-form deformation (FFD). The blue box is the framework for the machine learning and prediction procedure, which takes the results from coarser-scale registrations to label the model training data. The model prediction is then used to simulate HE based on IF features and thereby provides the reference image for the subsequent finer-scale FFD registration. The key feature of this framework is that both the learning and registration are carried out in multiple pyramidal levels. Please see the text for a detailed explanation of each step in this workflow.

2.1   IF and HE Affine Pre-alignment

As the three channels of fluorescence images are independent of each other, the average of the three channels was used to convert to the fluorescence gray-level image. HE images are true colour RGB images and thus were converted into gray-level images using a standard RGB to grey conversion by eliminating the hue and saturation information while retaining the luminance.

First, IF and HE grey-level images were aligned by affine registration using IF as a reference and HE as the moving image. As IF and HE are different modalities, the similarity measure for affine registration used is their normalized mutual information (NMI), a normalized variant of mutual information [12]. In our framework, the grey-level fluorescence image is only used in the affine pre-alignment, but not in the subsequent deformable registration.

2.2   HE Segmentation

Separating the Specimen from the Background. As shown in Figure 1, the background of our HE histological slices is white and has high luminosity intensities. The luminosity layer, L, was obtained by converting images from the RGB colour space into L*a*b color space. The Otsu's automatic threshold method [13] was then applied to the luminosity intensities to separate the specimen from the background.

Separation of Viable and Necrotic Regions. Unlike in the IF, where the fluorescence intensity is linearly related to the concentration of the fluorophore (amount of stain), the intensity I_r, I_g, I_b of each of the HE RGB channels depends on the color of the stain nonlinearly. The color deconvolution method has been proposed to convert RGB intensity in each pixel of a histological slice into the actual amount of Haematoxylin and Eosin stain [14]. The necrotic areas are stained for eosin (pink) but not for haematoxylin (blue), whereas the viable tissue is stained with both. Thus, the K-means cluster method is used to cluster the pixels in the specimen with H&E stain amount vectors into necrotic and live regions using the Euclidean distance metric. Together with the above mentioned specimen/background separation, the HE microscopic image is segmented into three regions - background, necrotic and viable tissue.

2.3   Simulation of HE from IF Based on a Robust Boosting Method

We simulated HE from IF features based on the Robustboost method proposed by Freund [15], which is designed to be particularly resistant to label noise. The normal boosting algorithm such as Adaboost aims to minimise the number of mistakes in training sets and could iteratively put large weights on mislabelled examples. In contrast, the goal of Robustboost is to minimise the number of examples whose normalised margin is smaller than a pre-set threshold. In our application, the threshold error margin is set to be 0.1. Below a brief description of the learning and prediction phases at each image scale of the pyramidal interactive registration-learning framework is given.

Training Phase: The HE segmentation label image is affinely aligned with IF using the above obtained affine transformation parameters. Let $S = \{s_1, s_2, ..., s_n\}$ denote the HE segmentation label image after alignment, where n is the number of pixels in the HE microscopic image and $s_i \in \mathcal{L} = \{$'background','necrotic','live'$\}$. Therefore, the fluorescence image $\mathbf{F} = \{f_1, f_2, ..., f_n\}$ is classified by S, where the feature vector for each pixel are the intensities of multichannel IF images, local range and entropy in a 3x3 neighbourhood (9 features in total). The three-class classification uses a multi-class extension of all boost methods proposed in [16]. The weak learner was chosen to be a decision stump because of its simple form, quick computation, as well as its superior performance in the presence of label noise compared to the deeper tree structure [15]. At resolution level i, a sample size of $100 * i^2$ pixels was used for as the training dataset.

Predicting Phase: The models obtained from the training phase were applied to all pixels of each IF for classification. To differentiate from the label nomenclature used in the training phase, the predicted region class was denoted with $P = \{p_1, p_2, ..., p_n\}$, which is the same as s_i, $p_i \in \mathcal{L} = \{$'background','necrotic','live'$\}$. The classifier was trained and tested on the same image, which overcomes the problem of staining variations across slices though the raw intensities was used as features without normalisation.

HE simulation: The spatial-averaged grey scale HE intensities in the background, necrotic and viable regions were assigned to the predicted region class P to synthesize a simulated HE image. A median filter was then applied to suppress possible spikes and to generate a smoother simulated HE image.

2.4   FFD Based Registration

To cope with local distortion caused by the HE image preparation procedure, the deformable registration of IF and HE images was posed as an energy optimization problem where energy functional, $\mathcal{E}$, is minimized for optimal alignment between the images. The energy is defined as:

$$\mathcal{E}(\mathbf{IF}, \mathbf{HE}|\mathbf{T}) = NCC(\mathbf{HE_{simu}}, \mathbf{HE}|\sigma) + \lambda\, \mathcal{R}_c(\mathbf{T}) \tag{1}$$

whereas **IF** and **HE** denotes the fluorescence and HE stained images, respectively, and **HE$_{simu}$** is the IF simulated HE image based on the supervised learning procedure described above. Instead of assessing the match between IF and HE (multimodality) directly, we use the normalized cross correlation to measure the similarity between the simulated HE and real HE images. We used two-dimensional free-form deformation (FFD) based on cubic B-splines [16] as our transformation model and regularisation term $\mathcal{R}_c(\mathbf{T})$ is the curvature regularisation function for elastic types of transformation and λ controls the amount of regularisation. The registration is completed using Medical Image Registration Toolbox provided by Andriy Myronenko (https://sites.google.com/site/myronenko/research/mirt). The original gradient descendent optimisation is replaced by an iterative quasi-newton optimization technique with Hessian update using Broyden-Fletcher-Goldfarb-Shanno (BFGS), which is available as MATLAB build-in function.

3   Results

3.1   Experiments and Image Acquisition

Tumour Line. Xenografted tumors were derived from an established human squamous cell carcinoma cell line of the head and neck: FaDu. The mouse experiments described here were approved according to national animal welfare regulations.

Fluorescence Image Acquisition. The individual whole tumor cyrosections were scanned at the same pixel size and photographed using the AxioVision 4.7 and the multi-dimensional and mosaix modules (Zeiss, Jena, Germany). In order to reflect fluorescent intensity changes of all three stains on a single image, each stain was given a particular colour: vessel stain CD31 as red, hypoxia stain Pimonidazole as green and perfusion stain Hoechst 3342 as blue.

HE Image Acquisition. After fluorescence images being taken, the cover slip needed to be removed in order to stain the same slice with HE to detect necrotic area. This procedure can sometimes cause severe tearing and folding in HE images. After HE staining, the HE whole tumour cross-sections were again scanned at the same pixel size and photographed with the same settings as the IF images. In total, 26 pairs of IF and HE images from five different tumours were processed.

Image Resolution. IF and HE images were processed as whole tumour cross-section images down-sampled to a resolution of 1000 x 1000 with each pixel size corresponding to 10μm.

3.2   Registration Results

Comparison Methods. The proposed registration framework, PIRLM, was compared to an IF-HE registration utilizing the classical multi-modality registration methods normalized mutual information (NMI). In order to incorporate multichannel information, we treat each IF channel as individual channel and replicate the HE grey-level image three times. The displacement field is taken as the average of the displacement field estimated from each channel independently [17]. Besides multi-channel mutual information based registration, we also performed an IF-HE registration without interactive HE simulation as a comparison (non-interactive learning and registration method, NILRM), in which case the learning-based simulation was only carried on one single scale (at the original resolution) using initial affine-aligned IF and HE images in the training phase. All three non-rigid registration methods are initialised using the results achieved by affine pre-alignment and are carried using the same pyramidal approach (The number of pyramidal level set to be 5).

Registration Parameter Setting. The regularisation term λ is chosen to be 0.01, which is found to be optimal for both normalised registration metrics. B-spline control point spacing is 16 pixels. The termination tolerance is set to be 1e-6 with a maximum iteration of 400 allowed. For mutual information, the bin size was set to be both 32 and 64, 32 bins achieve slightly better result, which is thus reported here.

Target Registration Error. We evaluate all the above registration methods based on the target registration error (TRE) of anatomical landmarks. Ten pairs of landmarks per image pair were manually extracted by two expert pathologists for all 26 pairs of images evaluated. The average inter-observer error of landmark extraction is around 1.5 pixels. Fig. 3 presents the registration results. Before registration, the mean landmark error was 19.2 pixels. The affine realignment reduced the mean landmark error to 6.6 pixels. Deformable registration using PILRM achieved both the minimum error mean (2.5 pixels) and median (2.1 pixels), which is significantly lower (p<0.05 with Wilcoxon signed rank test) than the registration results achieved by multichannel mutual information based registration (mean: 4.0 pixels, median: 2.5 pixels) and non-interactive registration framework (mean: 3.6 pixels, median: 2.7 pixels). An example of registration results achieved by PILRM and NMI is shown in Fig. 4.

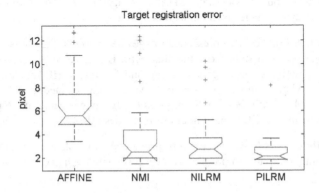

Fig. 1. Target registration error of different registration techniques. Landmark error before registration has a mean of 19.2 pixels and a median of 18.1 pixels.

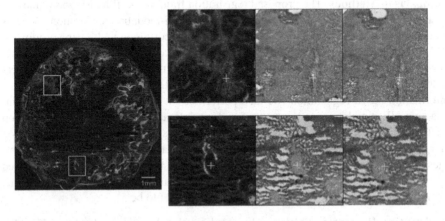

Fig. 4. An example of IF-HE registration results using PIRLM and NMI. Left: an overall IF view of the whole tumour cross-section. Right: top figure arrays showing a intersection of two vessels and bottom arrays showing a viable tissue island surrounded by necrotic regions are the enlarged view of the IF image (left), PIRLM registered HE (middle) and NMI registered HE (right), corresponding to the area within the yellow and purple rectangles, respectively. The yellow plus signs are the implemented landmarks in base image, IF.

When strong artefacts are present in the IF image (Fig. 5, top left), the learning quality of a single classifier is not sufficient, as shown in the poor predicted label image of HE (Fig. 5, bottom left). However, the interaction between learning and registration can improve the learning performance by iteratively updating the labels and retraining the classifier, as shown in the bottom right figure of Fig. 5.

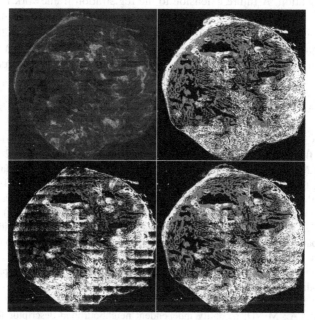

Fig. 5. An example of the difference in the learning-based prediction for the interactive learning and deformable registration (PILRM) and the non-interactive learning and registration (NILRM). Left top: IF with strong stitching artefacts; right top: HE segmentation: background (black), necrosis (grey) and viable tissue (white); left bottom: the predicted HE label based on NILRM; right bottom: the predicted HE label at highest scale based on PILRM.

4   Conclusion and Discussion

In this paper, we presented a framework for the multi-modal deformable registration of microscopy images using a supervised machine learning approach. Different from the conventional concept of supervised learning, no perfect labels (in our case 'perfect-registered' image pairs) were used in the training phase. Instead, 'roughly-registered' images were used to train the classifier and label noise that comes from the initial misalignment was rejected by the robust classifier as outliers in the learning phase. Moreover, we combine machine learning and deformable registration in a pyramidal registration framework, which uses deformable registration to update labels and hence the learning at the next pyramid level is improved. The comparison between the interactive and non-interactive approach well demonstrated the effect of using interactive learning and registration in a pyramidal setting on increasing registration accuracy.

In this presented application, a three-tissue class model is used to segment the HE image into viable, necrotic and background regions. When such a priori knowledge is not available, one can perform a principle component analysis to automatically segment the image into clusters without a predefined class number (e.g. [18]) and thus the proposed registration framework can be transferred to the new application with minor modification. A future extension to the registration framework is to simulate a full continuous grey-level image instead of a discrete label image, in which case the class probability of the Robustboost predictions would be used (as soft labels). Another potential approach is to use regression instead of classification to synthesize target modality [19], in which case the segmentation is no longer required.

References

1. Pitkeathly, W.T.E., Poulter, N.S., Claridge, E., Rappoport, J.Z.: Auto-align - multi-modality fluorescence microscopy image co-registration. Traffic 13, 204–217 (2012)
2. Wells, W.M., Viola, P., Atsumi, H., Nakajima, S., Kikinis, R.: Multi-modal volume registration by maximization of mutual information. Med. Image Anal. 1, 35–51 (1996)
3. Pluim, J.P.W., Maintz, J.B.A., Viergever, M.A.: Mutual-information-based registration of medical images: a survey. IEEE Trans. Med. Imaging 22, 986–1004 (2003)
4. Zhuang, X., Arridge, S., Hawkes, D.J., Ourselin, S.: A Non-rigid Registration Framework Using Spatially Encoded Mutual Information and Free-Form Deformations. IEEE Trans. Med. Imaging 30, 1819–1828 (2011)
5. Wachinger, C., Navab, N.: Entropy and Laplacian images: structural representations for multi-modal registration. Med. Image Anal. 16, 1–17 (2012)
6. Heinrich, M.P., Jenkinson, M., Bhushan, M., Matin, T., Gleeson, F.V., Brady, S.M., Schnabel, J.A.: MIND: modality independent neighbourhood descriptor for multi-modal deformable registration. Med. Image Anal. 16, 1423–1435 (2012)
7. Wein, W., Brunke, S., Khamene, A., Callstrom, M.R., Navab, N.: Automatic CT-ultrasound registration for diagnostic imaging and image-guided intervention. Med. Image Anal. 12, 577–585 (2008)
8. Burgos, N., et al.: Attenuation correction synthesis for hybrid PET-MR scanners. In: Mori, K., Sakuma, I., Sato, Y., Barillot, C., Navab, N. (eds.) MICCAI 2013, Part I. LNCS, vol. 8149, pp. 147–154. Springer, Heidelberg (2013)
9. Ou, Y., Sotiras, A., Paragios, N., Davatzikos, C.: DRAMMS: Deformable registration via attribute matching and mutual-saliency weighting. Med. Image Anal. 15, 622–639 (2011)
10. Tang, L.Y.W., Hamarneh, G.: Random Walks with efficient search and contextually adapted image similarity for deformable registration. In: Mori, K., Sakuma, I., Sato, Y., Barillot, C., Navab, N. (eds.) MICCAI 2013, Part II. LNCS, vol. 8150, pp. 43–50. Springer, Heidelberg (2013)
11. Warfield, S., Kaus, M., Jolesz, F.A., Kikinis, R.: Adaptive, template moderated, spatially varying statistical classification. Med. Image Anal. 4, 43–55 (2000)
12. Studholme, C., Hill, D.L.G., Hawkes, D.J.: An overlap invariant entropy measure of 3D medical image alignment. Pattern Recognit. 32, 71–86 (1999)
13. Ostu, N.: A Threshold Selection Method from Gray-Level Histograms. IEEE Trans. Syst. Man Cybern. 9, 62–66 (1979)
14. Ruifrok, A.C., Johnston, D.A.: Quantification of histochemical staining by color deconvolution. Anal. Quant. Cytol. Histol. 23, 291–299 (2001)

15. Freund, Y.: A more robust boosting algorithm. arXiv:0905.2138v1 (2009)
16. Allwein, E.L.: Reducing Multiclass to Binary: A Unifying Approach for Margin Classifiers. J. Mach. Learn. Res. 1, 113–141 (2000)
17. Avants, B.B., Duda, J.T., Zhang, H., Gee, J.C.: Multivariate normalization with symmetric diffeomorphisms for multivariate studies. In: Ayache, N., Ourselin, S., Maeder, A. (eds.) MICCAI 2007, Part I. LNCS, vol. 4791, pp. 359–366. Springer, Heidelberg (2007)
18. Song, Y., Treanor, D., Bulpitt, A., Wijayathunga, N., Roberts, N., Wilcox, R., Magee, D.: Unsupervised Content Classification Based Non-rigid Registration of Differently Stained Histology Images. IEEE Trans. Biomed. Eng. (2013)
19. Michel, F., Paragios, N.: Image transport regression using mixture of experts and discrete Markov Random Fields. In: 2010 IEEE International Symposium on Biomedical Imaging: From Nano to Macro, pp. 1229–1232. IEEE (2010)

A New Similarity Metric for Groupwise Registration of Variable Flip Angle Sequences for Improved T_{10} Estimation in DCE-MRI

Andre Hallack[1], Michael A. Chappell[1],
Mark J. Gooding[2], and Julia A. Schnabel[1]

[1] Institute of Biomedical Engineering, University of Oxford, Oxford, UK
[2] Mirada Medical, Oxford, UK

Abstract. Relaxation time (T_{10}) estimation using variable flip angle sequences is a key step for pharmacokinetic (PK) analysis of tumours in DCE-MRI exams. In this study, the effects of motion within flip angle sequences on the T_{10} and subsequent K_{trans} and k_{ep} estimation were examined. It was found that errors in T_{10} estimation caused by motion had a significant impact on subsequent PK analysis. A new similarity metric, based on the T_{10} regression error, for groupwise motion correction of variable flip angle sequences is proposed and compared against Groupwise Normalized Mutual Information (GNMI). In rigid registration experiments on simulated data, the new metric outperformed GNMI, showing an improvement alignment of over 14% in terms of average target registration error, which is also reflected by a lower T_{10} estimation error. Finally, registration was applied to 46 clinical sequences to identify the average amount of motion found in this type of acquisition; this showed an estimated displacement of 0.98mm, which could lead to over 25% K_{trans} estimation error if motion were not corrected.

1 Introduction

Pharamacokinetic (PK) analysis of tumours has a high potential to distinguish between malign and benign neoplasms and has recently shown promise to assess and predict antiangiogenic treatment response [11]. Dynamic contrast-enhanced magnetic resonance imaging (DCE-MRI) is one of the most suitable imaging techniques to acquire contrast agent (CA) uptake information within tumours. It consists of taking a dynamic MRI sequence over a short period of time upon the injection of a CA, which locally enhances the image intensities. These can then be analysed through PK models, providing quantitative information about the tissue microvascular properties. The most frequently used model, the Tofts model [10], provides physiologically relevant tissue information through permeability parameters K_{trans} and k_{ep}. Correlating intensity changes in DCE-MRI to CA concentration is one of the obstacles found in this type of analysis. Locally estimating the CA concentration requires the estimation of the relaxation time (T_{10}), a patient-specific tissue property, for the same region. Additional volumes

S. Ourselin and M. Modat (Eds.): WBIR 2014, LNCS 8545, pp. 154–163, 2014.
© Springer International Publishing Switzerland 2014

of images need to be acquired to estimate this property for each voxel of the DCE-MRI volumes. Several protocols have been developed for this task, such as inversion recovery and saturation-recovery [5]. In this work, T_{10} estimation is performed by the variable nutation angle method, which consists of acquiring a sequence of spoiled gradient echo (SPGR) volumes with several flip angles [5]. The tissue relaxation time at each voxel may then be estimated by analysing the MRI intensities at each voxel in all the different flip angle volumes. However, patient motion within these volumes may cause errors in the T_{10} estimation, which may then impact the accuracy of the PK analysis.

Even though a lot of effort has been put into analysing and correcting for motion within a DCE-MRI acquisition [2,4], little has been done to correct for motion within the variable flip angle SPGR sequence. The relation between T_{10} estimation errors on K_{trans} and k_{ep} was studied in [9], showing that inaccuracies in T_{10} resulted in even greater errors in K_{trans}. An image registration method using B-Spline free-form deformation with mutual information was applied in that work to correct for motion [9], but its effect and efficacy were not evaluated.

This paper is structured as follows. Sec. 2 presents the background for PK analysis from DCE-MRI studies and T_{10} estimation. In Sec. 3, a groupwise rigid registration framework is presented for motion correction of variable flip angle sequences, as well as the T_{10} regression error similarity metric, which is a new similarity metric that we propose for this type of MR sequences. This is followed by Sec. 4, which presents experiments that analyse the effects of motion on variable flip angle sequences in PK estimation and evaluate the motion correction framework and the new similarity metric. Finally, the conclusions and outlook of this work are discussed in Sec. 5.

2   Background

2.1   Pharmacokinetic Modelling

The two compartment Tofts model is one of the most popular models used for PK analysis[10]. It models the perfusion of the CA between the blood plasma and the extravascular extracellular space (EES). The leakage rate of the CA is described by two physiological parameters: K_{trans} and k_{ep}. In the Tofts model, the CA concentration C_e in the EES is given by:

$$C_e(t) = K_{trans} \exp(-k_{ep}t) * C_p(t) \tag{1}$$

$C_p(t)$, the arterial input function (AIF), is the CA concentration in the blood feeding the region being analysed. In this work we used a population model for the AIF, the Orton 3 model [7]. The main goal in the PK analysis is to extract relevant information from the tumour by estimating K_{trans} and k_{ep}.

2.2   Converting Concentration to Relaxation Time (T_1)

The Tofts model requires CA concentration uptake data to estimate K_{trans} and k_{ep}. The presence of CA causes a shortening of the T_1 relaxation time which

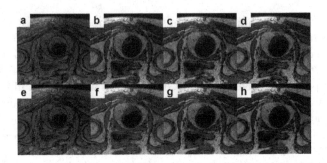

Fig. 1. MRI from SPGR sequences with variable flip angles; clinical data: (a) 3°, (b) 9°, (c) 12°, (d) 15°; simulated data: (e) 3°, (f) 9°, (g) 12°, (h) 15°. Despite all images presenting the same tissues and morphology, the MRI intensities change according to the acquired flip angle.

is reflected by an increase of the acquired MRI intensities. The relation between the CA concentration and the MRI intensity value[10] is given by:

$$T_1^{-1} = T_{10}^{-1} + r_1 C \qquad (2)$$

where r_1 is the relaxivity, a CA property, and C the tissue concentration. The estimation of T_{10}, the pre-injection relaxation time, plays a vital role in obtaining physiological information from DCE-MRI sequences. T_{10} may be computed from a sequence of variable flip angle SPGR volumes. Under the assumption of no motion, noise nor changes of the magnetic properties of the tissue, the intensity at any voxel i in these volumes will be given by [5]:

$$S(i) = M_0 \sin(\alpha) \left[1 - \exp\left(\frac{-T_R}{T_1(i)}\right)\right] \left[1 - \cos(\alpha)\exp\left(\frac{-T_R}{T_1(i)}\right)\right]^{-1} \qquad (3)$$

where T_R and α are respectively the sequence pulse repetition time and the flip angle. $M_0 = g\phi\exp\left(\frac{-T_E}{T_2^*(i)}\right)$, g is the MRI scanner gain, T_E the sequence echo time (both acquisition parameters) and ϕ the tissue proton density. By rearranging Eq. 3 into a linear function, T_{10} can be computed:

$$Y = AX + B$$

$$Y = \frac{S}{\sin(\alpha)}, X = \frac{S}{\tan(\alpha)}, A = \exp\left(\frac{-T_R}{T_{10}}\right), B = M_0\left(1 - \exp\left(\frac{-T_R}{T_{10}}\right)\right) \qquad (4)$$

At each voxel, A and B can be computed by a linear regression over the observed values on the variable flip angle volumes. However, this assumes that T_{10} remains fixed at each voxel over all the variable flip angle sequence, which is only true if there is no motion between the MRI acquisitions.

2.3 Pharmacokinetic Model Parameters Estimation

K_{trans} and k_{ep} can be estimated by finding the pair of parameters which generate concentration curves which best fit the observed DCE-MRI data. For a pair of candidate parameters $\hat{K}_{\text{trans}}$ and $\hat{k}_{\hat{e}p}$, a modeled CA concentration curve $(\hat{C}(\hat{K}_{\text{trans}}, \hat{k}_{\hat{e}p}, t))$ can be generated (Eq. 1). This can be converted into an estimated signal enhancement curve $\hat{S}_E(\hat{K}_{\text{trans}}, \hat{k}_{ep}, t)$:

$$\hat{S}_E(t) = \exp(-r_2 C(t) T_E) \left[\frac{1 - \exp\left(\frac{-T_R}{T_1(t)}\right)}{1 - \cos(\alpha) \exp\left(\frac{-T_R}{T_1(t)}\right)} \right] \left[\frac{1 - \cos(\alpha) \exp\left(\frac{-T_R}{T_{10}}\right)}{1 - \exp\left(\frac{-T_R}{T_{10}}\right)} \right]$$

$$(5)$$

Likewise, for each voxel i in the DCE-MRI sequence, a signal enhancement curve $(S_E(t(n)) = S(i, t(n))/S(i, t(0)))$ may be extracted as the signal intensity uptake after the injection of contrast. By minimizing the mean square error at each voxel i between the estimated and the acquired signal enhancement curves $(\hat{S}_E$ and $S_E)$, the PK parameters can be estimated. Computing T_{10} is essential for the computation of the estimated signal enhancement curve $\hat{S}_E$ and later in Sec. 4.3 we will analyse the effects of the use of incorrect T_{10} during PK analysis.

3 Methods

3.1 Groupwise Registration

A groupwise registration framework was used to evaluate different metrics for correcting motion within the SPGR volume sequence. It simultaneously registers all the N variable flip angles using a single similarity metric for the whole sequence of volumes. One of the variable flip angle volumes was considered as static, while the remaining ones were subjected to motion correction. A new similarity metric was created for groupwise registration of these volumes: the T_{10} regression error similarity metric, which is described in Sec. 3.2. A standard groupwise similarity metric, the Groupwise Normalized Mutual Information [1], was implemented as a commonly used similarity metric for comparison (Sec. 3.3). In this work, a Levenberg-Marquardt optimizer was used for similarity metric minimization (*alglib* library [3]). A pre-processing filtering stage was performed by applying a Gaussian blurring filter with a standard deviation of 1mm (close to in-plane voxel size). In this work, rigid registration was applied within this framework, however, other transformation model could be used.

3.2 T_{10} Regression Error Similarity Metric

We propose a new similarity metric for motion correction on variable flip angle SPGR volumes based on the T_{10} regression error. Estimating T_{10} consists in fitting a line through two or more points from the SPGR volume sequence at each voxel. In the presence of more than two points, this regression will yield a residual error which may be caused by motion between the volumes, noise and/or changes in the magnetic properties of the tissue. Hence, the misfit found can be used to assess the amount of patient motion between the MRI acquisitions.

Taking advantage of a modelled relationship between the intensities over a series of images has previously been proposed as a similarity metric. In [2,4], the

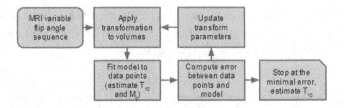

Fig. 2. Groupwise registration method by minimizing the T_{10} regression error in variable flip angle SPGR sequences

error between the data and the Tofts PK model was used as a non-linear motion correction similarity metric on DCE-MRI volumes.

In this work, a similar approach was taken to develop a similarity metric for the variable flip angle volume sequence. The T_{10} regression is expected to have a better fit when there is a better alignment. Hence, the proposed similarity metric is here defined as the error between the observed values for each flip angle volume $S(i, \alpha(n))$ and the fitted values $(\hat{S}(i, \alpha(n), \hat{T}_{10}(i), \hat{M}_0(i)))$:

$$
\text{sim}_{\text{reg}} = \frac{1}{NI} \sum_{i=1}^{I} \sum_{n=1}^{N} \left(S(i, \alpha(n)) - \hat{S}(i, \alpha(n), \hat{T}_{10}(i), \hat{M}_0(i)) \right)^2 \tag{6}
$$

where, I are the pixels within each volume and N the number of variable flip angle volumes within the sequence. An overview of the motion correction method using the T_{10} regression error similarity metric is shown in Fig. 2.

3.3   Groupwise Normalized Mutual Information

The Groupwise Normalized Mutual Information (GNMI) [1] was used for comparison for the simultaneous registration of variable flip angle sequences. It extends the Normalized Mutual Information (NMI) [8] for sets of volumes by summing the NMI of each volume I_n to a reference volume $\bar{I}$. The reference volume is generated by taking the mean intensity at each voxel of all the volumes being registered. Defining $H(I_1, I_2)$ as the joint entropy between I_1 and I_2 [6], the GNMI is given by: $\text{sim}_{\text{gnmi}} = (1/N) . \sum_{n=1}^{N} \left(\left(H(\bar{I}) + H(I_n) \right) / \left(H(\bar{I}, I_n) \right) \right)$

4   Results

4.1   Materials

Clinical Data. SPGR variable flip angle sequences from 27 patients with advanced colorectal adenocarcinomas were acquired on a 1.5T GE scanner using a T1-weighted, gradient-echo, fat-suppressed sequence (LAVA). Each sequence was composed of three or four volumes with different flip angles (3°, 9°, 12° and/or 15°) with $T_R = 4.5$ms and $T_E = 2.2$ms. Most of the patients were imaged twice, before and after chemoradiotherapy, thus there were 46 sequences.

The volumes had a resolution between 0.78 and 0.94mm in-plane, with a slice thickness between 4 and 5mm. All images had grid dimensions of 512 x 512 and the volumes contained between 20 to 28 slices. The colorectal region is the object of interest of these acquisitions and, to reduce computation time, this region was cropped from the original volumes. Each image was reduced to an in-plane 80 x 80 voxels region around the rectum and the upper and lower three slices were removed. Figs. 1 (a)-(d) show an example of a variable flip angle sequence.

Simulated Data. To assess the effects of motion on T_{10} estimation, ground truth volumes with known relaxation time and motion are required. However, from acquired clinical exams this is not possible, as the motion, which is the object of this study, will be present, but unknown. Thus, simulated ground truth variable flip angle volumes and T_{10} and M_0 maps were generated. These maps were created based on clinical data: for each variable flip angle sequence, T_{10} and M_0 were estimated according to the procedure shown in Sec. 2.2 and were considered as the ground truth. Creating such ground truth data ensures a similar distribution of values as found in clinical data. The variable flip angle volumes were generated by applying these maps to Eq. 3. For each ground truth generated sequence, the chosen flip angles were the same as the original sequence. Figs. 1 (e)-(h) show examples of these simulated images. Randomly generated known rigid motion was applied to the simulated volumes to evaluate the effects of motion in T_{10} estimation and compare different registration algorithms (Sec. 4.2). The rigid transformations were drawn from a normal distribution ($\mu = 0$) with σ_k standard deviation on each transformation parameter. For each motion level k, the amount of motion caused by the random transformations was computed as the mean level of motion introduced in the SPGR variable flip angle sequences. A volume size dependent scale was applied to normalize the motion on the rotation parameters, keeping the displacement caused by motion and translation on the same level.

4.2   Experiments

Evaluating the Effects of Motion on the Estimation of Pharmacokinetic Model Parameters. Two experiments were performed to assess the effects of motion within the SPGR volume sequence on T_{10} and subsequent PK model parameter estimation. Firstly, the error in T_{10} due to motion was estimated by applying varying levels of random levels of rigid deformations to simulated MRI variable flip angle sequences with known T_{10} values (Sec. 4.1). After applying the deformations, T_{10} was estimated and compared to the ground truth, providing a measure of the estimation error as a function of residual misalignment. The second experiment consisted of evaluating how motion corrupted T_{10} estimations affect subsequent PK model parameter estimation. Simulated DCE-MRI signals were generated with known K_{trans} and k_{ep} values and $T_{10} = 1.0s$. Erroneous T_{10} values were used to estimate these PK parameters and the obtained results were compared to the original ones, providing a measure of by how much T_{10} error propagates to PK analysis. In this experiment $\overline{K}_{trans}$ ranged from 0.01 to 2.00 and $\overline{k}_{ep}$ from 0.01 to 5, providing an average estimation error over different curves. Other parameters of this experiment were: $r_1 = 4.5$ (mM.s)$^{-1}$, $r_2 = 5.5$ (mM.s)$^{-1}$, $T_R = 4.5ms$, $T_E = 0.22ms$ and a 15° flip angle. The synthetic DCE-MRI curves were created with samples every 12 seconds for 5.2 minutes.

Evaluation and Comparison of Similarity Metrics for Rigid Body Motion Correction. The T_{10} regression and GNMI similarity metrics were tested using a rigid registration framework (Sec. 3.1) on 20 ground truth sequences of variable flip angle MRI volumes. The procedure to perform this test is presented below:

1. Ground truth parameter maps ($\overline{T}_{10}$ and $\overline{M}_0$) were created from the original clinical data, as explained in Sec. 4.1.
2. For each flip angle, a random rigid transformation was created and applied to the $\overline{T}_{10}$ and $\overline{M}_0$ volumes (Sec. 4.1).
3. The transformed maps were used to create motion corrupted MRI volumes with variable flip angles using Eq. 3.
4. The volumes were registered twice, once using the T_{10} regression error similarity metric and once using GNMI (Secs 3.1, 3.2 and 3.3).
5. The mean displacement and the T_{10} estimation error were computed before and after registration to assess the registration accuracy of each of the similarity metrics.

To complement this experiment, the robustness of these similarity metrics to noise was also evaluated. Several levels of Rician noise were applied to the motion corrupted synthetic sequences and registered using the T_{10} regression error similarity metric or GNMI.

Estimation of the Rigid Motion Found on SPGR Variable flip Angle Volume Sequences. The third experiment aims at estimating the amount of rigid motion found within the SPGR variable flip angle sequences. This provides, in conjunction with the other experiments, a lower bound to the error in PK parameter estimation caused by motion in T_{10} estimation. Rigid motion was quantified by applying the groupwise rigid registration method (Sec. 3.1) to several SPGR sequences. This was performed using both similarity metrics; the original motion was considered as the displacement caused by the obtained registration transforms.

4.3   Results and Discussion

Evaluating the Effects of Motion on the Estimation of Pharmacokinetic Model Parameters. The T_{10} estimation error as a function of the average motion is shown in Fig. 3 for each tested motion level. A linear relation between the amount of simulated motion and the T_{10} estimation error is observed. Fig. 4 shows how inaccuracies in T_{10} affect the estimation of K_{trans} and

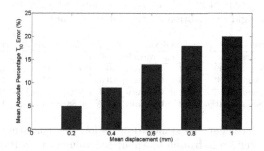

Fig. 3. Estimated T_{10} error due to motion within the SPGR sequence volumes. The average T_{10} error exceeds 15% for a motion equivalent to an in-plane voxel size (0.8mm).

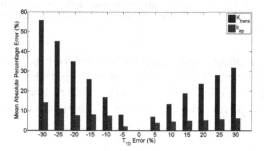

Fig. 4. K_{trans} and k_{ep} estimation error due to T_{10} inaccuracies. A magnification of the error occurs for underestimated T_{10} values.

k_{ep}. The most notable result is that underestimations of T_{10} have significantly greater effect on the PK model parameter estimation. Overall, T_{10} errors are amplified during K_{trans} estimation and reduced for k_{ep} estimation. These behaviours had already been reported on a similar experiment using a different AIF [9].

Evaluation of Similarity Metrics for Rigid Body Motion Correction.

The similarity metrics were evaluated by the mean displacement found between the original (pre-motion) and the registered volumes. The average amount of motion that was simulated, and the target registration and T_{10} estimation errors before and after registration are shown in Tab. 1. For all motion levels, the T_{10} regression metric showed a lower registration error than the GNMI metric and for each level a paired one-sided Wilcoxon signed test indicated that the new metric was statistically significantly better at correcting motion (p-level<0.01). The difference between the registration outcomes became more accentuated as the simulated motion increased. As for the T_{10} estimation, it almost always showed lower errors as the motion was corrected. In terms of PK model parameter estimation, when subjected to 1.23mm mean simulated motion, performing rigid

Table 1. Mean displacement and standard deviation and T_{10} estimation error before and after groupwise rigid registration on simulated volumes

Mean displacement ± standard deviation [mm] / Mean absolute T_{10} error [%]					
Pre-registration		T_{10} regression		GNMI	
0.46 ± 0.08mm	9%	**0.34 ± 0.15mm**	10%	0.38 ± 0.09mm	10%
0.68 ± 0.13mm	14%	**0.45 ± 0.19mm**	13%	0.55 ± 0.11mm	14%
0.92 ± 0.16mm	17%	**0.61 ± 0.38mm**	15%	0.69 ± 0.15mm	16%
1.23 ± 0.26mm	20%	**0.72 ± 0.39mm**	16%	0.88 ± 0.23mm	18%

Table 2. Mean displacement and standard deviation and T_{10} estimation error before and after groupwise rigid registration on simulated volumes with Rician noise

Noise level	Mean displacement ± standard deviation [mm] / Mean absolute T_{10} error [%]					
σ_n	Pre-registration		T_{10} regression		GNMI	
0		13%	**0.43 ± 0.10mm**	11%	0.55 ± 0.09mm	12%
15	0.72 ± 0.11mm	30%	**0.40 ± 0.10mm**	26%	0.59 ± 0.14mm	27%
30		46%	**0.42 ± 0.18mm**	44%	0.66 ± 0.14mm	44%

registration with the proposed similarity metric reduced the T_{10} estimation error by 4%, which would cause a decrease of similar magnitude on the K_{trans} error.

When evaluating the effects of noise on the registration of variable flip angle sequences, the results (presented in Tab. 2) show that both similarity metrics are robust to it.

Assessing the Rigid Motion Found on SPGR Variable Flip Angle Volume Sequences. A considerable discrepancy was found between the motion estimated using the T_{10} regression and the GNMI similarity metrics. The new metric indicated a mean rigid displacement of 0.98mm ± 0.41mm; when using GNMI, 0.53mm ± 0.45mm motion was observed. This result not only shows that considerable motion may occur within these volumes, but also that the choice of the metric when correcting for motion may have a relevant effect on the registration. Considering the lowest estimated motion (using the GNMI metric), an average error of around 12% may be expected for T_{10}, leading to about 15% K_{trans} error. Alternatively, the motion estimated using the T_{10} regression metric, 0.98mm, could indicate an estimation error of more than 25% on K_{trans}.

5   Discussion and Conclusion

This work has presented a novel method for correcting patient motion within variable flip angle sequences and studied how this may affect DCE-MRI analysis. A clear relation between motion and K_{trans} error was shown, quantifying how much misalignment may be present during relaxation time estimation without compromising the PK analysis. In contrast, k_{ep} estimation was much more robust to T_{10} error. Our experiments also showed that there exists a relevant amount of motion within variable flip angle MRI sequences, which would cause an error between 15% and 25% on K_{trans}, motivating the need for motion correction techniques when estimating T_{10} for PK analysis of DCE-MRI exams.

Our key contribution was the proposition of a new similarity metric for motion correction in SPGR variable flip angle sequences based on the T_{10} regression error. This novel metric consistently showed lower registration error on sets of simulated volumes with simulated motion when compared to the GNMI metric. However, further development is still needed for the validation of this technique in clinical variable flip angle sequences. The presence and correction of non-linear motion in these exams will be examined using the new similarity metric. Moreover, further experiments must be performed to analyse the effects of motion correction on clinical data to further establish whether flip angle sequence registration can improve the PK analysis results and the characterization of tumours.

Acknowledgements. AH gratefully acknowledges the support of the Research Council UK Digital Economy Programme grant number EP/G036861/1 (Oxford Centre for Doctoral Training in Healthcare Innovation) and the CAPES Foundation, process N° BEX 0725/12-9.

References

1. Bhatia, K.K., Hajnal, J., Hammers, A., Rueckert, D.: Similarity metrics for groupwise non-rigid registration. In: Ayache, N., Ourselin, S., Maeder, A. (eds.) MICCAI 2007, Part II. LNCS, vol. 4792, pp. 544–552. Springer, Heidelberg (2007)
2. Bhushan, M., Schnabel, J.A., Risser, L., Heinrich, M.P., Brady, J.M., Jenkinson, M.: Motion correction and parameter estimation in dceMRI sequences: Application to colorectal cancer. In: Fichtinger, G., Martel, A., Peters, T. (eds.) MICCAI 2011, Part I. LNCS, vol. 6891, pp. 476–483. Springer, Heidelberg (2011)
3. Bochkanov, S.: Alglib (2010), http://mloss.org/software/view/231/
4. Buonaccorsi, G.A., Roberts, C., Cheung, S., Watson, Y., O'Connor, J.B.P., Davies, K., Jackson, A., Jayson, G.C., Parker, G.J.M.: Comparison of the performance of tracer kinetic model-driven registration for dynamic contrast enhanced MRI using different models of contrast enhancement. Acad. Radiol. 13, 1112–1123 (2006)
5. Deoni, S.C.L., Rutt, B.K., Peters, T.M.: Rapid combined T1 and T2 mapping using gradient recalled acquisition in the steady state. Magn. Reson. Med. 49, 515–526 (2003)
6. Maes, F., Collignon, A., Vandermeulen, D., Marchal, G., Suetens, P.: Multimodality image registration by maximization of mutual information. IEEE Trans. Med. Imag. 16, 187–198 (1997)
7. Orton, M.R., D'Arcy, J.A., Walker-Samuel, S., Hawkes, D.J., Atkinson, D., Collins, D.J., Leach, M.O.: Computationally efficient vascular input function models for quantitative kinetic modelling using DCE-MRI. Phys. Med. Biol. 53, 1225–1239 (2008)
8. Studholme, C., Hill, D.L.G., Hawkes, D.J.: An overlap invariant entropy measure of 3D medical image alignment. Patt. Rec. 32, 71–86 (1999)
9. Tanner, L.N.: Functional Imaging Markers for Tumour Characterisation. PhD thesis, University of Oxford (2010)
10. Paul, S.T.: Modeling tracer kinetics in dynamic gd-dtpa mr imaging. J. Magn. Reson. Imaging 7, 91–101 (1997)
11. Yankeelov, T.E., Gore, J.C.: Dynamic contrast enhanced magnetic resonance imaging in oncology: theory, data acquisition, analysis, and examples. Curr. Med. Imaging Rev. 3, 91 (2009)

Motion Correction of Intravital Microscopy of Preclinical Lung Tumour Imaging Using Multichannel Structural Image Descriptor

Bartlomiej W. Papież[1], Thomas Tapmeier[2], Mattias P. Heinrich[3], Ruth J. Muschel[2], and Julia A. Schnabel[1]

[1] Institute of Biomedical Engineering,
Department of Engineering Science, University of Oxford, UK
[2] Gray Institute for Radiation Oncology and Biology
University of Oxford, UK
[3] Institute of Medical Informatics, Universität Lübeck, Germany

Abstract. Optical microscopy imaging techniques have enabled a wide spectrum of biomedical applications. Among visualization, a quantitative analysis of tumour cell growth in lungs is of great importance. The main challenges inherently linked with such data analysis are: local contrast changes related to tissue depth, lack of clear object boundaries due to the presence of noise, and cluttering with motion artefacts due to translational shift of the specimen and non-linear lung tissue collapse. This paper aims to address these problems by introducing a novel image registration framework specifically designed to correct for motion artefacts from optical microscopy of lung tumour cells imaging. For this purpose, a previously developed modality independent neighbourhood descriptor (MIND) was adapted to cope with multiple image channels for optical microscopy data. Two versions of this novel multichannel MIND (mMIND) are here presented. The proposed registration technique estimates both rigid transformations and non-linear deformations both common in the optical microscopy volumes and time-sequences acquisition. The performance of our registration technique based on a novel multichannel image representation is demonstrated using two distinctive optical imaging data sets of lung cells: 3D volumes with translation motion artefacts only, and time-sequences with both rigid and non-linear motion artefacts. Visual inspection of the registration outcomes and reported results of the qualitative evaluation show a promising improvement compared to images without correction.

Keywords: image registration, microscopy imaging, lung tumour cell imaging, structural image representation.

1 Introduction

Recent advances in optical microscopy methods in biomedical science have attracted active research in finding accurate and efficient tools for automated analysis of (usually large scale) imaging data sets. Such applications include but are

S. Ourselin and M. Modat (Eds.): WBIR 2014, LNCS 8545, pp. 164–173, 2014.

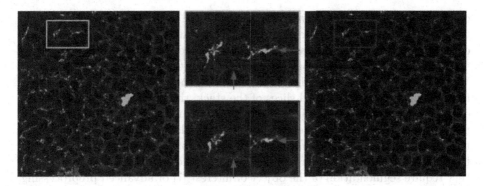

Fig. 1. Exemplar of intensity inconsistency for the mouse lung tumour tissue data. Areas depicted by the red arrows show the same anatomical structure taken from the neighbourhood slices of the entire stack, however the intensity values are different.

not limited to the following: variability of cell nuclei analysis [14], tumour cell migration analysis [5], classification of protein motion patterns [6], and vessel architecture and blood flow analysis [7].

In this paper, we consider intravital microscopy (IVM), which captures high-resolution image sequences and furthermore can be used for visualization of tumour cell growth and their interaction with host immune cells such as macrophages and T cells. The in vivo-model of choice is small rodents, and both whole organs (following explantation from the animal) as well as tumours *in situ* can be imaged. In our current experimental set-up, the acquisition protocol is specified for ex-vivo lung imaging as follows. Lungs that carry metastatic colonies are explanted to study the behaviour and phenotype of macrophages interacting with the colonies within the lungs. The lungs are kept at 37 °C for up to two hours while imaging. The protocol comes with a number of challenges, which this paper aims to address. The intrinsic regular motion patterns such as tissue movements (due to lung decompression) introduce motion artefacts; thus preventing stable image acquisition at high spatial resolution. In addition, the motion is not necessarily spatially and temporally uniform *i.e.* the whole lung might undergo motion, or parts of it only, and this may start at any time during image acquisition. This makes a high rate of abortive experiments and significantly limits the potential of intravital microscopy techniques.

1.1   Related Work

The majority of the applications using optical imaging data sets that have been investigated so far in the literature treat the registration between consecutive slices of the stack as a purely mono-modal registration problem. Such approaches proposed for stack motion correction usually use intensity based similarity measures *i.e.* the sum of the squared differences (SSD) or the sum of the absolute differences (SAD). However, usage of SSD (or SAD) based image registration implies the assumption that the corresponding structures in both input images have constant intensity values. However, this assumption is violated in the case of optical microscopy data, where changes in intensity are common due the artefacts caused by the optical characteristics of the microscopy system. One exemplar of such intensity inconsistency for mouse lung tumour tissue data is shown in Fig. 1. While the areas depicted by the red arrows show the same anatomical structure taken from the neighbourhood slices of the stack, the intensity values are different. [8] used mutual information based similarity measures but the results were not satisfactory as motion artefacts were not completely removed. This was due to the fact that mutual information is a global measure of image similarity, while the intensity inconsistencies are local. Other approaches tackling this problem either require segmentation of the object of interest [7] or advanced preprocessing using feature detection [6]. In our case, such segmentation or feature detection is not possible as it comes with extra segmentation of very irregularly shaped cells.

Here, we present an efficient post-acquisition image registration based technique to correct data corrupted by rigid and non-linear motion artefacts. In contrast to other approaches (e.g. [8]), our method directly integrates information from all channels of volume/sequence using a novel technique called multichannel modality independent neighbourhood descriptors (mMIND). These novel descriptors are robust to local contrast changes, and noise present in the acquired data. The proposed registration technique estimates both rigid and non-linear deformations inherently linked with the optical microscopy volumes or time-sequences acquisition. We demonstrate that the presented image registration framework is capable of correcting for motion artefacts apparent in the collected data sets.

The remainder of this paper is organized as follows. In Sec. 2 we briefly review the concept of the modality independent neighbourhood descriptor (Sec. 2.1) and then we introduce and explain in detail how to compute mMIND descriptors for multichannel data derived from MIND (Sec. 2.2). Finally, this section describes an adapted optimization scheme for rigid and non-linear registration. Section 3 presents the lung data set used for evaluation purposes (Sec. 3.1), and the employed experimental setup (Sec. 3.2). The obtained results for those data are presented in Sec. 3.3. The paper is summarized and concluded in Sec. 4.

2   Methodology

In this work, we consider registration for the multichannel images $I = [I_1, \ldots, I_c, \ldots, I_C]$ consisting of C channels of an entire stack $S = [I_1, \ldots, I_n, \ldots I_N]$ where N is the number of images in this stack acquired using optical microscopy. We start our registration by selecting this initial image from one of the images I_n from the stack to be a reference image (usually the first image of the stack I_1) and a consecutive image I_{n+1} of this stack is referred to as the moving image. Consequently, to remove rigid motion artefacts present in the entire stack S, we perform N-1 pairwise registrations minimizing a generally stated similarity function Sim in the following way:

$$\hat{p} = \arg\min_{p} \left(\sum_{n=1}^{N-1} \sum_{x} (Sim(\boldsymbol{I}_n(\boldsymbol{x}), \boldsymbol{I}_{n+1}(\boldsymbol{x} + \boldsymbol{p}))) \right) \tag{1}$$

where $\boldsymbol{p}$ denotes the estimated motion correction parameters (the parameters of adapted global transformation model), and $\boldsymbol{x}$ denotes a spatial position within the image domain. Similarly, to also remove any non-linear motion components in the entire stack, we perform N-1 pairwise deformable registrations combining the similarity measure and a regularisation term Reg:

$$\hat{u} = \arg\min_{u} \left(\sum_{n=1}^{N-1} \sum_{x} (Sim(\boldsymbol{I}_n(\boldsymbol{x}), \boldsymbol{I}_{n+1}(\boldsymbol{x} + \boldsymbol{u})) + \alpha Reg(\boldsymbol{u})) \right) \tag{2}$$

where $\boldsymbol{u}$ denotes the estimated displacement field, and α is a positive factor weighting the elements of the cost function.

Changing the reference image for each registration instead of using one pre-selected image was found to increase the quality of the stack reconstruction, as the corresponding neighbourhood slices of the stack contain the same anatomical structures [8].

2.1 MIND: Modality Independent Neighborhood Descriptor

The modality independent neighbourhood descriptor (MIND) was originally proposed by [3] for multimodal registration of CT/MRI lung data. Recently, this descriptor was also successfully applied to CT/Ultrasound rigid registration [1]. The modality independent neighbourhood descriptor is a vector defined as follows:

$$MIND(I(\boldsymbol{x}), \boldsymbol{r}) = \frac{1}{n} \exp \left(- \frac{d(I(\boldsymbol{x}), I(\boldsymbol{x} + r))}{v(I(\boldsymbol{x}))} \right) \tag{3}$$

where d is a distance measure between two local image patches within a spatial search range $r \in \boldsymbol{r}$, and v is a variance estimator. In case of grey-level images, the distance d between two points $\boldsymbol{x}$ and $\boldsymbol{x} + r$ was defined as the sum of the squared differences of all pixels within the two patches centred at $\boldsymbol{x}$ and $\boldsymbol{x} + r$.

The MIND descriptor (defined by Eq. (3)) cannot be used directly for our data, as it is defined for grey-level images (single channel images). Therefore, a particular channel needs to be chosen for the registration, or as suggested by [8] a single-channel composite image can be generated based on all image channels in the following way:

$$c(\boldsymbol{I}(\boldsymbol{x})) = \sum_{c=1}^{C} I_c(\boldsymbol{x}) \cdot \frac{\sum_{x} I_c(\boldsymbol{x})}{\sum_{x} I_1(\boldsymbol{x}) + \ldots + \sum_{x} I_C(\boldsymbol{x})} \tag{4}$$

While such linear combination of the image channels has no biological significance, however, it enables to process multichannel data without the need to discard any channel. However, the composite image $c(\boldsymbol{I})$ still suffers from any local contrast changes and presence of the noise.

2.2   mMIND: Multichannel Modality Independent Neighbourhood Descriptor

In order to extend the applicability of MIND for multichannel data, we propose two alternative approaches in order to avoid discarding information from any other channels. The first version of the multichannel MIND (mMIND) calculates the MIND descriptor for each channel separately and then merges those distances as elements of the new descriptor in the following way:

$$mMIND_a(\boldsymbol{I}(\boldsymbol{x}), r) = [MIND(I_1(\boldsymbol{x}), r), \dots, MIND(I_C(\boldsymbol{x}), r)] \qquad (5)$$

In case of four-neighbourhood spatial search space r, the $mMIND_a$ has $4 * C$ elements.

For the second version of the proposed mMIND descriptor we propose to use the sum of the squared differences between the vector-valued patches centred at $\boldsymbol{x}$ and $\boldsymbol{x} + r$.

$$mMIND_c(\boldsymbol{I}(\boldsymbol{x}), r) = \frac{1}{n} \exp \left(-\frac{\sum_{c=1}^{C} d(I_c(\boldsymbol{x}), I_c(\boldsymbol{x} + r))}{v(\boldsymbol{I}(\boldsymbol{x}))} \right) \qquad (6)$$

In case of four-neighbourhood spatial search space r, the $mMIND_c$ has same number of channels as the original single-channel MIND (4 elements).

2.3   Registration Framework

Rigid Registration. Following our previous formulation in Sec. 2 for stack motion correction, we restrict our parameters for the model of transformation $\boldsymbol{p} = [p_{t_x}, p_{t_y}]$ to be a translational part of the global rigid transformation. Our implementation of registration uses the traditional Levenberg-Marquardt (LM) algorithm for vector valued-images [11]. Different optimization methods can be used to find a local solution of the presented cost function (see [9]).

Non-Linear Registration. To estimate the non-linear components of motion artefacts in the data, we use the Demons approach [12], which is a widely used non-parametric registration framework. The original formulation of the Demons algorithm minimises the similarity Sim formulated as the sum of squared intensity differences and a diffusion based regularisation Reg of the deformation field is performed by Gaussian smoothing. The chosen framework can also be applied to vector-valued data using the multichannel Demons approach [10]. The particular choice of this registration is motivated by an efficient second order minimisation scheme (ESM) applied in the Demons algorithm where a second order approximation of the cost function is achieved by combining the image gradients of the reference image and the moving image. The novel representation of multichannel images using the proposed image descriptor, described in the previous section, produces images that can be treated as mono-modal, so that the multichannel Demons approach with ESM can be applied to a multichannel microscopy registration problem.

3   Evaluation

To demonstrate the functionality of our registration method with the new image descriptors, we apply it to the challenging application of correction for motion distortion from optical microscopy imaging.

3.1   Data Description

Images were acquired using a confocal laser scanning microscope (Zeiss 710 LSM, Carl Zeiss Jena, Germany) with a 20x objective and 845 nm 2P excitation. The in-plane dimension of the images is 1024×1024 with spatial resolution of $0.415 \times 0.415 \mu m^2$ with three 8 bit channels. There is variable stack size between 49 and 67 slices (with resolution of $1.0 \mu m$ in z direction). All acquisition procedures are in accordance with the ASPA (Animals Scientific Procedures Act) 1986 and ethical guidelines of the University of Oxford.

3.2   Experimental Setup

The particular registration parameters selected for our experiments are as follows. During registration a linear interpolation with a Neumann boundary condition is performed where pixel values outside the image domain are replaced by the values of the nearest pixel within the image boundary. Additionally, we employ a five level multi-resolution scheme to improve the convergence rate of the algorithms. Downsampling factors of $[16, 8, 4, 2, 1]$ are used for all experiments presented in this paper. To obtain mMIND descriptors for a lower resolution, we calculate appropriate distances between local patches in the original image resolution, and then down-sample this descriptor to the desired resolution. The mMIND parameters are $\sigma = 2.5$ for estimating the patch distance d and the four-neighbourhood spatial search region.

Due to the lack of ground truth, a surrogate criterion, the sum of the squared difference (SSD), was evaluated to quantify the performance of registration. We used the SSD to measure the similarity of the group of images in the registered stack computed as follows: $SSD = \frac{1}{N-1} \sum_{n=1}^{N-1} \sum_{x} (I_n(x) - I_{n+1}(x))^2$ Additionally, we also calculated the peak signal-to-noise ratio (PSNR) [2].

3.3   Results

Data with Translation Motion Distortions. Figure 2 shows a z-stack sum projection for one of the data sets with translation distortions before and after rigid registration. The translational motion is apparent as a smooth image blur reducing sharpness of object details. The effective elimination of translational motion was achieved by both presented descriptors $mMIND_a$ and $mMIND_c$. As an example Fig. 2(right) shows a reduction of motion artefacts after registration using the $mMIND_a$ descriptor. The sum of the squared differences (SSD) before registration is $9.88 * 10^3$, while after registration using the $mMIND_a$ and $mMIND_c$ was reduced to $3.88 * 10^3$ and $3.86 * 10^3$, respectively. The PSNR before

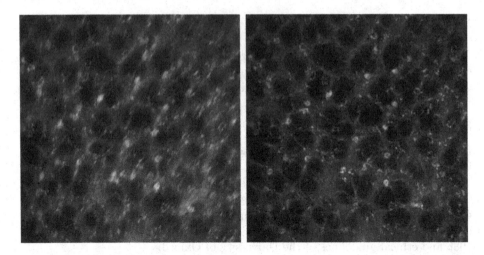

Fig. 2. Example of rigid registration results for a lung tissue data set with translational motion distortions. (left) z-stack sum projection of entire volume before registration, (right) z-stack sum projection of entire volume after rigid registration using mMIND$_a$. The effectiveness of rigid motion artefacts reduction can be clearly seen, and it is possible to distinguish and evaluate individual cells (green).

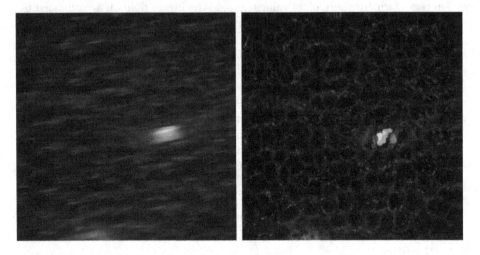

Fig. 3. Example of rigid registration results for very challenging lung tissue data with translational motion distortions. (left) z-stack sum projection of entire volume before registration, (right) z-stack sum projection of entire volume after rigid registration using mMIND$_a$. Before registration, the image is unusable for analysis; however, rigid motion artefacts reduction clearly improves the quality of the image.

registration was $27.2 \pm 4.5dB$ while after registration using the mMIND$_a$ was $29.2 \pm 3.9dB$, and using the mMIND$_c$ was $29.2 \pm 4.1dB$.

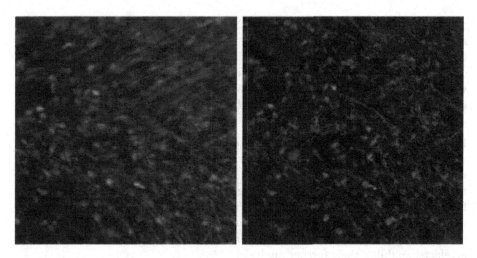

Fig. 4. Example of deformable registration results for lung tissue data with non-linear motion distortions. (left) z-stack sum projection of entire volume before registration, (right) z-stack sum projection of entire volume after non-linear registration. The correction for non-linear motion renders a larger area of the sample image suitable for analysis.

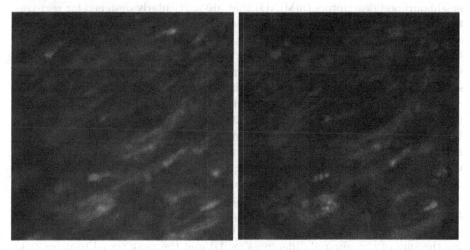

Fig. 5. Example of deformable registration results for lung tissue data with non-linear motion distortions. (left) z-stack sum projection of entire volume before registration, (right) z-stack sum projection of entire volume after non-linear registration. The image quality is improved and the outline of blood vessels (green) can be traced. Also, cells (red) can be evaluated. However, the quality of underlying data limits the effectiveness of non-linear motion artefact correction.

Similarly, Fig. 3 shows the sum z-stack projection for a very challenging example of the collected data set with translational distortions before and after rigid registration using $mMIND_a$. As before, the proposed registration techniques based on image descriptors $mMIND_a$ and $mMIND_c$ were able to reduce motion distortions. The SSD before registration for data shown in Fig. 3 is $6.25 * 10^3$, while after registration using the $mMIND_a$ and $mMIND_c$ was reduced to $2.07 * 10^3$ and $2.04 * 10^3$, respectively. The PSNR before registration was $26.5 \pm 4.6 dB$ while after registration using the $mMIND_a$ was $34.2 \pm 5.1 dB$, and using the $mMIND_c$ was $34.1 \pm 5.2 dB$.

Data with Non-Linear Motion Distortions. Fig. 4 and Fig. 5 show a sum z-stack projections for two data sets with non-linear distortions before (left) and after deformable registration (right). The proposed registration was able to reduce both translational and non-linear motion artefacts apparent due to the lung collapse as indicated by Fig. 4 (right) and 5 (right). This demonstrate the potential of our proposed image registration method using mMIND descriptors to restore data sets that were severely distorted by rigid and non-linear motion artefacts, enabling their further analysis.

4   Discussion and Conclusions

In this paper, we have presented a set of new multichannel modality independent neighbourhood descriptors (mMIND) that are particularly designed for registration of multichannel image data. The crucial step of mMIND generation in terms of the calculation of the neighbourhood patch distances, was performed in two different ways: between the patches of each channel separately, and between vector-valued patches integrating all channels of these data. The obtained results indicate that registration with either of the presented descriptors is able to cope well with motion artefacts. The rigid and non-linear components of motion artefacts were estimated via efficient optimisation schemes: the Levenberg-Marquardt algorithm for rigid registration and the Demons framework with the efficient second order minimisation scheme (ESM). In the examples presented, image registration visually improved the quality of the data sets acquired. Due to the registration based on the proposed multichannel extension of MIND, the motion correction framework is not sensitive to the data noise, and removes blurry information only related to the motion artefacts. The visual inspection of image registration outcomes is further supported by quantitative results comparing the sum of the squared differences (SSD) and the peak signal-to-noise ratio (PSNR) before and after registration. From the biological perspective, the presented method renders formerly unusable data open to quantitative analysis and salvages work that otherwise would have had to be discarded by the scientists.

Future work will focus on further development of image registration methods suitable for intravital microscopy (IVM), facilitating detailed and automated analysis of tumour cell growth and migration. This type of analysis requires the development of a computationally efficient framework in order to be able to upscale to large biomedical experiments. Therefore, we plan to investigate descriptors with near real-time performance such as the quantized self-similarity descriptor with a similarity measure based on the Hamming distance [4]. Further improvement of the presented descriptors might also be possible. The multichannel MIND are not rotationally invariant which could be a limitation in some applications. Therefore, the use of the other image descriptors such entropy or Laplacian image representation [13] could address such specific requirements.

Acknowledgements. We would like to acknowledge funding from the CRUK/ EPSRC Cancer Imaging Centre at Oxford.

References

1. Cifor, A., Risser, L., Heinrich, M.P., Chung, D., Schnabel, J.A.: Rigid registration of untracked freehand 2D ultrasound sweeps to 3D CT of liver tumours. In: Yoshida, H., Warfield, S., Vannier, M.W. (eds.) Abdominal Imaging 2013. LNCS, vol. 8198, pp. 155–164. Springer, Heidelberg (2013)
2. Gonzalez, R.C., Woods, R.E.: Digital image processing. Prentice Hall (2008)
3. Heinrich, M.P., Jenkinson, M., Bhushan, M., Matin, T., Gleeson, F.V., Brady, M., Schnabel, J.A.: MIND: Modality independent neighbourhood descriptor for multi-modal deformable registration. Med. Image Anal. 16(7), 1423–1435 (2012)
4. Heinrich, M.P., Jenkinson, M., Papież, B.W., Brady, S.M., Schnabel, J.A.: Towards realtime multimodal fusion for image-guided interventions using self-similarities. In: Mori, K., Sakuma, I., Sato, Y., Barillot, C., Navab, N. (eds.) MICCAI 2013, Part I. LNCS, vol. 8149, pp. 187–194. Springer, Heidelberg (2013)
5. Kedrin, D., Gligorijevic, B., Wyckoff, J., Verkhusha, V.V., Condeelis, J., Segall, J.E., van Rheenen, J.: Intravital imaging of metastatic behavior through a mammary imaging window. Nat. Methods 5(12), 1019–1021 (2008)
6. Kim, I.-H., Chen, Y.-C.M., Spector, D.L., Eils, R., Rohr, K.: Nonrigid registration of 2-D and 3-D dynamic cell nuclei images for improved classification of subcellular particle motion. IEEE Trans. Image Process. 20(4), 1011–1022 (2011)
7. Kumar, A.N., Short, K.W., Piston, D.W.: A motion correction framework for time series sequences in microscopy images. Microsc. Microanal. 19, 433–450 (2013)
8. Lorenz, K.S., Salama, P., Dunn, K.W., Delp, E.J.: Digital correction of motion artefacts in microscopy image sequences collected from living animals using rigid and nonrigid registration. J. Microsc. 245(2), 148–160 (2012)
9. Modersitzki, J.: FAIR: Flexible Algorithms for Image Registration. SIAM, Philadelphia (2009)
10. Peyrat, J.-M., Delingette, H., Sermesant, M., Xu, C., Ayache, N.: Registration of 4D cardiac CT sequences under trajectory constraints with multichannel diffeomorphic Demons. IEEE Trans. Med. Imag. 29, 1351–1368 (2010)
11. Thevenaz, P., Ruttimann, U.E., Unser, M.: A pyramid approach to subpixel registration based on intensity. IEEE Trans. Image Process. 7(1), 27–41 (1998)
12. Vercauteren, T., Pennec, X., Perchant, A., Ayache, N.: Diffeomorphic Demons: Efficient non-parametric image registration. NeuroImage 45, S61–S72 (2009)
13. Wachinger, C., Navab, N.: Entropy and laplacian images: structural representations for multi-modal registration. Med. Image Anal. 16(1), 1–17 (2012)
14. Yang, S., Kohler, D., Teller, K., Cremer, T., Le Baccon, P., Heard, E., Eils, R., Rohr, K.: Nonrigid registration of 3-D multichannel microscopy images of cell nuclei. IEEE Trans. Image Process. 17(4), 493–499 (2008)

Registration of Image Sequences from Experimental Low-Cost Fundus Camera

Radim Kolar[1,2], Bernhard Hoeher[3,4], Jan Odstrcilik[1,2],
Bernhard Schmauss[3,4], and Jiri Jan[1]

[1] Department of Biomedical Engineering, Faculty of Electrical Engineering
and Communication, Brno University of Technology, Brno, Czech Republic
kolarr@feec.vutbr.cz
[2] International Clinical Research Center, Center of Biomedical Engineering,
St. Anne's University Hospital, Brno, Czech Republic
[3] Institute of Microwaves and Photonics,
Friedrich-Alexander University of Erlangen-Nuremberg, Erlangen, Germany
[4] Erlangen Graduate School in Advanced Optical Technologies (SAOT),
University of Erlangen-Nuremberg, Erlangen, Germany

Abstract. This paper describes new registration approach for registration of low SNR retinal image sequences. We combine two approaches - Fourier-based method for large shift correction and Lucas-Kanade tracking for small shift and rotation correction. We also propose method for evaluation of registration results, which uses spatial variation of minimum value in intensity profiles through blood-vessels. We achieved precision of registration below 2.1 pixels, which is acceptable with regards to image SNR (around $10dB$). The final averaging of registered sequence leads to improvement of image quality and improvement in SNR over 10 dB.

1 Introduction

Digital fundus camera is a fundamental diagnostic device, which is widely utilized in ophthalmology for assessment of the human retina. Nowadays, two branches in developing of fundus camera instrumentations can be identified. One is focused on development of an advanced imaging devices using adaptive optics to eliminate eye aberrations. The second branch focuses on development of low-cost fundus camera enabling to acquire single-shot or video sequences. Motivation to develop such low-cost devices is to extend the use of fundus cameras into different fields of medical examination as there are promising non-ophthalmic applications, e.g. vascular applications [1]. Another motivation factor is telemedicine - these cameras are intended for being used in developing countries with off-site image reading.

Several authors described low-cost fundus camera and alternative camera design. Guyomard at el. [2] has described endoscope for small animal retinal imaging including fluorescein angiography video acquisition. Tran et al. [3] used Panasonic Lumix G2 with commercially available optics to acquire single-shot

S. Ourselin and M. Modat (Eds.): WBIR 2014, LNCS 8545, pp. 174–183, 2014.

50° field of view human fundus images. There is also an increasing effort to use smart phones for retinal imaging. Haddock et al. [4] used hand held ophthalmic lens and iPhone with Filmic Pro application for controlling the illumination, focus and exposure to acquire video sequences. Similar approach with special lens smart phone adapter was used in [5]. This effort is connected also with development of appropriate image processing techniques for acquired sequences, which are usually more noisy, non-uniformly illuminated and containing different artefacts. One of the main (pre)processing method is registration of acquired retinal sequences.

There are many journal publications, which describe different approaches for retinal image registration. Major part of these techniques are based on utilization of blood vessel tree as a source of landmarks, e.g. [6], [7]. Some authors also used intensity based approaches with different optimization criteria, e.g. [8], [9]. Current approaches combines intensity- and landmarks-based methods, e.g. [10], [11]. Detailed state-of-the-art including comparison of different approaches can be found in [12]. In a spite of these published papers there are still applications, where image registration is challenging task. These applications include low SNR images, multimodal registration (e.g. near infrared imaging, angiographic imaging, fundus laser scanning modalities, optical coherence tomography), sub-pixel registration or registration of long-term retinal images with different morphological changes. These specific applications need to modify existing approaches.

This paper deals with registration of low SNR fundus temporal sequences from experimental low-cost fundus camera. We used phase correlation approach (as in our our previous work [12]) together with Lucas-Kanade (LK) tracking. We found only two relevant papers, where LK method has been applied in retinal application, which are close to ours. The first paper used LK method for estimation of macular disparity map in multiple view fundus imaging [13]. The second paper used LK tracking for processing of 1° field of view sequences from adaptive optics confocal scanning laser ophthalmoscope [14]. Here we show that LK method can be satisfactorily applied also for registration of sequences from low-cost experimental fundus camera.

The paper is organized as follows: Section 2 introduces our camera and image sequences, Section 3 describes the registration approach. The evaluation of registration is described in Section 4. Last two sections discuss our results and conclude the paper.

2   Image Acquisition and Image Properties

The fundus camera that was used to acquire the image data is designed as a low-cost device consisting of some components that are available on the mass market. It is a mobile lab demonstrator including a computer with a custom software for data recording, displaying of a live preview and controlling the fundus camera.

A new method called "stripe field imaging" [15] was realized and proved by the demonstrator. Compared to conventional fundus cameras based on ring illumination methods, there are improvements that partially compensate the loss in quality caused by the use of low-cost components. The demonstrator is capable of capturing colour images and videos from the human eye at pupil size of only 2 mm. Even with such small pupils it is possible to acquire a very large field of view (FOV). The geometry of the FOV is a square with a length of 68° and width of 18° (viewing angles). Such large FOVs at only 2 mm pupil diameter are not possible with the common used ring illumination method where only a circular FOV with a diameter of around 20° would be possible at a pupil diameter of 1.58 mm [16]. An eye piece intended for amateur telescopes was used to image the retina to an internal image plane. This plane was imaged by a C-mount lens ($f = 16$ mm) to an industry standard CCD (Sensor: Sony ICX274, monochrome, 1628x1236 pixels). The illumination was realized by a power LED module with three emitters producing red (625 nm), green (527 nm) and blue (470 nm) light, which are used sequentially for capturing three monochrome images. These are then combined to one colour image by image post-processing.

Several image artifacts were identified during acquisition of some "dark frames", where an absorber is placed instead of the eye. These frames can be averaged and typical artifacts caused by the optics inside the fundus camera can be identified and consequently eliminated using this "dark frames".

We tested the intensity SNR in different uniform areas and different acquired fundus images and sequences. We obtained values around 10 dB (evaluated as intensity SNR = 20log(mean/standard deviation)). The image SNR in fundus images acquired from professional camera is typically over 20 dB, as we tested on images from Canon CR-1 with Canon EOS 40D digital camera. Four examples of acquired images from different acquisitions (eyes) are given in Fig. 1. Typical image as well as very noisy, non-uniformly illuminated, as well as image with specific reflection artefacts are shown.

We tested our method on 5 experimental sequences with the number of frames from 39 to 179. We also checked the quality visually and we excluded images without any fundus structures (due to very strong reflections from cornea or because the object moved out of optical axis or out of focus).

3   Registration Approach

The registration approach consists of preprocessing and two main steps. The first step compensates the large shifts between consecutive images and the second step tracks blood vessels using basic optical flow method and compensates for small shift and rotation.

3.1   Sequence Preprocessing

The first necessary step is preprocessing of each frame in the sequence due to presence of non-uniform illumination and noise. The noise is eliminated using median filter with 3×3 kernel and is followed by contrast limited adaptive histogram equalization (CLAHE [17]), which has been successfully used in retinal applications dealing with fundus image processing, e.g. [18], [19]. This helps to

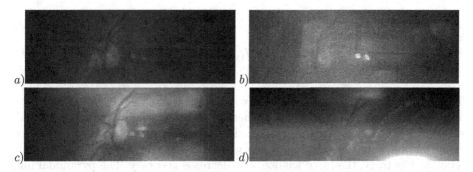

Fig. 1. a) Standard image quality with apparent low illumination; b) Noisy image with low reflection and high noise level; c,d) Images with artefacts due to light reflections from structures apart from retina.

increase the contrast of the blood vessels and equalize image illumination, see Fig. 4. We observed that using this preprocessing has positive influence on both registration steps.

3.2 Phase-Correlation Based Alignment

The first step of registration is based on phase correlation, which employs Fourier shift theorem [20]. Let $f_1(x, y)$ and $f_2(x, y)$ be two functions, which differ only by displacements x_0 and y_0. The normalized cross spectrum is computed using a complex conjugate (*) of one of the spectra (denoted as $F_1(u, v)$ and $F_2(u, v)$, respectively):

$$\frac{F_2(u, v)F_1(u, v)^*}{|F_2(u, v)F_1(u, v)^*|} = e^{-j(ux_0+vy_0)}. \tag{1}$$

Taking the inverse FT of the right hand side term leads to Dirac function $\delta(x - x_0, y - y_0)$ at the coordinates (x_0, y_0) defining the spatial shift [21]. This method has been used for long-term fundus image registration in our previous work together with model for rotation and scaling transformation [12]. Nevertheless, here we use only translation, because we suppose that rotation between frames is low. Furthermore, due to low SNR, it is difficult to estimate rotation by this method (as we had tested in preliminarily stage of this project).

3.3 Blood Vessels Tracking

Lucas-Kanade Tracking. After large shift compensation, Lucas-Kanade tracking is applied [22]. The goal of the tracking is to find, for given point $X_j = (x_j, y_j)$ in image I_i, corresponding point $X'_j = (x'_j, y'_j) = X_j + D_j$ in image I_{i+1}, using the assumption that the neighborhood of the point X_j is similar to the neighborhood of the point X'_j. The vector $D_j = (dx_j, dy_j)$ is referred as the optical flow at X_j and can be different for specific points X_j for $j = 1, 2, ...N$. Vector D_j minimizes the function:

$$\epsilon(D_j) = \sum_{x=x_j-w_{x_j}}^{x_j+w_{x_j}} \sum_{y=y_j-w_{y_j}}^{y_j+w_{y_j}} [I_i(x,y) - I_{i+1}(x+dx_j, y+dy_j)]^2 \; for \; j = 1,2,...N.$$

(2)

The w_x and w_y define the summation window of size $2w_x + 1, 2w_y + 1$ and usually (for isotropic pixel) $w_x = w_y$. There is a trade-off between accuracy and robustness when choosing the window size. Smaller window leads to capturing small motion, but the tracking is lost when the movement exceeds the search window. Contrary, the large window size decrease accuracy. The pyramidal implementation can partially reduce this drawback. Nevertheless, in our approach we used the basic version, because the large movements have been compensated by Fourier approach as described in previous section. Hence, the choice of w_x, w_y is not so critical. We set the windows size as $w_x = w_y = 10$, which corresponds to the estimated precision of Fourier-based alignment. This value also corresponds to the thickest blood vessels in acquired retinal scenes.

It should be noted that tracking only the blood vessels has some advantages. First, it should be more robust then tracking all pixels in the image, because there are various artefacts through the sequence (reflections of illumination light source, nonuniformity in illumination) and the noise level is relatively high. Second, there are regions without some (significant) structures, which would be difficult to track. And third, blood vessel tracking is faster than tracking of all pixels. The main disadvantage of this approach is a need of correctly segmented vascular tree (see next section).

Detection of Tracking Points. The detection of tracking point is crucial for successful optical flow registration. We apply this detection on randomly selected image in aligned sequence obtained in the first step, after application of median filter and CLAHE method.

Since the blood vessels appear in the filtered image mainly as a valley (darker than background), we can determine their position using Hessian matrix. This matrix of the second derivatives is defined as [23]:

$$H_{ij} = \begin{pmatrix} \partial_{xx}I(x,y) \; \partial_{xy}I(x,y) \\ \partial_{yx}I(x,y) \; \partial_{yy}I(x,y) \end{pmatrix}.$$

(3)

The Hessian has two real eigenvalues because $\partial_{yx}I(x,y) = \partial_{xy}I(x,y)$. This matrix and corresponding eigenvalues are computed for each pixel using Sobel difference operator. Since we are interested in image valleys, we take only the higher positive eigenvalue. This *parametric* (eigenvalue) image is further thresholded. The selection of threshold has been finally adjusted empirically (after testing several methods - Kittler, Otsu etc.). As the next step, the thresholding approach will be modified to be fully automatic. Small segmented regions are consequently removed as we assume that segmented blood vessels should create longer (i.e. larger) structures. Morphological thinning is finally used to obtain *skeleton* of the blood vessels. An example of segmentation results and skeleton image is shown in Fig. 2. White arrow indicates an artifact due to acquisition geometry, which has been masked out using "dark frames" as mentioned in Section 2. The number of tracking points is finally reduced by decimation of skeleton coordinates as there are hundreds of pixels to track in the vascular skeleton.

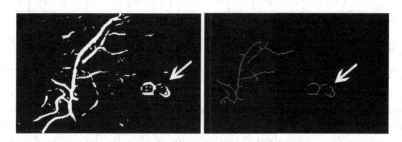

Fig. 2. Results of blood vessel segmentation in one frame (left) and corresponding skeleton image (right). The white arrows indicates position of segmented artefacts.

Spatial Transformation. Once the optical flow for each tracking point is determined, the transformation must be performed. We used shift and rotation:

$$\begin{bmatrix} x'_j \\ y'_j \end{bmatrix} = \begin{bmatrix} cos(\varphi) & -sin(\varphi) \\ sin(\varphi) & cos(\varphi) \end{bmatrix} \times \begin{bmatrix} x_j \\ y_j \end{bmatrix} + \begin{bmatrix} t_{x_j} \\ t_{y_j} \end{bmatrix}. \tag{4}$$

The minimization of:

$$\sum_{j=1}^{N} \left| \begin{pmatrix} x_j \\ y_j \end{pmatrix} - \begin{pmatrix} x'_j \\ y'_j \end{pmatrix} \right|^2 \to \min \tag{5}$$

is employed with respect to transformation parameters $\varphi, t_{x_j}, t_{y_j}$. This leads to overestimated set of linear equations, which can be easily solved by Gauss elimination method.

These steps provide estimation of transformation parameters, which are consequently applied on moving registered image. This minimization is iteratively applied on currently registered image until there is only small change in the value of transformation parameters (the minimum required change is 0.1 pixel for shifts and 0.01 radians for rotation).

3.4   Registration Evaluation

Proper evaluation is usually critical part of image registration techniques, in a case where gold standard datasets are not available. Here we evaluated the registered sequences with the help of intensity profiles extracted from the selected blood vessels. For registered sequence, the centre of the blood vessels should remain on the same position (denoted as a point P_{min}) and only small variation of

Table 1. Standard deviations computed for each sequence from positions of the minimum intensity point of blood vessel located in the central (Pc), inferior (Pi) and superior (Ps) part of the sequence. 'Final' row stands for final sequences; 'DFT' row stands for sequences after phase correlation.

	Sequence 1			Sequence 2			Sequence 3			Sequence 4			Sequence 5		
	Pc	Pi	Ps	Pc	Pi	Ps	Pc	Pi	Ps	Pc	Pi	Ps	Pc	Pi	Ps
Final	1.13	0.82	0.78	2.10	0.89	1.26	1.65	1.36	1.79	1.20	1.43	0.43	1.64	1.02	0.54
DFT	1.34	1.31	1.38	2.80	1.58	3.10	2.54	1.95	2.22	2.21	1.84	1.35	2.91	2.63	1.35
	39 frames			82 frames			179 frames			82 frames			95 frames		

thickness due to blood pulsation is observed. Therefore, we manually defined the position of intensity profiles through the blood vessels with high image contrast in each sequence and we evaluated the variation of P_{min} by the means of standard deviation. To be able to capture subpixel variations, interpolation with factor 8 has been applied on each profile. This has been evaluated in the three different positions of fundus - in optic disc (Pc) and in superior (Ps) and inferior (Pi) part of the blood vessel tree.

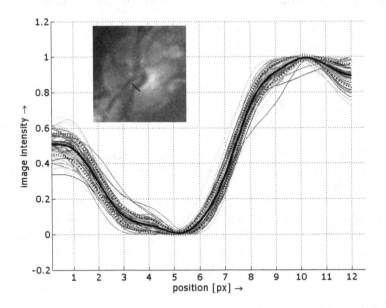

Fig. 3. Intensity profiles through one blood vessel from the centre of the optic disc (colour curves) as depicted on RGB image by blue line. The black profile represents the mean spatial profile with standard deviation (dotted black curves).

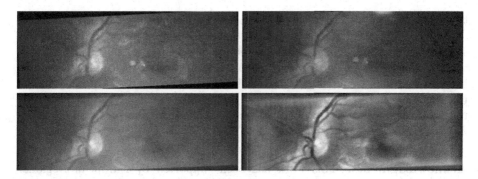

Fig. 4. Two images from Sequence 3 are shown at the top row. Averaged image after registration (left bottom) followed by CLAHE method application (right bottom) is presented.

4 Results and Discussion

We tested our method on five sequences of different length. The standard deviation of P_{min} is shown in Table 1 for registered sequence ('Final' row) and sequence after large shift compensation ('DFT' row). The values are below 2.1 pixels and the total mean value of standard deviations is 1.20 pixels for final sequences. The sequences after large shift compensation are under 3.1 pixels and the mean value is 2.03. This mean value of standard deviations can be viewed as the mean precision of registration. Therefore, we can conclude that the LK method improves the registration up to 1 pixel.

We can also observed from the Table 1 that there are not significant differences between different positions (Pc, Pi, Ps), which means that there is no systematic error. This also implies that selected spatial transformation is convenient for this task. The intensity profiles with the mean profile has also been plotted for subjective assessment of the registration results (see Fig. 3 as an example).

The registered sequences were averaged and SNR has been evaluated in each sequence within homogeneous regions. We obtained values around 20dB, which indicates 10dB improvement. An example of averaged sequence 2 is shown in Fig. 4. Small blurring is present due to limited precision of our method. However, it is obvious that more structures can be seen in averaged image, particularly after CLAHE method application.

5 Conclusion

The main purpose of this work was to prove that the proposed approach is convenient for the sequence from our experimental fundus camera. We showed that combination of Fourier approach together with basic Lucas-Kanade tracking method can be used with acceptable precision. There are still some parts, which must be solved to make this method more robust. The most important part in tracking is detection of tracking points, which utilizes segmentation of vascular tree using manually selected threshold in this work. In a spite of many published methods in retinal vessel segmentation, the segmentation in low SNR images is still challenging task. The automatic detection of 'bad' frames must also be solved to exclude the images with barely visible retinal structures from registration, because they don't contribute to overall quality of sequences. The selection of the reference or starting frame must also be included in the next step to improve the robustness. It is also probably possible to improve the precision by using different LK-based approaches, e.g. [24].

Acknowledgments. This work has been supported by European Regional Development Fund - Project FNUSA-ICRC (No.CZ.1.05/1.1.00/02.0123) under Ministry of Education, Youth and Sports. The authors also gratefully acknowledge funding of the Erlangen Graduate School in Advanced Optical Technologies (SAOT) by the German Research Foundation (DFG) in the framework of the German excellence initiative.

References

1. Kumar, D.K., Aliahmad, B., Hao, H., Che Azemin, M.Z., Kawasaki, R.: A method for visualization of fine retinal vascular pulsation using nonmydriatic fundus camera synchronized with electrocardiogram. ISRN Ophthalmology 2013, Article ID 865834 (January 2013)
2. Guyomard, J.L., Rosolen, S.G., Paques, M., Delyfer, M.N., Simonutti, M., Tessier, Y., Sahel, J.A., Legargasson, J.F., Picaud, S.: A low-cost and simple imaging technique of the anterior and posterior segments: eye fundus, ciliary bodies, iridocorneal angle. Investigative Ophthalmology & Visual Science 49(11), 5168–5174 (2008)
3. Tran, K., Mendel, T.A., Holbrook, K.L., Yates, P.A.: Construction of an inexpensive, hand-held fundus camera through modification of a consumer "point-and-shoot" camera. Investigative Ophthalmology & Visual Science 53(12), 7600–7607 (2012)
4. Haddock, L.J., Kim, D.Y., Mukai, S.: Simple, inexpensive technique for high-quality smartphone fundus photography in human and animal eyes. Journal of Ophthalmology 2013, Article ID 518479, 5 pages (2013)
5. Myung, D., Jais, A., He, L., Blumenkranz, M.S., Chang, R.T.: 3D Printed Smartphone Indirect Lens Adapter for Rapid, High Quality Retinal Imaging. Journal of Mobile Technology in Medicine 3(1), 9–15 (2014)
6. Ryan, N., Heneghan, C., de Chazal, P.: Registration of digital images using landmark correspondence by expectation maximization. Image and Vision Computing 22, 883–898 (2004)
7. Deng, K., Tian, J., Zheng, J., Zhang, X., Dai, X., Xu, M.: Retinal Fundus Image Registration via Vascular Structure Graph Matching. International Journal of Biomedical Imaging 2010, Article ID 906067, 13 pages (2010)
8. Ritter, N., Owens, R., Cooper, J., Eikelboom, R.H., Saarloos, P.P.: Registration of Stereo and Temporal Images of the Retina. IEEE Transaction on Medical Imaging 18(5), 404–418 (1999)
9. Kolar, R., Kubecka, L., Jan, J.: Registration and Fusion of the Autofluorescent and Infrared Retinal Images. International Journal of Biomedical Imaging 2008, Article ID 513478, 11 pages (2008)

10. Chanwimaluang, T., Fan, G., Fransen, S.R.: Hybrid Image Registration. IEEE Transactions on Information Technology in Biomedicine 10(1), 129–142 (2006)

11. Wang, W., Chen, H., Li, J., Yu, J.: A Registration Method of Fundus Images Based on Edge Detection and Phase-Correlation. In: International Conference on Innovative Computing, Information and Control, vol. 3, pp. 572–576. IEEE Computer Society, Los Alamitos (2006)

12. Kolar, R., Harabis, V., Odstrcilik, J.: Hybrid retinal image registration using phase correlation. The Imaging Science Journal 61(4), 369–384 (2013)

13. Giancardo, L., Meriaudeau, F., Karnowski, T.P., Tobin, K.W., Grisan, E., Favaro, P., Ruggeri, A., Chaum, E.: Textureless macula swelling detection with multiple retinal fundus images. IEEE Transactions on Biomedical Engineering 58(3), 795–799 (2011)

14. Li, H., Lu, J., Shi, G., Zhang, Y.: Tracking features in retinal images of adaptive optics confocal scanning laser ophthalmoscope using KLT-SIFT algorithm. Biomedical Optics Express 1(1), 31–40 (2010)

15. Hoeher, B., Voigtmann, P., Michelson, G., Schmauss, B.: Non-mydriatic, wide field, fundus video camera. In: Proc. SPIE 8930, Ophthalmic Technologies XXIV, p. 89300K (February 2014)

16. Pomerantzeff, O., Webb, R., Delori, F.C.: Image formation in fundus cameras. Investigative Ophthalmology and Visual Science 18(6), 630–637 (1979)

17. Pizer, S.M., Amburn, E.P., Austin, J.D., Cromartie, R., Geselowitz, A., Greer, T., ter Haar Romeny, B., Zimmerman, J.B., Zuiderveld, K.: Adaptive histogram equalization and its variations. Computer Vision, Graphics, and Image Processing 39(3), 355–368 (1987)

18. Bae, J.P., Kim, K.G., Kang, H.C., Jeong, C.B., Park, K.H., Hwang, J.M.: A study on hemorrhage detection using hybrid method in fundus images. Journal of Digital Imaging 24(3), 394–404 (2011)

19. Kolar, R., Tornow, R.P., Laemmer, R., Odstrcilik, J., Mayer, M.A., Gazarek, J., Jan, J., Kubena, T., Cernosek, P.: Analysis of Visual Appearance of Retinal Nerve Fibers in High Resolution Fundus Images: A Study on Normal Subjects. Computational and Mathematical Methods in Medicine 2013, Article ID 134543, 10 pages (2013)

20. Jan, J.: Digital signal filtering analysis and restoration. IEE Telecommunications Series 44 (2000)

21. Murat, B., Hassan, F.: Subpixel registration directly from the phase difference. EURASIP Journal on Applied Signal Processing 2006, Article ID 60796, 11 pages (2006)

22. Lucas, B.D., Kanade, T.: An Iterative Image Registration Technique with an Application to Stereo Vision. In: Proceedings of Imaging Understanding Workshop, vol. 130, pp. 121–130 (1981)

23. Trujillo, L., Olague, G.: Automated Design of Image Operators that Detect Interest Points. Evolutionary Computation 16(4), 483–507 (2008)

24. Dowson, N., Bowden, R.: Mutual information for Lucas-Kanade Tracking (MILK): an inverse compositional formulation. IEEE Transactions on Pattern Analysis and Machine Intelligence 30(1), 180–185 (2008)

Non-rigid Groupwise Image Registration for Motion Compensation in Quantitative MRI

Wyke Huizinga[1], Dirk H.J. Poot[1,2], Jean-Marie Guyader[1], Henk Smit[1],
Matthijs van Kranenburg[3,4], Robert-Jan M. van Geuns[3,4], André Uitterdijk[4],
Heleen M.M. van Beusekom[4], Bram F. Coolen[5], Alexander Leemans[6],
Wiro J. Niessen[1,2], and Stefan Klein[1]

[1] Biomedical Imaging Group Rotterdam, Depts. of Radiology & Medical Informatics,
Erasmus MC, Rotterdam, The Netherlands
[2] Quantitative Imaging Group, Dept. of Imaging Physics, Faculty of Applied
Sciences, Delft University of Technology, Delft, The Netherlands
[3] Department of Radiology, Erasmus MC, Rotterdam, The Netherlands
[4] Department of Cardiology, Erasmus MC, Rotterdam, The Netherlands
[5] Department of Radiology, Academic Medical Center, Amsterdam, The Netherlands
[6] Image Sciences Institute, University Medical Center Utrecht, The Netherlands

Abstract. Quantitative magnetic resonance imaging (qMRI) aims to extract quantitative parameters representing tissue properties from a series of images by modeling the image acquisition process. This requires the images to be spatially aligned but, due to patient motion, anatomical structures in the consecutive images may be misaligned. In this work, we propose a groupwise non-rigid image registration method for motion compensation in qMRI. The method minimizes a dissimilarity measure based on principal component analysis (PCA), exploiting the fact that intensity changes can be described by a low-dimensional acquisition model. Using an unbiased groupwise formulation of the registration problem, there is no need to choose a reference image as in conventional pairwise approaches. The method was evaluated on three applications: modified Look-Locker inversion recovery T_1 mapping in a porcine myocardium, black-blood variable flip-angle T_1 mapping in the carotid artery region, and apparent diffusion coefficient (ADC) mapping in the abdomen. The method was compared to a conventional pairwise alignment that uses a mutual information similarity measure. Registration accuracy was evaluated by computing precision of the estimated parameters of the qMRI model. The results show that the proposed method performs equally well or better than an optimized pairwise approach and is therefore a suitable motion compensation method for a wide variety of qMRI applications.

Keywords: groupwise image registration, quantitative MRI, motion compensation, T_1 mapping, ADC mapping, principal component analysis.

1 Introduction

Magnetic resonance images (MRI) can be acquired with different contrast weightings and together these images provide information about the anatomy, function

S. Ourselin and M. Modat (Eds.): WBIR 2014, LNCS 8545, pp. 184–193, 2014.
© Springer International Publishing Switzerland 2014

and pathology. In qMRI, quantitative parameters reflecting magnetic resonance tissue properties are estimated by fitting a parametric acquisition model to a series of contrast-weighted images. Examples are diffusion tensor MRI, ADC mapping, dynamic contrast-enhanced MRI and MR relaxometry (T_1 and T_2 mapping) [1].

Patient motion, e.g. breathing and heart pulsations, cause anatomical structures in consecutive images to be misaligned. However, the qMRI model assumes that the same tissue is present at a specific voxel in each of the images. If this is not the case, estimation of the tissue parameters will be corrupted. Therefore, aligning the images prior to parameter estimation is necessary and for this purpose image registration techniques can be employed.

Alignment is commonly achieved by a pairwise registration of all images to a reference image [2, 3]. The downside is that the result of the registration depends on the choice of reference image. Therefore, in case of a series of images, a groupwise registration, in which all images are aligned simultaneously, is preferable. It has previously been shown that groupwise image registration leads to more consistent results than a pairwise approach [4, 5], because a groupwise approach avoids a bias towards a reference image and takes into account the intensity information of all images simultaneously.

In literature several different groupwise registration approaches have been proposed, e.g. [4–8]. Metz et al. proposed a groupwise measure based on voxelwise variance [4]. Marsland et al. proposed minimum description length as a dissimilarity measure for groupwise image registration [5]. Wachinger et al. introduced a framework for multivariate similarity measures, in which the sum for all image pairs of a pairwise measure is used as a groupwise measure [6]. Miller et al. proposed a stack entropy cost function in which the sum of voxelwise entropies is used as an alignment criterion [8]. In previous work, we proposed a groupwise registration method for diffusion MRI data, using a dissimilarity measure based on PCA which minimizes a sum of eigenvalues [7]. Hamy et al. also used PCA for motion correction, but they used PCA to obtain the low-rank data components and used a residual complexity measure for registration [9].

In this article, we propose a groupwise non-rigid registration method for motion compensation in qMRI. In our approach we exploit that intensity changes are expected to behave according to a low-dimensional acquisition model, which is typically the case in qMRI. Because of the groupwise formulation of the registration, the need for choosing a reference image is eliminated. The method is based on our previous work [7], which focused on diffusion tensor MRI. We investigate whether the method can be applied to other types of qMRI, as in theory the method is not bound to a certain qMRI model. The method was applied to modified Look-Locker inversion recovery (MOLLI) T_1 mapping in an infarcted porcine myocardium, black-blood variable flip-angle (VFA) T_1 mapping in the carotid artery region, and ADC mapping in the abdomen. Whereas in [7] only used affine transformations were used, we use a B-spline transformation model that can account for the non-rigid deformations.

2   Method

2.1   Groupwise Registration Framework

We use a parametric registration approach, where the transformation is modeled by a set of parameters $\boldsymbol{\mu}$. Let $M_g(\boldsymbol{x})$ be a series of G images, acquired in a qMRI experiment, with $g \in \{1 \ldots G\}$ and $\boldsymbol{x}$ a 2D or 3D spatial coordinate and let $\mathbf{T}_g(\boldsymbol{x}; \boldsymbol{\mu}_g)$ be a transformation applied to image $\mathrm{M}_g(\boldsymbol{x})$, parameterized by parameters $\boldsymbol{\mu}_g$. The transform parameters for each separate volume $\boldsymbol{\mu}_g$ are concatenated into one parameter vector $\boldsymbol{\mu} = \left(\boldsymbol{\mu}_1^{\mathrm{T}}, \boldsymbol{\mu}_2^{\mathrm{T}}, \ldots, \boldsymbol{\mu}_G^{\mathrm{T}}\right)^{\mathrm{T}}$. We formulate groupwise registration as the minimization of a dissimilarity measure $\mathcal{D}$ with respect to $\boldsymbol{\mu}$:

$$\hat{\boldsymbol{\mu}} = \arg \min_{\boldsymbol{\mu}} \mathcal{D}(\boldsymbol{\mu}). \tag{1}$$

In this process all images M_g are aligned simultaneously. The transformation is modeled with a cubic B-spline [10], in which the parameter vector $\boldsymbol{\mu}_g$ is formed by the elements of the B-spline control point coefficients. The control point spacing ν is application dependent and defined by the user.

2.2   qMRI Acquisition Models

In qMRI the intensity at $\boldsymbol{x}$ for each image M_g is predicted by an acquisition model m_g:

$$M_g(\boldsymbol{x}) = m_g(\boldsymbol{\theta}(\boldsymbol{x})), \tag{2}$$

where $\boldsymbol{\theta}$ is a vector with l tissue parameters at coordinate $\boldsymbol{x}$. The m_g functions for the three different datasets used in this paper are given below. The first dataset is acquired with a MOLLI sequence and hence the expected intensity is governed by a inversion recovery T_1 model [11] (T1MOLLI), which is given by:

$$m_g(\boldsymbol{\theta}(\boldsymbol{x})) = \left| A(\boldsymbol{x}) - B(\boldsymbol{x}) e^{-TI_g/T_1^*(\boldsymbol{x})} \right| \text{ with } \boldsymbol{\theta}(\boldsymbol{x}) = (A(\boldsymbol{x}), B(\boldsymbol{x}), T_1^*(\boldsymbol{x})), \tag{3}$$

where TI_g is the inversion time for image M_g. The parameter of interest, $T_1(\boldsymbol{x})$ can be calculated from A, B and T_1^* [11]. The second dataset is acquired with a black-blood VFAT1 sequence [12] with predicted intensity:

$$m_g(\boldsymbol{\theta}(\boldsymbol{x})) = \left| A(\boldsymbol{x}) \sin(\alpha_g) \frac{1 - e^{-TR/T_1(\boldsymbol{x})}}{1 - \cos(\alpha_g) e^{-TR/T_1(\boldsymbol{x})}} e^{-TE_g/T_2(\boldsymbol{x})} \right|, \tag{4}$$

with $\boldsymbol{\theta}(\boldsymbol{x}) = (A(\boldsymbol{x}), T_1(\boldsymbol{x}), T_2(\boldsymbol{x}))$. α_g is the flip-angle and TE_g the echo time per image M_g and TR the repetition time. The last dataset is acquired with an ADC sequence, with the predicted intensity:

$$m_g(\boldsymbol{\theta}(\boldsymbol{x})) = B_0(\boldsymbol{x}) e^{-b_g \boldsymbol{u}_g^{\mathrm{T}} \mathbf{D}(\boldsymbol{x}) \boldsymbol{u}_g} \tag{5}$$

with $\boldsymbol{\theta}(\boldsymbol{x}) = (B_0(\boldsymbol{x}), D_{11}(\boldsymbol{x}), D_{22}(\boldsymbol{x}), D_{33}(\boldsymbol{x}))$ and $\boldsymbol{u}_g$ is a vector in the direction of the applied gradient. $\mathbf{D}(\boldsymbol{x})$ is a 3×3 symmetric diffusion tensor, where for the purpose of ADC mapping only its diagonal needs to be considered, b_g is the so-called b-value and the ADC is given by ADC = trace($\mathbf{D}$)/3.

For all models, the qMRI parameters $\theta(x)$ are estimated by fitting the model m_g to the measured intensities M_g. The number of images acquired for qMRI is usually higher than the number of qMRI model parameters that need to be estimated. This is done to obtain a more precise estimation of the qMRI model parameters.

2.3 Dissimilarity Measure

In this section the groupwise dissimilarity measure is presented. Let the images M_g be represented as columns of an $N \times G$ matrix $\mathbf{M}$, where N is the number of voxels in one image M_g. A row of $\mathbf{M}$ can be considered as a data point in a G-dimensional space. In a zero noise setting it is expected that these data points actually lie in a non-linear l-dimensional subspace, where l is the number of free qMRI model parameters (the dimension of θ). The correlation matrix of the data points in $\mathbf{M}$ is defined as:

$$\mathbf{K} = \frac{1}{N-1}\mathbf{S}^{-1}\left(\mathbf{M} - \overline{\mathbf{M}}\right)^{\mathrm{T}}\left(\mathbf{M} - \overline{\mathbf{M}}\right)\mathbf{S}^{-1}, \tag{6}$$

where $\mathbf{S}$ is a diagonal matrix with the standard deviations of each column of $\mathbf{M}$ as diagonal elements and $\overline{\mathbf{M}}$ is a matrix with in each column the column-wise average of $\mathbf{M}$. The dimension of the subspace can be determined by an eigenvalue decomposition of $\mathbf{K}$ i.e., by a PCA. The key idea behind the proposed dissimilarity measure is that, when motion is present in the images, the data no longer adheres to the presumed acquisition model and the eigenvalue spectrum of $\mathbf{K}$ changes.

To illustrate how motion can affect the eigenvalue spectrum of $\mathbf{K}$, we created a synthetic image based on the T1MOLLI model. The relative eigenvalue spectrum of $\mathbf{K}$ is shown in Fig. 1 for both a perfectly aligned series of images and for the same series artificially deformed. In the aligned case the first 3 eigenvectors capture 100% of the data variance, but in the misaligned case, the first 3 eigenvectors capture only 88% of the data variance.

The aim is to transform the images M_g such that the eigenvalue spectrum of $\mathbf{K}$ approaches the spectrum of an aligned set of images. Let λ_j be the jth eigenvalue of $\mathbf{K}$, then our dissimilarity measure is defined as:

$$\mathcal{D}_{\mathrm{PCA}}(\boldsymbol{\mu}) = \sum_{g=1}^{G} \mathrm{K}_{gg}(\boldsymbol{\mu}) - \sum_{j=1}^{L} \lambda_j(\boldsymbol{\mu}) = G - \sum_{j=1}^{L} \lambda_j(\boldsymbol{\mu}), \tag{7}$$

where the dependence on $\boldsymbol{\mu}$ has been made explicit to clarify that $\mathbf{K}$ (and thus λ_j) is computed based on the deformed images $M_g(\mathbf{T}_g(x;\boldsymbol{\mu}_g))$. The constant $1 \leq L \leq G$ is a user-defined parameter. For different models, a different value of L must be chosen. A good initial guess is $L = l$, assuming that the non-linear l-dimensional subspace can be approximated by an l-dimensional hyperplane.

2.4 Optimization

For minimization with gradient-based optimizers the derivative of $\mathcal{D}$ with respect to $\boldsymbol{\mu}$ must be known, which was derived in [7]. An adaptive stochastic gradient

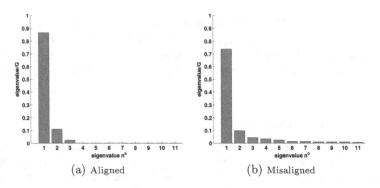

(a) Aligned   (b) Misaligned

Fig. 1. Eigenvalue spectra for aligned and misaligned synthetic T1MOLLI data

descent optimization method is used [13], which randomly samples positions in image space at each iteration in order to reduce computation time and interpolation artifacts [14]. A conventional multi-resolution strategy is used. The number of random samples, the number of resolution levels, and the number of iterations per resolution level are user-defined parameters. The average deformation of the images is constrained to be zero by the approach of Balci *et al.* [15]: the average derivative of the dissimilarity measure with respect to its parameters μ_g is subtracted from each derivative to μ_g, i.e. the derivatives are centered to zero mean.

$$\frac{\partial \mathcal{D}^*}{\partial \mu_g} = \frac{\partial \mathcal{D}}{\partial \mu_g} - \frac{1}{G} \sum_{g'} \frac{\partial \mathcal{D}}{\partial \mu_{g'}}. \tag{8}$$

where $\partial \mathcal{D}^*/\partial \mu_g$ is the zero-centered derivative. Linear interpolation is used to interpolate the images during registration, to limit computation time. Cubic B-spline interpolation was used to produce the final deformed images.

3 Experiments

3.1 Data

Experiments were performed with three qMRI applications: T_1 mapping in the myocardium of a porcine heart (T1MOLLI-HEART), T_1 mapping in the carotid artery region (VFAT1-CAROTID) and ADC mapping in the abdomen (ADC-ABDOMEN). Figure 2 shows example images.

The T1MOLLI-HEART datasets were obtained using single-slice acquisition, from porcine hearts with transmural myocardial infarction of the lateral wall. For each of the nine subjects 11 images were acquired, with inversion times $TI_g \in \{94, 784, 1473, 163, 853, 1542, 266, 956, 1646, 2335, 3025\}$ ms. The voxel spacing was 0.70×0.70 mm^2 with slight differences between the datasets due to changes in field of view. The acquisition matrix was equal to 128×128 and the slice thickness of 6 mm.

The VFAT1-CAROTID data was acquired with a 3D iMSDE prepared black-blood TFE sequence [12]. For each acquisition, five images were acquired with an isotropic voxel spacing of 0.7mm: one anatomical reference TFE scan and four

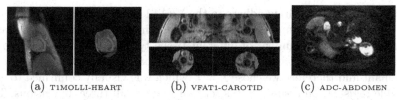

(a) T1MOLLI-HEART   (b) VFAT1-CAROTID   (c) ADC-ABDOMEN

Fig. 2. Example images and registration masks. (a) a short axis slice of a T1MOLLI-HEART dataset, (b) a slice of a VFAT1-CAROTID dataset, (c) a slice of an ADC-ABDOMEN dataset

scans with varying α_g and TE_g. The echo times were $TE_g \in \{11.5, 11.5, 26, 45\}$ ms, the flip-angles were $\alpha_g \in \{4, 15, 15, 15\}$ and the repetition time was $TR = 10$ ms for $g = 2\dots5$. The acquisition matrix was equal to $224{\times}223{\times}36$. Unfortunately, it proved difficult to perform accurate voxelwise T_2 fits on the variable TE data, regardless of the registration strategy, therefore we only report evaluations of T_1 values. The anatomical scan was not used for T_1 quantification. Four subjects were scanned twice, resulting in eight VFAT1-CAROTID datasets.

The ADC-ABDOMEN data was acquired using multi-slice acquisition, with three orthogonal gradient directions, aligned with the read, phase and slice directions. In each acquisition $b_g \in \{0, 100, 150, 200, 300, 500, 900\}$ [mm^2/s]. The voxel spacing was $1.48{\times}1.48{\times}5.00$ mm^3 and the acquisition matrix was equal to $128{\times}112{\times}40$. Five subjects were scanned four times in a single scan session, providing 20 ADC-ABDOMEN datasets. Before further processing, within-image motion artifacts due to interleaved acquisition were corrected [16]. All volumes except the $b_g = 0$ [mm^2/s] were used in ADC quantification.

3.2   Image Registration Settings

All datasets were registered with the proposed groupwise method using the measure $\mathcal{D}_{\mathrm{PCA}}$ and with a pairwise approach using the MI measure $\mathcal{D}_{\mathrm{MI}}$. The proposed method was implemented in the publicly available registration package Elastix [14]. For both methods the number of iterations per resolution was 1000 and the number of spatial samples was 2048.

The T1MOLLI-HEART data was registered with a mask (see Fig. 2(a)), loosely drawn around the cardiac region, to reduce influence of surrounding organs. For $\mathcal{D}_{\mathrm{PCA}}$ we chose $L = l = 3$, and ν was set to 32 mm in both dimensions. We observed that the choice of reference image was of high influence on the results when using $\mathcal{D}_{\mathrm{MI}}$. Therefore, we repeated all experiments using M_g with $g \in \{1, 4, 7, 11\}$ as reference images, and report the results for all cases.

The VFAT1-CAROTID data was registered with two different masks, around the left and right carotid artery (see Fig. 2(b)). For $\mathcal{D}_{\mathrm{PCA}}$ we chose $L = l = 3$. Visual inspection of the registration results of the VFAT1-CAROTID data showed that $\mathcal{D}_{\mathrm{PCA}}$ led to misregistrations with $L = 3$. Possible explanations for this are the following. Firstly, the range of used echo times was small compared to the typical T_2 in both ROIs, which affects the expected eigenvalue spectrum of $\mathbf{K}$. Secondly, the anatomical scan, which was taken into account in the groupwise registration, does not entirely adhere to the VFAT1 model, which can give a different eigenvalue spectrum of $\mathbf{K}$ than expected. Finally, the registration masks were small causing the number of different tissue types within the masks to be limited. All these issues can cause the first principal component of the data to be dominant and therefore we chose $L = 1$, which was visually confirmed to give acceptable registration results. ν was set to 15 mm in all three dimensions. The chosen reference image for $\mathcal{D}_{\mathrm{MI}}$ was the anatomical scan.

For the ADC-ABDOMEN data $L = l = 4$ was used for $\mathcal{D}_{\mathrm{PCA}}$. ν was set to a relatively coarse setting of 150 mm in all three dimensions, because the $\mathcal{D}_{\mathrm{MI}}$ approach lead to misregistrations for a lower value of ν. The chosen reference image for $\mathcal{D}_{\mathrm{MI}}$ was the $b_g = 0$ image. No mask was used for registration.

3.3   Evaluation Method

In all experiments the result of $\mathcal{D}_{\mathrm{PCA}}$ was transformed to the space of the $\mathcal{D}_{\mathrm{MI}}$ reference image, using the inverse transformation $T_{g^\dagger}(\boldsymbol{x}; \mu_{g^\dagger})$ with $g^\dagger$ indicating the reference image. In this space, $\boldsymbol{\theta}$ was estimated with a maximum-likelihood (ML) estimator that takes the Rician noise of MRI data into account [17]. The uncertainty of $\boldsymbol{\theta}$ was quantified by the Cramér–Rao lower bound (CRLB), which gives a lower bound for the variance of the ML estimated parameters [17–19]. To use the CRLB as indicator of misalignment we adopt the measure proposed by Bron *et al.* [3], which is the 90% percentile of the square root of the CRLB (90%CRLB$_\sigma$) over a region of interest (ROI). This measure identifies misalignment, since, especially at tissue boundaries, misalignment may result in biologically implausible values of the estimated parameters. Additionally, the model will fit less accurately to the data, resulting in a higher estimated noise level and thus CRLB [3]. The 90%CRLB$_\sigma$ for all datasets and all three cases (no registration (-), $\mathcal{D}_{\mathrm{MI}}$ and $\mathcal{D}_{\mathrm{PCA}}$) were calculated in manually specified ROIs.

In the T1MOLLI-HEART data the myocardial region of interest (ROI) was drawn on each image that was chosen as a reference image for the $\mathcal{D}_{\mathrm{MI}}$ measure. In the VFAT1-CAROTID data the walls of both arteries were annotated as ROIs. The mean of the 90%CRLB$_\sigma$ over the two ROIs is reported. In the

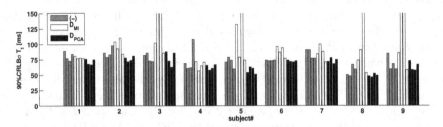

Fig. 3. 90%CRLB$_\sigma$ results for the T1MOLLI-HEART data in the myocardium. Note that the maximum of the y-axis is 500 ms, but some bars are higher. The four bars with equal color for each subject correspond to the four reference spaces. The typical T_1 in the ROI was 859 ms.

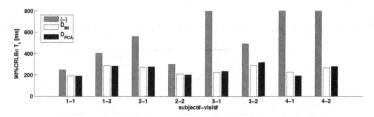

Fig. 4. The mean 90%CRLB$_\sigma$ for T_1 estimation over the two carotid artery wall regions of the VFAT1-CAROTID data. The typical T_1 was 901 ms. Note that the maximum of the y-axis is 800 ms, but some bars are higher in case of not using registration.

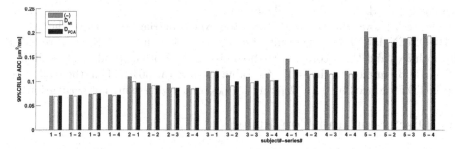

Fig. 5. 90%CRLB$_\sigma$ results with ADC-ABDOMEN data for a ROI at the boundary of the liver and the kidney. ADC values in the ROI ranged between $0.70 - 2.40$ $\mu m^2/ms$.

ADC-ABDOMEN a spherical region at the boundary of the kidney and the liver was annotated as ROI. Note that the ROIs where the alignment was evaluated were different from the masks that were used for registration.

For the ADC-ABDOMEN four series per acquisition session were available, providing the opportunity to measure the experimental reproducibility of the model fit. The experimental reproducibility was quantified by evaluating the 90% percentile of standard deviation (90%STD) of the ADC values in the ROI over the four series of the abdomen. To this end all series were registered to the space of the scans of the first series, using an additional pairwise registration between the $b_g = 0$ images.

4   Results

Figure 3 shows the 90%CRLB$_\sigma$ of the T_1 for the three cases (no registration (-), $\mathcal{D}_{MI}$ and $\mathcal{D}_{PCA}$) of the T1MOLLI-HEART data of the nine subjects in the annotated ROIs. The results show that 90%CRLB$_\sigma$ for the results of $\mathcal{D}_{MI}$ highly depends on the chosen reference image. Visually, the scan with the longest inversion time, i.e. image M_{11}, depicts anatomy most clearly. In most cases, the best result is indeed obtained when the 11th image in the series is set as a reference image. In most cases the best result is obtained when the 11th image in the series is set as a reference image. The $\mathcal{D}_{PCA}$ shows the most stable results over the four reference spaces and it also shows the lowest overall 90%CRLB$_\sigma$.

Table 1. Experimental reproducibility of the ADC value in the ROI of the ADC-ABDOMEN data

	subject#				
	1	2	3	4	5
90%STD (-) [μm^2/ms]	0.32	0.92	0.74	0.78	0.48
90%STD $\mathcal{D}_{MI}$ [μm^2/ms]	0.29	0.48	0.61	0.57	0.41
90%STD $\mathcal{D}_{PCA}$ [μm^2/ms]	0.31	0.43	0.64	0.40	0.41

Figure 4 shows the mean 90%CRLB$_\sigma$ of the T_1 in the annotated ROIs for the eight cases of the VFAT1-CAROTID data. The mean 90%CRLB$_\sigma$ is reduced by both $\mathcal{D}_{MI}$ and $\mathcal{D}_{PCA}$ compared to using no registration. Both methods led to a similar 90%CRLB$_\sigma$ in almost all subjects.

Figure 5 shows the 90%CRLB$_\sigma$ of the ADC for the 20 cases of the ADC-ABDOMEN data. From the results it can be seen that the 90%CRLB$_\sigma$ is reduced by both $\mathcal{D}_{MI}$ and $\mathcal{D}_{PCA}$ compared to no registration. Both methods led to a similar 90%CRLB$_\sigma$ in most of the subjects. Table 1 shows the 90%STD in the ROI. The 90%STD is reduced by both $\mathcal{D}_{MI}$ and $\mathcal{D}_{PCA}$ compared to using no registration.

5   Discussion and Conclusion

The results of the T1MOLLI-HEART data showed that $\mathcal{D}_{MI}$ failed for some reference images, whereas the proposed method $\mathcal{D}_{PCA}$ consistently performed well, which is an advantage of the groupwise approach. The results of the VFAT1-CAROTID and the ADC-ABDOMEN data showed that both $\mathcal{D}_{MI}$ and $\mathcal{D}_{PCA}$ led to a (similar) improvement in precision of the fitted tissue parameters, compared to using no registration.

For the VFAT1-CAROTID data the initial $L = l = 3$ was changed to $L = 1$ since apparently the chosen acquisition settings and relatively small registration mask led to only 1 dominant eigenvector. On all qMRI datasets the other registration settings (ν, number of spatial samples, number of iterations) were optimized for $\mathcal{D}_{MI}$ and it is a question for further research to investigate if settings optimized for $\mathcal{D}_{PCA}$ can further improve the results of the proposed approach.

In this work, a B-spline transformation model was used, however, the proposed method can be implemented with other transformation models as well.

In conclusion, we presented a groupwise image registration method using a PCA-based dissimilarity measure that was designed for the alignment of qMRI images. It has been shown that the approach performs as good as or better than a MI-based pairwise approach. Notably, the result of the pairwise method highly depends on the chosen reference image. This disadvantage is eliminated in the groupwise approach. The proposed method is therefore a suitable model-free approach for the registration of qMRI data.

Acknowledgments. We would like to thank L. Bernardin and N. Douglas for providing the ADC-ABDOMEN data. This project has received funding from the European Union's Seventh Framework Programme for research, technological development and demonstration under grant agreement no. 601055.

References

1. Tofts, P.: Quantitative MRI of the Brain: Measuring Changes Caused by Disease. John Wiley & Sons (2003)
2. Mangin, J.F., et al.: Distortion correction and robust tensor estimation for MR diffusion imaging. Med. Image Anal. 6, 191–198 (2002)
3. Bron, E., et al.: Image registration improves human knee cartilage T1 mapping with delayed gadolinium-enhanced MRI of cartilage (dGEMRIC). Eur. Radiol. 23, 246–252 (2013)
4. Metz, C.T., et al.: Nonrigid registration of dynamic medical imaging data using nD+t B-splines and a groupwise optimization approach. Med. Image Anal. 15, 238–249 (2010)
5. Marsland, S., et al.: A minimum description length objective function for groupwise non-rigid image registration. Image Vis. Comput. 26, 333–346 (2008)
6. Wachinger, C., et al.: Simultaneous registration of multiple images: Similarity metrics and efficient optimization. IEEE Trans. Pattern Anal. Mach. Intell. 7, 667–674 (2012)
7. Huizinga, W., et al.: Groupwise registration in diffusion weighted MRI for correcting subject motion and eddy current distortions using a PCA based dissimilarity metric. In: Computational Diffusion MRI and Brain Connectivity - MICCAI Workshops, pp. 163–174 (2013)
8. Miller, E., et al.: Learning from one example through shared densities on transforms. In: Proceedings of the IEEE Conference on Computer Vision and Pattern Recognition, vol. 1, pp. 464–471 (2000)
9. Hamy, V., et al.: Respiratory motion correction in dynamic MRI using robust data decomposition registration - Application to DCE-MRI. Med. Image Anal. 18, 301–313 (2013)
10. Rueckert, D., et al.: Nonrigid registration using free-form deformations: Application to breast MR images. IEEE Trans. Med. Imag. 18, 712–721 (1999)
11. Messroghli, D.R., et al.: Modified Look-Locker Inversion recovery (MOLLI) for high-resolution T1 mapping of the heart. Magn. Reson. Med. 52, 141–146 (2004)
12. Coolen, B.F., et al.: 3D carotid wall T1 quantification using variable flip angle 3D merge with steady-state recovery. In: Proc. Annu. Meet. ISMRM (2013)
13. Klein, S., et al.: Adaptive stochastic gradient descent optimization for image registration. Int. J. Comput. Vis. 81, 227–239 (2009)
14. Klein, S., et al.: Elastix: a toolbox for intensity based medical image registration. IEEE Trans. Med. Imag. 29, 196–205 (2010)
15. Balci, S., et al.: Free-form B-spline deformation model for groupwise registration. In: Proc. Stat. Regis. Workshop - MICCAI, pp. 23–30 (2007)
16. Guyader, J.M., Bernardin, L., Douglas, N., Poot, D., Niessen, W., Klein, S.: Influence of image registration on adc images computed from free-breathing diffusion mris of the abdomen. In: SPIE Medical Imaging (2014)
17. Sijbers, J., et al.: Parameter estimation from magnitude MR images. Int. J. Imag. Syst. Tech. 10, 109–114 (1999)
18. Cavassila, et al.: Cramér-Rao bounds: an evaluation tool for quantitation. NMR Biomed. 14, 278–283 (2001)
19. Rao, C.R.: Minimum variance and the estimation of several parameters. Proc. Cambridge Phil. Soc. 43, 280–283 (1946)

4D Liver Ultrasound Registration

Jyotirmoy Banerjee[1,2], Camiel Klink[1], Edward D. Peters[2], Wiro J. Niessen[1,2], Adriaan Moelker[1], and Theo van Walsum[1,2]

[1] Dept. of Radiology, Erasmus MC, Rotterdam, The Netherlands
[2] Dept. of Medical Informatics, Erasmus MC, Rotterdam, The Netherlands
{j.banerjee,t.vanwalsum}@erasmusmc.nl

Abstract. In this paper we present a rigid registration approach for 4D ultrasound (US) datasets, where images are registered over time. The 3D registration approach preceding the 4D registration consists of two main steps - block-matching and outlier rejection. The outlier rejection step removes the spurious matchings' from the block-matching module and ensures inverse consistency. For 4D registration, we perform registration of consecutive US volumes over the time series. Transformation between any two frames is estimated by taking the product of all the intermediate transforms. To avoid accumulation of error over the series of transformations, a long range feedback mechanism is proposed. A mean total registration error of 1 mm is achieved across six 4D ultrasound sequences of human liver with an execution speed of 10 Hz.

1 Introduction

Motivation : Ultrasound (US) is a unique imaging modality. Unlike computed tomography (CT) and magnetic resonance imaging (MRI), it is mobile and real-time. This is a desired combination in diagnostic and interventional setup. With the advent of 4D ultrasound, volumes of human anatomy can be visualized in real-time. Interoperative imaging using 4D ultrasound has huge potential in minimally invasive surgery of the liver. Image registration is a basic requirement in these applications and they aid in image stabilization for better visualization. A group wise 4D registration approach takes a stack of US volumes to perform the registration over the time series [1]. This approach is benefited from looking at US volumes in hindsight and is suited for offline processes as they have high computational and storage cost. A more dynamic approach would be to register images in streaming 4D US data. In this scenario, registrations are required to be up to date until the current time point, appending the registration results of the subsequent US frame. Given the registration results for the left half of the time axis the challenge is to move forward in time, keeping the registration up to date. A typical 3D US registration method when extended in the time domain is likely to face the following challenges -

- Due to motion (probe, patient or breathing), the region of interest might undergo large displacements, resulting in small overlap between the US frames.

S. Ourselin and M. Modat (Eds.): WBIR 2014, LNCS 8545, pp. 194–202, 2014.

- Over time small errors in the 3D registration could accumulate, yielding widely diverging outcomes.
- Continuous input stream of US volumes induces heavy computational and storage burden on the registration approach.

Related work : Image registration is the process of determining the geometrical transformation that aligns the moving image to the fixed image. 4D registration extends this notion in the temporal domain. Group wise 4D US registration was addressed by Vijayan et al. [1], where spatial and temporal smoothness of the transformations are enforced by using a temporal free-form deformation (TFFD) model. Shi et al. [2] extend the TFFD model with a sparse representation and use it to recover smooth motion from time sequence of cardiac US images. Øye et al. [3] propose a method to perform real time image registration on streaming 4D ultrasound data, and use it to deduce the positioning of each ultrasound frame in a global coordinate system. In this paper, the 3D registration framework which is precursor to our 4D registration approach is part of an existing work submitted to a journal. In this work we extend the previous registration framework, to address the issues related to the 4D US registration problem.

Our Contributions : In this paper we present a 4D registration approach which unlike the group wise approaches performs registration dynamically. First, to maximize the chance of overlap between the contents of the frames, we register consecutive frames in time. In order to have a robust registration an inverse consistency criteria is enforced. This ensures consistency between the forward backward transforms. Second, the inverse consistency criteria helps the preprocessing (which in our case is the block-matching scheme) done in a parallel fashion. Third, to neutralize or reduce the accumulation of registration errors over the time series, we propose a feedback mechanism over a time gap.

2   Method

2.1   3D Registration

The 3D registration approach is based on block-matching [4]. For a collection of points from the fixed images the block-matching gives a set of correspondences in the moving image. As US images are poor in quality, the correspondences may have lots of spurious matches. We remove the false matches using an outlier rejection module. A game-theoretic matching approach, similar to [5], is employed to reject the false matches[1]. The true matches are further used to estimate the rigid transformation using Arun's et al. least-squares registration algorithm [6].

---

[1] This approach of performing registration {a) point selection b) block-matching and c) game theory based outlier rejection} is part of an existing work (submitted). Our contribution in this paper is to extend the method to forward-backward (or inverse consistency based) registration.

2.2   4D Registration

Let $P = \{p_i\}$ and $Q = \{q_i\}$ where $0 < i \leq n$, be the set of locations from fixed volume and moving volume, respectively. We have a one to one correspondence between the point sets from the block-matching. Let a mapping $M \subseteq P \times Q$ represent potential correspondence from the point set P to Q; and similarly in the reverse direction a mapping $N \subseteq Q' \times P'$ represent potential correspondence from the point set $Q' = \{q'_i\}$ to $P' = \{p'_i\}$. Ideally if all the points are tracked well both in the forward and the backward directions then $\forall i \; p'_i = p_i \Rightarrow q'_i = q_i$ and vice-versa (*Inverse consistency*). Note that we choose the point sets P and Q', independently. This has two advantages, first, inverse consistency is not enforced explicitly, and second, the block-matching can be executed in parallel. Later we show how we incorporate the inverse consistency in an implicit way. Further as the point sets are from volumes representing the same anatomical structure, the geometric distance between the points should be preserved (*Geometric consistency*). A point q_i in the moving volume that preserves the geometric distances with most of the other points in the same set Q and their corresponding p_i and p'_i are in close proximity, have a better chance of being an inlier. The criteria of preserving the geometric distances, similar to [7] and the inverse consistency criteria forms the basis of our outlier rejection scheme.

The geometric consistency information can be embedded in a graph structure and can be represented as two affinity matrices (*forward*):

$$A_{i,j} = \begin{cases} e^{-\delta_{ij}^2/2\sigma^2} & \text{if } i \neq j \\ 0 & \text{else} \end{cases}, \tag{1}$$

where $\delta_{ij} = (\|q_i - q_j\| - \|p_i - p_j\|)$; and (*backward*),

$$B_{i,j} = \begin{cases} e^{-\delta'^2_{ij}/2\sigma^2} & \text{if } i \neq j \\ 0 & \text{else} \end{cases}, \tag{2}$$

where $\delta'_{ij} = (\|p'_i - p'_j\| - \|q'_i - q'_j\|)$.

For ensuring an inverse consistency in an implicit way, we combine the forward and backward block-matching information into a single graph. This is done by combining the matrix A and B into a symmetric matrix G as follows (*forward-backward*):

$$G = \begin{bmatrix} A \mid C^T \\ - \quad - \\ C \mid B \end{bmatrix}, \tag{3}$$

where the matrix C is given as:

$$C_{i,j} = e^{-\delta''^2_{ij}/2\sigma^2}, \tag{4}$$

where $\delta''_{ij} = (\|q_i - q'_j\| - \|p_i - p'_j\|)$.

Given a vector $\mathbf{x}$ defining the probability of points in $\{P, Q'\}$ being an inlier, we try to find a vector $\mathbf{x}$ that maximizes $\mathcal{F}$:

$$\max \mathcal{F}(\mathbf{x}) = \mathbf{x} \cdot G \mathbf{x} \qquad \text{subject to} \quad \mathbf{x} \in \Delta, \tag{5}$$

where $\Delta = \{\mathbf{x} \in \mathbb{R}^n : x_i \geq 0$ and $\sum_{i=1}^{n} x_i = 1\}$. Finding the internal nodes or the inliers corresponds to the notion of a dominant set [8].

Equation 5 can be optimized (local optimum) using replicator dynamics [8][9]. The replicator dynamics update equation to maximize a energy term of the form $\mathbf{x} \cdot G\mathbf{x}$, subject to $\mathbf{x} \in \Delta$ is:

$$x_i(t+1) = x_i(t) \frac{(G\mathbf{x}(t))_i}{\mathbf{x}(t) \cdot G\mathbf{x}(t)} \, , \qquad (6)$$

where x_i is the ith term of $\mathbf{x}$. The equation ensures that $\forall t, \mathbf{x}(t) \in \Delta$. Equation 1, Equation 2 and Equation 6 are part from our previous work (submitted).

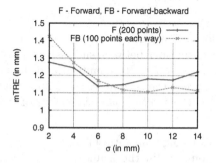

Fig. 1. Pairwise 3D Registration for various values of σ (See equation 1, 4)

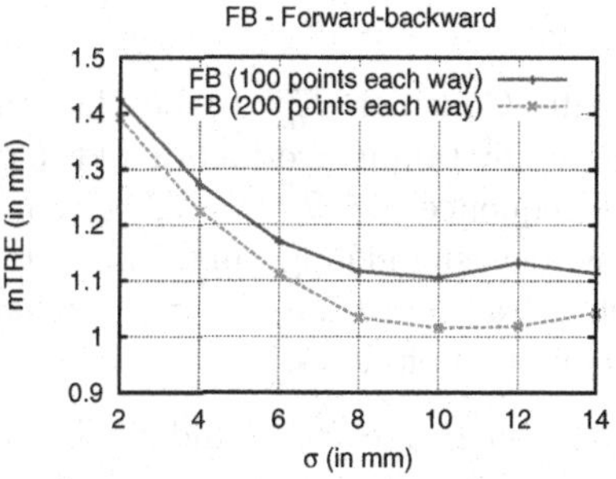

Fig. 2. Pairwise Forward-Backward 3D Registration for two grid spacings

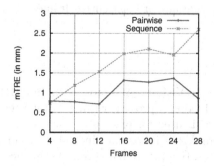

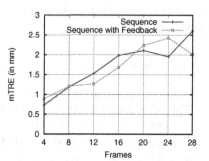

Fig. 3. Pairwise 3D vs. 4D Registration error

Fig. 4. 4D vs. 4D with feedback

2.3 Penalizing Drift

Registration over consecutive frames in a time series is likely to accumulate errors. To address this issue we bring a strategy that would help in reducing

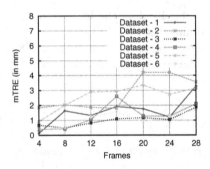 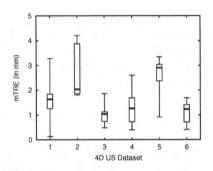

Fig. 5. 4D Registration error per dataset over the time series

Fig. 6. Boxplot: 4D Registration error per dataset

the drift. Consider $\mathcal{T}_{\tau_0}^{\tau_n}$ to be the transformation from frame $\tau_0 \to \tau_n$. It is estimated by taking product of all the transformations between successive frames in the sequence, i.e. $\mathcal{T}_{\tau_0}^{\tau_n} = \mathcal{T}_{\tau_{n-1}}^{\tau_n} \times \mathcal{T}_{\tau_{n-2}}^{\tau_{n-1}} \times \cdots \times \mathcal{T}_{\tau_0}^{\tau_1}$. To counter the drift we propose occasional long range interaction between the current frame τ_n and some previous frame in time, say τ_{n-d}, where d is the *feedback gap*. The steps of the strategy are as follows:

1. Register frames τ_{n-d} and τ_n. Let the resulting transform be $\mathcal{F}_{\tau_{n-d}}^{\tau_n}$.
2. Let the pointsets $P_{\tau_{n-d}}$ and P_{τ_n} be pointsets in the frames τ_{n-d} and τ_n, respectively. These pointsets are related by the transform $\mathcal{F}_{\tau_{n-d}}^{\tau_n}$, i.e. $P_{\tau_n} = \mathcal{F}_{\tau_{n-d}}^{\tau_n} * P_{\tau_{n-d}}$.
3. The projection of the pointsets $P_{\tau_{n-d}}$ over the frame τ_{n-1} is $P_{\tau_{n-1}}$, and is estimated as $P_{\tau_{n-1}} = \mathcal{T}_{\tau_{n-d}}^{\tau_{n-1}} * P_{\tau_{n-d}}$.
4. Include the additional points $P_{\tau_{n-1}}$ and P_{τ_n}, in their respective frames, during the registration (outlier rejection module) of consecutive frames τ_{n-1} and τ_n.

3   Experiments

The code was implemented in C++ and MeVisLab. A laptop with Intel(R) Core(TM) i7-2720QM CPU @ 2.20 G Hz, 4 Core(s) processor using 64-bit Windows 7 operating system and 8 GB of RAM is used for processing the code.

The 4D US data is acquired at 6 Hz from iU22 Philips machine. Three volunteers were used. From each of the volunteers, two (axial and coronal) sequences of 4D US were captured. The probe was kept steady during the acquisition. We use Elastix registration toolbox [10] to generate the reference standard. Different grids were used in the method and the evaluation. From the six 4D US datasets, systematically pairs of US volumes were selected to evaluate the performance. For all the experiments, we use the same set of parameters: block-size of $(11, 11, 11)$ mm and grid spacing of 14 mm (which translates to around 200 points). The sum of square distance (SSD) is the similarity metric using in block-matching. The first two experiments are performed to evaluate the registration

approach. The third experiment is performed to evaluate the feedback mechanism.

1. The purpose of the experiment is to study the parameter σ (given in equation 4) and its effect on pairwise 3D registration. The two pairwise registrations evaluated are a) Forward registration (using affinity matrix in
   equation 1) and b) Froward Backward registration (using affinity matrix in
   equation 4). The range of σ values evaluated are $\{2, 4, 6, 8, 10, 12, 14\}$. We
   systematically select pairs of 3D US volumes from the six 4D US dataset. The
   pairs correspond to the following time points $\{(0, 4), (0, 8), (0, 12), (0, 16),$
   $(0, 20), (0, 24), (0, 28)\}$ are used in the evaluation. Based on the registration
   results, we choose the best σ value for our application and report the corresponding registration error. We use mean total registration error (mTRE)
   as the registration error metric. The mTRE is given as:

$$mTRE(\widehat{\mathcal{T}}_{\tau_1}^{\tau_2}, \mathcal{T}_{\tau_1}^{\tau_2}) = \frac{1}{n} \sum_{i=1}^{n} \|\widehat{\mathcal{T}}_{\tau_1}^{\tau_2} p_i - \mathcal{T}_{\tau_1}^{\tau_2} p_i\|, \tag{7}$$

   where $\widehat{\mathcal{T}}_{\tau_1}^{\tau_2}$ is the reference standard transformation from time point τ_1 to τ_2.
2. Next we evaluate the performance of our registration approach over a se-
   quence of US volumes. The 4D registration between the time points $(2, 5)$,
   for example is estimated by registering $2 \rightarrow 3$, $3 \rightarrow 4$, $4 \rightarrow 5$ time points
   and then multiplying the respective transformation sequentially to derive the
   final transform. 4D registration and the pairwise 3D registration are compared with the reference standard, for the time points $\{(0, 4), (0, 8), (0, 12),$
   $(0, 16), (0, 20), (0, 24), (0, 28)\}$.
3. In the third experiment we evaluate the feedback mechanism. Sequential
   registration similar to the previous experiment is performed for the time
   points $\{(0, 4), (0, 8), (0, 12), (0, 16), (0, 20), (0, 24), (0, 28)\}$. Additionally, a
   feedback is used to counter the drift. The feedback gap d is set to 4.

Results :

1. Figure 1 shows the forward and forward-backward registration results for
   various σ values and two different grid space settings. The grid spacing of
   14 mm, 18 mm correspond to 200, 100 sample points, respectively. For a
   fair comparison between the forward and forward-backward approach, the
   total number of points used for registration should be equal. In terms of
   the number of points, the forward approach with 200 points is equivalent to
   the forward-backward approach with 100 points each way. Figure 1 shows
   that the forward-backward registration approach performs better than the
   forward registration approach, given the number of points are same in the
   two methods. For grid spacing of 14 mm, the forward-backward approach
   performs best at $\sigma = 10$ mm with mTRE of 1 mm. Figure 2 shows the
   forward-backward registration results for various σ values and two different grid space settings. Increase in sample points improves the registration
   results.

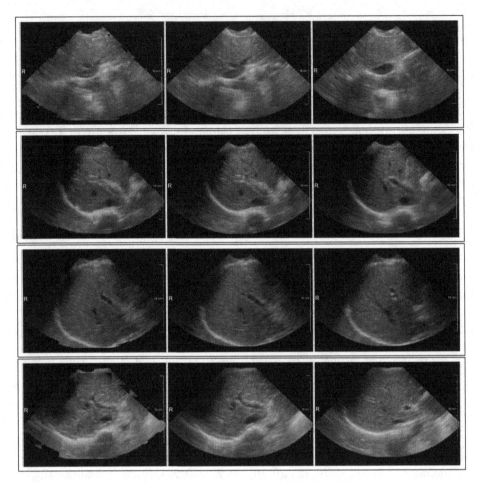

Fig. 7. 4D Registration results for four datasets: Left - Registration result in checker box view, Middle - Fixed image, Right - Moving Image. First Row - Registration between time points 0 and 8, Second Row - Registration between time points 0 and 12, Third Row - Registration between time points 0 and 20, Last Row - Registration between time points 0 and 28.

2. In Figure 3 we study the performance of the registration approach when applied between consecutive frames over the time series. For the first consecutive eight frames the mTRE is below 1.2 mm. Beyond these initial frames the registration performance diverge gradually. The results for all the six 4D US datasets are plotted in Figure 6. These results are also compared to the pairwise 3D registration results and are shown in Figure 3. Figure 5 and Figure 6 show the registration results on all the datasets.

3. In Figure 4 the 4D registration is evaluated with and without the feedback mechanism. The 4D registration without feedback graph diverges. The 4D registration with feedback curve descends and moves closer to the reference standard. Some representative registration results are shown in Figure 7.

4   Discussion and Conclusion

In this work we present a registration framework to perform registration over a time series, and demonstrate its application on 4D US liver dataset. The method consists of two parts - the first part performs a 3D registration between subsequent volumes and ensures inverse consistency, the second part uses an feedback mechanism to counter accumulation of registration error.

Figure 3 shows that the pairwise registration performs well with mTRE of 1 mm. When applied sequentially, the registration results in Figure 3 show that the sequential registration works well for the first eight to ten frames. However after that the registration diverges and performance gradually deteriorates. Hence it is advisable to register back with the original frame after every tenth frame to maintain good registration accuracy. We further apply a feedback criterion to counter the accumulation of registration error over a time series. The initial results as shown in Figure 4 are encouraging. The feedback gap parameter d is data dependent. In our experiments we select $d = 4$ as for $d - 1$ consecutive frames the accumulated registration error is below (1 mm) a tolerable limit, see Figure 3. More in-depth analysis is part of future work.

The block-matching and forward-backward outlier rejection was additionally implemented in OpenCL. The implementation was run on a NVIDIA GTX 780 Ti graphics processing unit. For block-size of $(11, 11, 11)$ mm, grid spacing of 18 mm (i.e. 100 points) and search range of $(20, 20, 20)$ mm the block-matching algorithm takes 0.045 seconds. The outlier rejection module with the forward-backward condition takes 0.05 seconds for grid spacing of 18 mm each way. Adding both the modules results in an execution speed of 10 Hz.

To conclude, we present a forward-backward transformation based registration approach for 4D US data. We evaluate a strategy to counter the accumulation of registration error using a feedback mechanism applying long range interaction. The approach is evaluated using six 4D US sequences with satisfactory results.

References

1. Vijayan, S., Klein, S., Hofstad, E., Lindseth, F., Ystgaard, B., Langø, T.: Validation of a non-rigid registration method for motion compensation in 4D ultrasound of the liver. In: IEEE ISBI2013 (2013), Work done in collaboration with NTNU/SINTEF, Trondheim, Norway
2. Shi, W., Jantsch, M., Aljabar, P., Pizarro, L., Bai, W., Wang, H., O'Regan, D.P., Zhuang, X., Rueckert, D.: Temporal sparse free-form deformations. Medical Image Analysis 17(7), 779–789 (2013)
3. Øye, O.K., Wein, W., Ulvang, D.M., Matre, K., Viola, I.: Real time image-based tracking of 4D ultrasound data. In: Ayache, N., Delingette, H., Golland, P., Mori, K. (eds.) MICCAI 2012, Part I. LNCS, vol. 7510, pp. 447–454. Springer, Heidelberg (2012)
4. Commowick, O., Wiest-Daesslé, N., Prima, S.: Block-matching strategies for rigid registration of multimodal medical images. In: ISBI, pp. 700–703 (2012)
5. Albarelli, A., Bulò, S.R., Torsello, A., Pelillo, M.: Matching as a non-cooperative game. In: ICCV, pp. 1319–1326 (2009)

6. Arun, K.S., Huang, T.S., Blostein, S.D.: Least-squares fitting of two 3-D point sets. IEEE Trans. Pattern Anal. Mach. Intell. 9(5), 698–700 (1987)

7. Torresani, L., Kolmogorov, V., Rother, C.: A dual decomposition approach to feature correspondence. IEEE Trans. Pattern Anal. Mach. Intell. 35(2), 259–271 (2013)

8. Pavan, M., Pelillo, M.: Dominant sets and pairwise clustering. IEEE Trans. Pattern Anal. Mach. Intell. 29(1), 167–172 (2007)

9. Weibull, J.W.: Evolutionary Game Theory. MIT Press (1995)

10. Klein, S., Staring, M., Murphy, K., Viergever, M.A., Pluim, J.P.W.: Elastix: A toolbox for intensity-based medical image registration. IEEE Trans. Med. Imaging 29(1), 196–205 (2010)

An Adaptive Multiscale Similarity Measure for Non-rigid Registration

Veronika A. Zimmer and Gemma Piella

Simulation, Imaging and Modelling in Biomedical Systems (SIMBioSys),
Department of Information and Communication Technologies,
Universitat Pompeu Fabra, Barcelona, Spain

Abstract. Popular intensity-based similarity measures such as (normalized) mutual information estimate statistics over the entire image, neglecting spatial relationships and local image properties. In this work, we present an adaptive multiscale image similarity measure for non-rigid registration which combines image statistics at multiple scales for a multiscale representation of regional image similarities. We validated the proposed similarity measure on simulated and clinical MR brain datasets. Results show that our approach achieves higher registration accuracy and robustness than conventional global measures or their local variations at a single scale.

1 Introduction

Image registration is an essential image processing technique for the analysis of medical images in various applications, ranging from computer-aided diagnosis to interventional planning and guidance, that may require spatial normalization. The objective of image registration is to find a spatial transformation which aligns corresponding (anatomical) structures in two or more images.

Similarity measures based on voxel intensities often rely on the assumptions of independence and stationarity of the intensities from voxel to voxel. As a consequence, such measures cannot capture the complex interactions between voxel intensities (e.g. local structures), and they are not robust against spatially-varying intensity distortions.

Popular intensity-based similarity measures are mutual information (MI) [21] and its normalized version, normalized mutual information (NMI) [19]. They estimate the shared information between the images to be registered by constructing intensity histograms over the entire images, assuming a global statistical relationship between them and neglecting spatial relationships. To take spatial information into account, a common approach is to consider spatial location as an additional channel [18] or to weight intensities with local spatial kernels to vary the contributions of voxels to the joint statistics [15,20,7,9,25].

Such local methods have shown to significantly improve the registration results compared to the standard (global) ones. However, one problem of such regional approaches is that local statistics are only effective within a small image region, which may create numerous local minima of the objective function. Additionally,

S. Ourselin and M. Modat (Eds.): WBIR 2014, LNCS 8545, pp. 203–212, 2014.

local measures are less robust to noise and outliers than global measures. Only using local statistics on small regions of the image may lead to poor estimates of joint probabilities and therefore to poor registration results. To overcome this, some approaches have proposed to combine global and local statistics [6,24], where in the latter the combinations weights are dependent on the local statistics around individual voxels. One drawback common to all the aforementioned approaches is the selection of the region size for statistics computations. In medical images, regions of interest may appear in various sizes and contain features of different granularity. Hence, deformation to be captured by image registration may occur at a variety of scales. In this paper, we address this issue by combining similarity measures at different levels of granularity. This involves computing regional similarities on a hierarchy of image patches and combining them across the hierarchical levels to obtain a multiscale similarity mesure. Our approach encodes the notion of scales directly into the hierarchy, thus enabling a multiscale representation of regional similarities.

The idea of considering multiple scales in the similarity measure is somewhat related to the classical approach of registering images at several scales using a multiresolution representation for the images [3,5,12]. Following this coarse to fine strategy, Likar $et\ al$ [8] proposed a hierarchical approach for elastic registration. Images were divided into subimages at different scales, locally affine registered and elastically interpolated. In [22], a wavelet-based multiresolution strategy was used to combine MI with spatial information obtained from the high-frequency coefficients of the wavelet transform at each resolution. In the framework of large deformation diffeomorphic metric mapping (LDDMM), Risser $et\ al$ [13] included scale in the regularization metric by adding kernels of different scales. Recently, Sommer $et\ al$ [17] developed a multiscale extension of the LDDMM, the kernel bundle framework, which allows multiple kernels at multiple scales. These latter approaches, however, are computationally expensive and are not well adapted to multimodal images. We will show that our measure using NMI and free-form deformations is particularly well adapted to multimodal image registration while maintaining manageable computation cost.

2   Method

2.1   Image Registration

Registration of two differentiable images $F, M : \mathbb{R}^d \to \mathbb{R}$ with dimension $d \in \{2, 3\}$ can be formulated as an optimization of a cost function (a distance measure plus a regularization term) over a space of transformations:

$$\hat{\mu} = \arg \min_{\mu} \left(-\mathcal{S}(F, M \circ T_\mu) + \gamma \mathcal{R}(T_\mu) \right),$$

where F, M are respectively the fixed and moving images, $\mathcal{S}$ is a similarity measure, $T_\mu : \mathbb{R}^d \to \mathbb{R}^d$ is a transformation with parameterization μ, $\mathcal{R}$ is a regularizer and γ is a regularization penalty weight.

In this work, we focus on the similarity measure $\mathcal{S}$ that quantifies the degree of match between the images. Information-theoretic similarity measures, such as MI and NMI, are among the most popular measures used in intensity-based image registration:

$$\mathcal{S}_{\mathrm{MI}}(F, M; T_\mu) = \mathrm{H}(F) + \mathrm{H}(M \circ T_\mu) - \mathrm{H}(F, M \circ T_\mu), \tag{1}$$

$$\mathcal{S}_{\mathrm{NMI}}(F, M; T_\mu) = \frac{\mathrm{H}(F) + \mathrm{H}(M \circ T_\mu)}{\mathrm{H}(F, M \circ T_\mu)}, \tag{2}$$

where $\mathrm{H}(F), \mathrm{H}(M)$ are the Shannon's marginal entropies of the fixed and moving images, and $\mathrm{H}(F, M \circ T_\mu)$ is their joint entropy.

We choose NMI as similarity measure because, unlike MI, it is robust to changes in the region of overlap between the images, and its range is bounded between 1 and 2, which is an interesting property for the definition of our adaptive multiscale similarity measure in Section 2.2.

In this work, the negative NMI is minimized using the L-BFGS algorithm [1]. The implementation of NMI is based on a Parzen-window method to estimate the probability density functions such that the entropy of an image F is computed with $\mathrm{H}(F) = -\sum_x p_F(x) \log p_F(x)$, where p_F is the histogram of F estimated using Parzen-windows [12,23]. With this estimation, NMI is differentiable and the gradient with respect to the parameters μ of T_μ, which is needed by the optimization algorithm, is given by $\nabla_\mu \mathcal{S}_{\mathrm{NMI}} = \left[\frac{\partial \mathcal{S}_{\mathrm{NMI}}}{\partial \mu_1}, \ldots, \frac{\partial \mathcal{S}_{\mathrm{NMI}}}{\partial \mu_n} \right]$ with

$$\frac{\partial \mathcal{S}_{\mathrm{NMI}}}{\partial \mu_i} = \frac{1}{A^2(\mu)} \sum_{x,y} \left(A(\mu) \log p_M(y; \mu) - B(\mu) \log p(x, y; \mu) \right) \frac{\partial p(x, y; \mu)}{\partial \mu_i},$$

where $p_M(y; \mu)$ is the histogram of image $M \circ T_\mu$, $p(x, y; \mu)$ is the joint histogram of F and $M \circ T_\mu$, and $A(\mu) = \mathrm{H}(F, M \circ T_\mu)$, $B(\mu) = \mathrm{H}(F) + \mathrm{H}(M \circ T_\mu)$ using the Parzen-window estimation for the entropies. More details on the gradient computation can be found in [23].

As transformation model, we choose a free-form transformation modeled using B-splines [14]. By deforming an underlying grid of uniformly spaced control points, the moving image is transformed iteratively. The parameters of the transformation are the control points μ of the grid. We used a multiresolution approach by varying the control point spacing of the B-spline grid in a coarse to fine manner [14]. Our implementations are based on the Insight Segmentation and Registration Toolkit[1] (ITK).

2.2   Adaptive Multiscale Similarity Measure

Encoding local spatial information into the NMI and MI measures has been shown to improve their performance. One drawback of this approach is the lack of a systematic method to select the region size over which to compute the local statistics. Different regions can contain information at different scales, and

---

[1] http://www.itk.org/

choosing a single scale may miss deformations occuring at other levels. The idea of measuring image similarity on multiple levels at spatially-varying locations aims at addressing this issue.

The methodology is inspired from the idea of multiscale patch representation [2,4,16]. In particular, in the context of manifold learning, this was used in [2] to construct manifold embeddings that take into account local properties of the image. We construct an image partition similar to a quadtree structure, i.e., the full image is divided into four (or eight in 3D) regular quadrants or patches, which in turn are recursively divided into four (or eight) subquadrants until the desired number of levels is obtained (see Fig. 1). Thus, for each input image, a set of hierarchical patches is obtained. Each level in the quadtree corresponds to a different spatial resolution level, with the lowest level $l = 0$ corresponding to the whole image (coarsest level) and the highest level $l = L$ to the finest one. At each level l there are up to $2^{d \cdot l}$ patches (4^l for 2D and 8^l for 3D images).

For each patch p at level l, we can compute a local similarity measure $\mathcal{S}^{l,p}$ and a matching measure $\mathcal{M}^{l,p}$ that combines the current local similarity $\mathcal{S}^{l,p}$ with a more global one (derived from all or a set of patches from previous levels). On the coarsest level $l = 0$, there is only one patch $p = 1$, and the matching measure is $\mathcal{M}^{0,1} = \mathcal{S}^0$, which is the similarity measure over the entire image. On the subsequent levels, the matching measure of each patch is computed by

$$\mathcal{M}^{l,p} = (1 - \lambda_l)\mathcal{S}^{l,p} + \lambda_l \sum_{p'=1}^{2^{d(l-1)}} \alpha_{p'} \mathcal{M}^{l-1,p'}, \tag{3}$$

where $\lambda_l \in [0, 1]$, $\alpha_{p'} \in \mathbb{R}$ are weighting parameters that determine the influence of each term. Note that for each patch at a given level, the matching measure $\mathcal{M}^{l,p}$ takes into account both local and global statistics, respectively measured by $\mathcal{S}^{l,p}$ and a combination of matching measures at the previous coarser level $l - 1$. For a given number of levels L, the proposed adaptive multiscale similarity measure is then computed as

$$\mathcal{M}^{(L)} = \frac{1}{2^{dL}} \sum_{p=1}^{2^{dL}} \mathcal{M}^{L,p}, \tag{4}$$

which is a function of all patches and levels. This allows capturing the local structure of the images at different levels of granularity along with the global image structure.

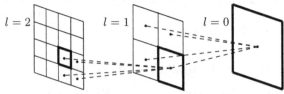

Fig. 1. Division of a 2D image into hierarchical patches to obtain image information at different levels. Each subdivision at a given level l is contained within one parent patch at level $l - 1$.

For the computation of the proposed similarity measure, we introduced two weighting parameters: $\lambda_l \in [0, 1]$, to determine the influence of the current local patch similarity over the coarser ones, and $\alpha_{p'} \in \mathbb{R}$, to weight the different contribution of the coarser parent patches.

The choice of the weighting parameters is important to adapt the similarity measure to both local and global stastistics, and hence to allow for a higher accuracy of the registration algorithm. Here, we define an adaptive weight for each patch, i.e., $\lambda_l = \lambda_l(p)$, such that the lower the local similarity measure $\mathcal{S}^{l,p}$, the higher its weight is. In this way, local dissimilarities are emphasized during optimization and the registration is guided to correct for such local mismatches. On the other hand, when local similarity is high, a larger weight is assigned to the most global similarity term $(\sum_{p'=1}^{2^{d(l-1)}} \alpha_{p'} \mathcal{M}^{l-1,p'}$, computed from patches at previous levels). This behavior can be obtained by defining $\lambda_l(p)$ as an increasing function of $\mathcal{S}^{l,p}$. Since we use NMI as local similarity, which is bounded between 1 and 2, we set $\lambda_l(p) = \mathcal{S}^{l,p} - 1$; hence $\lambda_l(p) \in [0,1]$. For example, if images are very similar in patch p of level l, $\mathcal{S}^{l,p}$ will be close to 2 and the local weight $1 - \lambda_l = 2 - \mathcal{S}^{l,p}$ in Eq. (3) will be close to zero. Hence, only the more global statistics will be considered for the patch matching measure $\mathcal{M}^{l,p}$.

In [24], the authors combine local and global similarities at a single scale using a weighting strategy opposite to ours: the higher the local statistics, the higher its contribution to the overall similarity. They argued that if the local similarity term is low, it means that local statistics do not provide sufficient information for matching and therefore a global measure should be used. However, with this weighting approach, the registration algorithm could fail in correcting small local dissimilarities when the global similarity is already high. Experiments in Section 3.1 demonstrate that this affects the correct alignment.

The weighting parameter $\alpha_{p'}$ determines the influence of each of the parents patch similarities to the more global similarity term that is combined with the local similarity $\mathcal{S}^{l,p}$ of the current patch. Since each patch p is contained in exactly one patch p' at the previous level (Fig. 1), a simple way to define the weighting parameter would be to set $\alpha_{p'} = 1$ for the patch p' which contains patch p at the next level, and $\alpha_{p'} = 0$ otherwise. However, especially when patch p lays on the border of patch p' (as illustrated in Fig. 1 for the black-border patch at level 2), the statistics of p' may not capture the whole neighborhood of p. Thus, we propose to take into account all parent patches p' at the previous level, with a weighting $\alpha_{p'} = \frac{1}{d_{p'}} / \sum_{p'=1}^{2^{d(l-1)}} \frac{1}{d_{p'}}$, where $d_{p'}$ is the Euclidean distance between the center of patch p' at level $l-1$ and the current patch p at level l. This weighting was also used in [2] to align patches with their parent patches.

3   Results

We validated the proposed adaptive multiscale image similarity measure on two synthetic datasets (2D phantoms and simulated 3D brain images from BrainWeb database[2]) and on a clinical brain dataset obtained from The Alzheimer's Disease NeuroImaging Initiative[3] (ADNI) [11].

---

[2] http://www.bic.mni.mcgill.ca/brainweb/
[3] http://www.adni-info.org

The similarity measures to evaluate are: (i) NMI: the global NMI (i.e., $\mathcal{S}^0$), (ii) L-NMI: a local NMI that computes the NMI value in local regions at a single scale (here with a local region size of 32), (iii) LG-NMI: a combination of local and global NMI at a single scale, using an adaptive weight as in [24], and with a local region size of 32, (iv) LG*-NMI: LG-NMI but with the adaptive weight proposed in this work (opposite to [24]), and (v) AM-NMI: the proposed adaptive multiscale similarity measure on three scales ($L = 2$, i.e., $\mathcal{M}^{(2)}$, which corresponds to one global and two local scales).

3.1   Synthetic Data

We start with a simple synthetic example to illustrate the advantages of considering both local and global statistics at multiple levels in the presence of high intensity differences and intensity gradients. We used synthetic phantoms (shown in Fig. 2) similar to those employed in [10]. Both images contain a circle, which is black with a white background in one image and with an intensity gradient in the other image. We examined the changes of the studied different similarity measures with respect to horizontal translations. Similarity curves are plotted in Fig. 2. It can be seen that global NMI fails in detecting a minimum for minimal translation (Fig. 2b). A minimum is reached using only local information at a fixed scale (Fig. 2c) but with translation of $t = (-1, 0)$. Combining local and global information with LG-NMI leads to the correct minimum of $t = (0, 0)$, but the similarity plot is not symmetric around the minimum. If we use a weighting as proposed in section 2.2, the symmetry is restored and the correct minimum is reached (Fig. 2g). Computing the local information only at one scale is sensitive to the selected region size, as seen in Fig. 2f, where instead of 32 a region size of 64 was set. The similarity plot still shows a minimum but with a translation of $t = (4, 0)$. This also happens using L-NMI or LG*-NMI with a local region size of 64. AM-NMI detects the correct translation corresponding to the ground truth registration and provides smooth and symmetric similarity plot without being dependent on the selected region size (Fig. 2h).

Second, we evaluated the accuracy of registration with our approach on simulated normal brain images from the BrainWeb database. Triplets of pre-registered T1-, T2- and proton density- (PD) weighted MR images were generated with a slice thickness of 1 mm, a noise level of 3% and intensity non-uniformity (INU) fields of 0 %, 20% and 40 %. We created five random deformations (maximal voxel displacement of 4 mm) using random displacements of the control points of a dense B-Spline grid and used them to deform the three modalities. The inverse deformation field was used as ground truth. Next, we performed pairwise registrations with the deformed T1, T2 and PD as moving images and the undeformed T1 as fixed image. Each image pair used for registration had the same INU. The error of the registration was computed as the root mean square error (RMSE) between the ground truth deformation and the estimated one. Results are shown in Table 1. For monomodal registrations (T1-T1), the error is small for all measures. For registrations with an INU field of 0 %, the errors are very similar for all measures, although L-NMI, LG*-NMI and AM-NMI have the

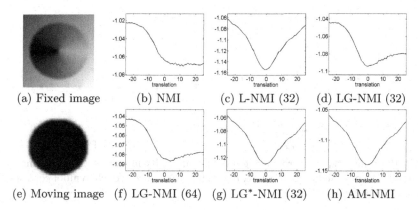

(a) Fixed image   (b) NMI   (c) L-NMI (32)   (d) LG-NMI (32)

(e) Moving image   (f) LG-NMI (64)   (g) LG*-NMI (32)   (h) AM-NMI

Fig. 2. Similarity plots on synthetic phantoms (left). Similarity curves are obtained from horizontally translating the moving image over the fixed image using different similarity measures. The local region sizes, if needed, are given in brackets.

smallest errors. For multimodal registrations (T1-T2, T1-PD), errors are bigger than those for T1-T1. However, results show that AM-NMI achieves the best performance.

The distribution of errors is shown in Fig. 3 for each deformation. The difference in the performance of the different similarities becomes more evident when INU field increases. For monomodal registration, INU does not affect too much the results (see Table 1), whereas for multimodal registrations (Fig. 3) results are sensitive to increasing INU. NMI is adversely affected when the INU fields become stronger (error increases from 0.446 mm for 0 % INU level up to 1.269 mm for 40 % level). In contrast, using local information alleviates the effect of INU, being the AM-NMI the more robust. Note that the registration errors with LG*-NMI are always smaller than with LG-NMI.

Table 1. Root mean square error of the displacement error using different similarity measures. Five pairwise registrations are conducted between T1 (fixed image) and each deformed T1, T2 and PD (moving images). For each modality pair class, mean error and standard deviation are shown. Errors are in mm.

Mod.	INU	NMI	L-NMI	LG-NMI	LG*-NMI	AM-NMI
T1-T1		0.459 ± 0.012	$\mathbf{0.415 \pm 0.013}$	0.440 ± 0.018	$\mathbf{0.415 \pm 0.012}$	0.419 ± 0.013
T1-T2	0 %	0.965 ± 0.012	0.931 ± 0.005	0.937 ± 0.03	0.932 ± 0.002	$\mathbf{0.929 \pm 0.012}$
T1-PD		0.821 ± 0.009	$\mathbf{0.796 \pm 0.009}$	0.799 ± 0.013	0.804 ± 0.015	0.806 ± 0.010
T1-T1		0.465 ± 0.011	$\mathbf{0.413 \pm 0.014}$	0.501 ± 0.159	0.419 ± 0.006	0.420 ± 0.020
T1-T2	20 %	1.164 ± 0.011	0.974 ± 0.005	1.067 ± 0.004	1.001 ± 0.006	$\mathbf{0.940 \pm 0.026}$
T1-PD		1.237 ± 0.031	0.962 ± 0.012	1.053 ± 0.021	0.983 ± 0.020	$\mathbf{0.913 \pm 0.025}$
T1-T1		0.468 ± 0.010	$\mathbf{0.420 \pm 0.011}$	0.449 ± 0.019	0.427 ± 0.009	0.421 ± 0.007
T1-T2	40 %	1.329 ± 0.016	1.089 ± 0.015	1.149 ± 0.030	1.084 ± 0.016	$\mathbf{1.007 \pm 0.046}$
T1-PD		1.485 ± 0.050	1.060 ± 0.022	1.194 ± 0.021	1.080 ± 0.022	$\mathbf{0.972 \pm 0.025}$

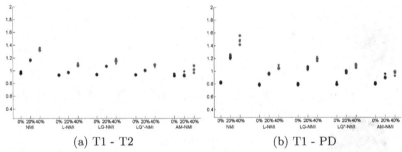

(a) T1 - T2   (b) T1 - PD

Fig. 3. Root mean square errors using different similarity measures with different intensity non-uniformity fields (black: 0 %, blue: 20 %, red: 40 %). Each symbol corresponds to one random deformation.

3.2   Clinical Data

We applied the proposed AM-NMI image similarity measure on a clinical dataset of longitudinal MR brain images from the ADNI database [11]. This database contains subjects with normal cognition, mild cognitive impairment and with Alzheimer's disease. We registered T2-weighted MR images of the same patient at two different timepoints (with a time difference of twelve months) using as similarity measures the standard global NMI and the proposed AM-NMI. In Fig. 4 the difference images between the fixed and the registered images for two axial slices are shown. By visually inspecting the registered images, one can see that global NMI leads to misregistrations in some local regions, while registration artifacts are diminished when using AM-NMI.

4   Discussion

We have proposed an adaptive multiscale image similarity measure based on NMI for non-rigid image registration. The AM-NMI similarity measure combines image information across hierarchical levels to capture differences in image features of varying granularity. We validated our measure on simulated and clinical MR brain images. Results show that, especially for multimodal registration, the AM-NMI is an accurate and robust similarity measure for non-rigid image registration. AM-NMI registration results outperform the ones obtained with the typically global NMI, the local NMI and the combination of local and global statistics at a single scale, in terms of registration accuracy measured by the RMSE of the voxel displacements. Additionally, the AM-NMI is more robust to intensity non-uniformities than the aforementioned measures.

For the definition of local regions in our measure, we do not need to select a region size a priori for statistics computation, which is an advantage over other methods that use local information. In our approach, the region size is automatically set by the number of levels used for the AM-NMI computation. However, the selection of the finest level is important, since too small regions may lead to poor histogram estimations, and therefore to poor registration results. In [8], the authors found that if the local region size is too small, the probabilities

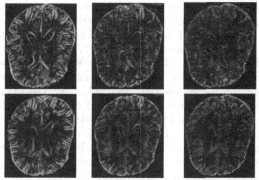

Fixed - Moving   Fixed - NMI   Fixed - AM-NMI

Fig. 4. Registration example from the ADNI dataset. Difference images between fixed and moving image (left) and fixed and registered image using NMI (middle) and AM-NMI (right) are displayed in fake colors for an easier visualization of the errors. Each row corresponds to a different axial slice. Red arrows show misregistered regions using global NMI, while AM-NMI leads to more accurate results.

estimations may not be correct. Additionally, the finest patch level should be also related to the finest deformation scale. If there is a large non-rigid deformation between the images to be registered, the region size on the finest level should be smaller than if the deformation between the images is small. In this work, we used regular patches and a fixed number of levels $L = 2$ (corresponding to a minimum patch size of $32 \times 32 \times 32$ for the BrainWeb and $32 \times 32 \times 16$ for the ADNI data). For a better adaptation to the underlying anatomy and image properties, one could define non-regular patches, which capture specific features of the images at different scales, and dynamically adapt the number of levels during the registration process.

Acknowledgements. V. A. Zimmer is supported by the grant FI-DGR 2013 (2013 FI_B00159) from the Generalitat de Catalunya. This research was partially funded by the Spanish Ministry of Economy and Competitiveness (TIN2012-35874) and by the European Union FP7 grant agreement no. HEAR-EU 304857.

References

1. Byrd, R., Lu, P., Nocedal, J., Zhu, C.: A limited memory algorithm for bound constrained optimization. SIAM J. Sci. Comput. 16, 1190–1208 (1995)
2. Bhatia, K.K., Rao, A., Price, A.N., Wolz, R., Hajnal, J.V., Rueckert, D.: Hierarchical manifold learning for regional image analysis. IEEE Trans. Med. Imag. (2013)
3. Li, D., Wang, H., Yin, Y., Chen, J.: A new multiscale registration method for medical image. In: Proc. ICCSIT, vol. 3, pp. 10–13 (2010)
4. Zhu, P., Zhang, L., Hu, Q., Shiu, S.C.K.: Multi-scale patch based collaborative representation for face recognition with margin distribution optimization. In: Fitzgibbon, A., Lazebnik, S., Perona, P., Sato, Y., Schmid, C. (eds.) ECCV 2012, Part I. LNCS, vol. 7572, pp. 822–835. Springer, Heidelberg (2012)

5. Haber, E., Modersitzki, J.: Cofir: Coarse and fine image registration. SIAM Real-Time PDE-Constrained Optimization, 37–49 (2007)
6. Hermosillo, G., Faugeras, O.: Dense image matching with global and local statistical criteria: a variational approach. In: Proc. CVPR, pp. 73–78 (2001)
7. Klein, S., van der Heide, U.A., Lips, I.M., van Vulpen, M., Staring, M., Pluim, J.P.W.: Automatic segmentation of the prostate in 3-D MR images by atlas matching using localized mutual information. Med. Phys. 35, 1407–1417 (2008)
8. Likar, B., Pernuš, F.: A hierarchical approach to elastic registration based on mutual information. Image & Vis. Comput. 19, 33–44 (2001)
9. Loeckx, D., Slagmolen, P., Maes, F., Vandermeulen, D., Suetens, P.: Nonrigid image registration using conditional mutual information. IEEE Trans. Med. Imag. 29 (2010)
10. Mellor, M., Brady, M.: Phase mutual information as a similarity measure for registration. Med. Image Anal. 9, 330–343 (2005)
11. Mueller, S.G., Weiner, M.W., Thal, L.J., Petersen, R.C., Jack, J., Jagust, W., Trojanowski, J.Q., Toga, A.W., Beckett, L.: The Alzheimer's disease neuroimaging initiative. Neuroimaging Clinics of North America 15, 869–877 (2005)
12. Thévenaz, P., Unser, M.: Optimization of mutual information for multiresolution image registration. IEEE Trans. Imag. Proc. 9, 2083–2099 (2000)
13. Risser, L., Vialard, F.X., Wolz, R., Murgasova, M., Holm, D.D., Rueckert, D.: Simultaneous multi-scale registration using large deformation diffeomorphic metric mapping. IEEE Trans. Med. Imag. 30, 1746–1759 (2011)
14. Rueckert, D., Sonoda, L.I., Hayes, C., Hill, D.L.G., Leach, M.O., Hawkes, D.J.: Non-rigid registration using free-form deformations: application to breast MR images. IEEE Trans. Med. Imag. 18, 712–721 (1999)
15. Russakoff, D.B., Tomasi, C., Rohlfing, T., Maurer Jr., C.R.: Image similarity using mutual information of regions. In: Pajdla, T., Matas, J. (eds.) ECCV 2004. LNCS, vol. 3023, pp. 596–607. Springer, Heidelberg (2004)
16. Said, A., Pearlman, W.A.: A new fast and efficient image codec based on set partitioning in hierarchical trees. IEEE Trans. Circuits & Syst. for Video Technol. 6, 243–250 (1996)
17. Sommer, S., Lauze, F., Nielsen, M., Pennec, X.: Sparse multi-scale diffeomorphic registration: The kernel bundle framework. J. Math. Imag. & Vis. 46, 292–308 (2013)
18. Studholme, C., Hill, D.L.G., Hawkes, D.J.: Automated 3D registration of MR and CT images of the head. Med. Image Anal. 1, 163–175 (1996)
19. Studholme, C., Hill, D.L.G., Hawkes, D.J.: An overlap invariant entropy measure of 3D medical image alignment. Pattern Recogn. 32, 71–86 (1999)
20. Studholme, C., Drapaca, C., Iordanova, B., Cardenas, V.: Deformation-based mapping of volume change from serial brain MRI in the presence of local tissue contrast change. IEEE Trans. Med. Imag. 25, 626–639 (2006)
21. Viola, A.P.: Alignment by maximization of mutual information. Ph.D. thesis, Massachusetts Institute of Technology (1995)
22. Xu, R., Chen, Y.-W.: Wavelet-based multiresolution medical image registration strategy combining mutual information with spatial information. Int. J. Innov. Comput., Info. & Control 3, 285–296 (2007)
23. Xu, R., Chen, Y.-W., Tang, S.-Y., Morikawa, S., Kurumi, Y.: Parzen-window based normalized mutual information for medical image registration. IEICE Trans. on Inf. & Syst. E91-D, 132–144 (2008)
24. Yi, Z., Soatto, S.: Nonrigid registration combining global and local statistics. In: Proc. CVPR, pp. 2200–2207 (2009)
25. Zhuang, S., Arridge, D., Hawkes, D., Ourselin, S.: A nonrigid registration framework using spatially encoded mutual information and free-form deformations. IEEE Trans. Med. Imag. 30, 1819–1828 (2011)

Registration Fusion Using Markov Random Fields

Tobias Gass, Gabor Szekely, and Orcun Goksel

Computer Vision Lab, Swiss Federal Institute of Technology (ETH) Zurich, Switzerland
{gasst,szekely,ogoksel}@vision.ee.ethz.ch

Abstract. Image registration is a ubiquitous technique in medical imaging. However, finding correspondences reliably between images is a difficult task since the registration problem is ill-posed and registration algorithms are only capable of finding local optima. This makes it challenging to find a suitable registration method and parametrization for a specific application. To alleviate such problems, multiple registrations can be fused which is typically done by weighted averaging, which is sensitive to outliers and can not guarantee that registrations improve. In contrast, in this work we present a Markov random field based technique which fuses registrations by explicitly minimizing local dissimilarities of deformed source and target image, while penalizing non-smooth deformations. We additionally propose a registration propagation technique which combines multiple registration hypotheses which are obtained from different indirect paths in a set of mutually registered images. Our fused registrations are experimentally shown to improve pair-wise correspondences in terms of average deformation error (ADE) and target registration error (TRE) as well as improving post-registration segmentation overlap.

1 Introduction

Image registration is at the core of a multitude of medical image analysis techniques. It enables ubiquitous methods such as atlas generation, atlas-based segmentation, multimodal information fusion, pre-operative planning and intra-operative guidance. High registration reliability and accuracy are critical for the success of any applied method. However, it is well known that the registration problem is ill-posed [1] when anatomical correspondences are established using image similarity. Artefacts from the imaging process (noise, bias) and from discretizing the continuous spatial domain into pixels/voxels further complicate the image registration process. Numerous techniques have been developed to cope with these challenges. Firstmost, registration algorithms typically include regularization terms that penalize anatomically unreasonable deformations such as due to folding or tearing. For example, Markov random field (MRF) based registration penalizes deformations with large Euclidean distance between displacements of neighboring points [2]. Other approaches include Gaussian smoothing of velocity and update fields [3], or they restrict the type of deformation to be diffeomorphic (smoothly invertable) [4]. A comprehensive overview of registration regularization is given in [5]. Higher-level prior knowledge can also be used to regularize registration algorithm. For example, it is reasonable to expect that the outcome of registering image A to B should be the same as inverting the registration from B to A. Such registration *symmetry* has

S. Ourselin and M. Modat (Eds.): WBIR 2014, LNCS 8545, pp. 213–222, 2014.

been succesfully enforced for example in the demons [6] and SyN registration algorithms [7]. One key challenge of regularized registration is that the resulting elastic matching problem is NP-complete [8] and therefore solutions can be found only approximatively, typically following the gradient of the objective function. To avoid poor local optima in such optimizations, most non-rigid registration methods require a suitable initialisation from another robust rigid or affine registration algorithm. Multi-resolution pyramids are frequently used to prevent algorithms from falling into local minima due to fine detail in early stages of the registration [9]. Despite these advances, medical image registration is still an open problem.

It is known from information theory that many weak information sources can be combined into strong information for example via boosting [10]. This is reflected by the trend in medical image segmentation, where state-of-the art results are achieved by *fusing* segmentation hypotheses obtained from multiple atlases [11]. Optical flow can be computed by fusing multiple hypotheses using a mixed continuous-discrete approach [12]. There also exist studies that present methods to fuse multiple hypotheses for landmark detection [13,14], which can be seen as a sparse registration problem. Some of the fusion methods are specific to the chosen detection method, for example choosing landmarks based on the cumulative score of multiple support vector machines that are independently trained [14]. A more general technique was presented in [13], where multiple landmark hypotheses obtained from different atlases were fused using similarity weighted averaging. Such averaging can be also applied to dense registration fusion, but has two drawbacks: First, averaging can give no *guarantee* that the result improves the registration fidelity, or that it even improves any image-to-image similarity. Second, the average may easily result in anatomically unreasonable deformations since there is no straight-forward way to regularize the result.

In this paper, we formulate the registration fusion as an optimization problem where the objective function is designed such that post-registration image similarity is maximized while non-smooth deformations are penalized. We cast this as a discrete energy minimization problem, which can be solved using a Markov random Field (MRF). Our MRF-based registration fusion (MRegFuse) then locally *selects* one of the candidate displacement hypotheses, while penalizing non-smooth deformations in a first-order neighborhood system. We show experimentally that MRegFuse is capable to successfully fuse *independent* registrations obtained from randomly selected registration algorithms and parametrizations, alleviating the common need to carefully select those. In order to avoid explicitly calculating multiple registrations for a pair of images, we also adapt a technique presented to generate multiple segmentation hypotheses from a single image in a *population* of mutually registered images [11,15]. Similarly to this method, we generate multiple *registration* hypotheses by composing deformations along indirect paths from a source to a target image, and subsequently fuse them using our algorithm.

2   Registration Fusion Using an MRF

Let image X be a function that maps points in the D-dimensional spatial domain Ω to a space $\mathcal{F}$ of image intensities, e.g. CT Hounsfield units. A non-rigid deformation $\mathcal{T}$ is a mapping from Ω to Ω which is based on a displacement field $\mathcal{D}$ such that $\mathcal{T}(p) = p +$

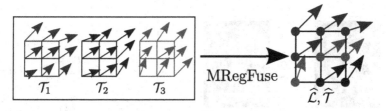

Fig. 1. Schematic of the proposed MRF fusion (MRegFuse). The MRF computes a labelling $\widehat{\mathcal{L}}$ (colored disks, right) which locally selects displacements from the input registrations $\mathcal{T}_n$ according to a joint image similarity and deformation smoothness criterion. $\widehat{\mathcal{L}}$ is then converted to the fused deformation $\widehat{\mathcal{T}}$ (arrows). Best viewed in color.

$\mathcal{D}(p)$ for all points p in Ω. Note that both X and $\mathcal{D}$ are commonly defined on a discrete (Cartesian) regular grid, where non-grid values can be obtained by interpolation. In this notation, deforming an image is a function composition $X \circ \mathcal{T} = X(\mathcal{T})$. A *set of* registrations $\mathcal{R}(X, Y) = \{\mathcal{T}_1, \ldots, \mathcal{T}_N\}$ may contain N different registrations between images X and Y. The goal of registration fusion is then to combine such registrations into a new registration estimate. Ideally, such fused registrations should maximize post-registration image similarity while penalizing anatomically unreasonable deformations.

We propose a discrete optimization method which locally *selects* one displacement of N hypotheses based on local image similarity and global registration smoothness (Fig. 1). To this end, we define a discrete label domain $L = \{1, \ldots, N\}$, such that each label l uniquely refers to a registration $\mathcal{T}_l \in \mathcal{R}(X, Y)$. Then, a labelling $\mathcal{L} : \Omega \to L$ assigns a label l_p to every pixel/voxel p of an image. Finally, such labelling defines the corresponding registration $\mathcal{T}_{\mathcal{L}}$ as follows:

$$\mathcal{T}_{\mathcal{L}} : \Omega \to \Omega \quad : p \to \mathcal{T}_{l_p}(p). \tag{1}$$

This allows us to define the discrete optimization problem as energy minimization in a first-order Markov random field (MRF), for which efficient solvers exist. The MRF energy is commonly defined as a sum of potential functions defined on a graph which typically is the lattice of pixels/voxels in computer vision. The goal of the MRF is then to assign a label l_p to each graph node p such that an energy-criterion is minimized. The registration fusion problem can then be formalized as follows:

$$\widehat{L} = \arg\min_{L'} \sum_{p \in \Omega} \left(\mathcal{V}_p(l_p) + \lambda \sum_{q \in \mathcal{N}(p)} \mathcal{V}_{pq}(l_p, l_q) \right), \tag{2}$$

where the unary term $\mathcal{V}_p(l_p)$ is the data fitness at point p for label l_p, and $\mathcal{V}_{pq}$ is a pairwise energy term which allows implementing prior knowledge about the spatial smoothness of the solution, and λ is the weighting for the latter.

Unary Term $\mathcal{V}_p$. This term penalizes choosing labels that result in low similarity Φ of image X and deformed image $Y(\mathcal{T}_{l_p})$ at location p as follows:

$$\mathcal{V}_p(l_p) = 1 - \Phi\left(X, Y(\mathcal{T}_{l_p}), p\right). \tag{3}$$

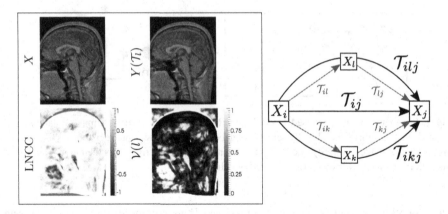

Fig. 2. Left: Unary potential computation for one label l, $\sigma=4$ and $\gamma=10$. Right: Generating registration hypotheses by composing deformations along indirect paths in a population-based setting (c.f. Sec. 2.2).

We use local normalized cross correlation (LNCC) [16] as a robust similarity metric, which was successfully utilized earlier to locally rank segmentation hypotheses in [17]. LNCC is smooth, and can be efficiently computed using convolutions with Gaussian kernels of size σ. From the LNCC metric, we compute the similarity

$$\Phi\left(X, Y(\mathcal{T}_{l_p}), p\right) = \left(\frac{1 + \text{LNCC}_\sigma(X, Y(\mathcal{T}_{l_p}), p)}{2}\right)^\gamma, \qquad (4)$$

which normalizes LNCC to the range $[0, 1]$. γ is used to scale the similarity such that contributions from individual registrations are well spread [13]. An example of such unary potentials is shown in Fig. 2(left).

Pair-wise Term $\mathcal{V}_{pq}$. We penalize non-smooth deformations based on squared Euclidean distance between the displacements of neighboring points:

$$\mathcal{V}_{pq}(l_p, l_q) = ||\mathcal{T}_{l_p}(p) - \mathcal{T}_{l_q}(q)||^2. \qquad (5)$$

Solving the MRF. Although the number of labels is typically relatively small, the underlying MRF graph can become huge, which makes solving (2) on the lattice of image pixels prohibitive. Since registrations can be represented on a coarse grid of control points [9], we define our MRF over a coarse graph $\mathcal{G}$, and interpolate displacements at non-grid locations using B-splines after $\widehat{\mathcal{R}}$ is estimated. Since there is no guarantee that the pairwise potential in (5) satisfies any metricity or submodularity criteria, it is not possible to use common discrete optimization methods such as α-expansion [18]. We thus use tree-reweighted message passing TRW-S, which allows using arbitrary pairwise potentials [19] and additionally gives a lower bound on the energy which can be used to assess the quality of the solution. If the energy of the solution is equal to the lower bound, TRW-S arrives at the globally optimal solution.

2.1   MRegFuse with Folding Removal (MRegFuseR)

Since labels and hence deformations are selected in a locally discrete fashion, displacement continuity at label seams cannot be guaranteed. We therefore propose the following post-processing step to remove folding if the minimum of the Jacobian determinant, $\min(|J|)$, of a deformation field $\widehat{\mathcal{T}}$ is smaller than zero: $\widehat{\mathcal{T}}$ is smoothed with K Gaussian kernels each of size $\sigma_k=0.5 \cdot 2^k$ mm, resulting in K deformation fields $\widehat{\mathcal{T}}_{\sigma_k}$. K is increased sequentially until $\widehat{\mathcal{T}}_{\sigma_K}$ has a positive $\min(|J|)$. We then fuse the resulting set of registration $\{\widehat{\mathcal{T}}, \widehat{\mathcal{T}}_{\sigma_1}, \ldots, \widehat{\mathcal{T}}_{\sigma_K}\}$ using MRegFuse as before. If the $\min(|J|)$ is still negative, we repeat the fusion step with an increased pair-wise potential weight $\lambda \leftarrow 2\lambda$ until folding is removed. To avoid *over-smoothing* the result and to increase computational efficiency, we update any labels for folding removal solely for nodes that are in the vicinity (3σ) of negative Jacobian determinants.

2.2   Pair-Wise and Population-Based Registration Fusion

For a given pair of images, the proposed MRegFuse can fuse multiple registration hypotheses obtained from running different registration algorithms or parametrizations thereof. This can, for example, be useful when a universally optimal registration algorithm/parametrization is difficult to find or does not exist.

MRegFuse can also be used when a *population* of images is to be mutually registered. Here, it is possible to obtain multiple registration hypotheses by composing deformations along indirect paths between images. This principle was used succesfully to generate and fuse *segmentation* hypotheses in [11,15]. Formally, if a registration $\mathcal{T}_{ij}$ registers images X_i and X_j, an indirect registration $\mathcal{T}_{ikj}$ is the composition of $\mathcal{T}_{ik}$ and $\mathcal{T}_{kj}$, i.e. $\mathcal{T}_{ikj}=\mathcal{T}_{kj} \circ \mathcal{T}_{ik}$. The set of registration hypotheses is then $\mathcal{R}(X_i, X_j)=\{\mathcal{T}_{ij}, \mathcal{T}_{ikj}, \mathcal{T}_{ilj}, \ldots\}$, which we illustrate in Fig. 2(right). For a set of N images, it is therefore possible to obtain N-1 registration hypotheses per image pair without explicitly re-computing registrations. It is also possible to iteratively improve the results by using the fused pairwise registrations themselves to compute new hypotheses, which can then again be fused. We perform this iterative improvement until the average post-registration image similarity stops improving significantly.

3   Experimental Results

We evaluate our method in two experiments on two datasets. First, we fuse registrations obtained from running different registration algorithms with several different parametrizations each. Then, we evaluate the performance of MRegFuse in a group-wise registration approach.

Data Sets. To evaluate the accuracy of dense registrations, we generated a dataset of medical images with known dense correspondences as follows: We used 19 mid-saggital slices of brain MRI with 481×374 px^2 resolution and 0.3 mm spacing. We first registered one randomly chosen image to the remaining 18 images using Markov-random field (MRF) based registration [2]. The computed registrations were then used to deform the source image, and the 18 deformed images plus the source image were

Table 1. Results using independently computed registrations and their fusion. Different parameter sets p were obtained for each registration method, and the resulting registrations then fused using globally and locally weighted averaging (GWA and LWA) and our proposed MRegFuse and MRegFuseR. mJD denotes the minimum Jacobian determinant of all pair-wise registrations, while ADE and NCC are averaged over the set.

			Independent Registrations									Fusion	
Demons				MRF-reg						GWA	LWA	MRegFuse	MRegFuseR
p_{d_1}	p_{d_2}	p_{d_3}	p_{d_4}	p_{m_1}	p_{m_2}	p_{m_3}	p_{m_4}	p_{m_5}	p_{m_6}				
ADE	4.00	4.44	3.50	3.61	2.64	2.43	2.96	4.05	1.92	2.28	1.91	1.68	**1.11**	**1.11**
NCC	0.77	0.81	0.84	0.81	0.91	0.88	0.91	0.78	0.94	0.94	0.94	0.96	**0.97**	**0.97**
mJD	0.64	-165	0.05	0.36	0.03	0.09	0.02	0.28	0.05	0.01	**0.09**	-229.06	-9.25	$3e^{-4}$

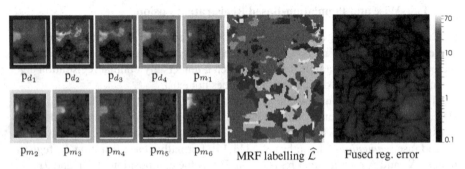

Fig. 3. Example fusion result for independently computed registrations for the 2D MR image pair shown in Fig. 2(left). The small images on the left side show the local deformation error magnitude of the computed registration with regard to the known ground-truth (log-scale). The frame of each image is colored such that the resulting MRF labelling (center) locally selects one of the registrations based on its color. The right-most image then shows the deformation error magnitudes of the fused registration.

used as a new dataset. This dataset then exhibits true anatomical variability, and ground-truth registrations can be inferred from the deformation process.

The second dataset consists of 15 clinical 3D CT scans of the head of different individuals, with $160 \times 160 \times 129 \, \text{px}^3$ resolution and unit spacing. The presence and the number of teeth vary substantially in this dataset. To evaluate registration accuracy, landmarks were placed at anatomically identifiable locations on the jawbone and the skull for all images. Additionally, the jawbone was manually segmented by experts, which allows us to also report post-registration segmentation overlap for this dataset.

Pair-Wise Registration Fusion. In this experiment, we evaluated the fusion of multiple independently computed pair-wise registrations. This is a relevant scenario, as it is frequently not known a-priori which registration algorithm with which parametrization would be best suited for a given registration problem. We registered each image pair of the 2D MR dataset multiple times using different parametrizations of well-known

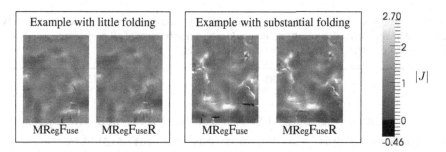

Fig. 4. Two registration examples showing the Jacobian determinant values for MRegFuse and MRegFuseR, with little folding (left) and substantial folding (right). The left example also corresponds to the images/results presented both in Figs. 2 and 3. In both examples, MRegFuseR is seen to completely remove folding.

demons- and MRF-based registrations [4,2]. For each image pair, we fuse all available registrations using globally and locally weighted averaging (GWA and LWA) in addition to the proposed MRegFuse. For each method we report the average (dense) deformation error (ADE), average post-registration image similarity (NCC), and the minimum of the local determinants of the Jacobian, which indicates folding [20]. The free parameters were optimized for each fusion method separately, yielding $\gamma=20$ for GWA, $\gamma=16$ and $\sigma=8$ for LWA, and $\gamma=10$, $\sigma=4$ and $\lambda=0.02$ for our MRegFuse. For our MRF fusion, we used MRFs with 4 px spacing, resulting in control grids of size 121×94 in 2D. Results are reported in Tab. 1. MRegFuse is seen to achieve lower ADE compared to both averaging-based registration fusion techniques, meanwhile leading to less folding compared to locally weighted averaging. Note that globally weighted averaging leads to no folding overall, as the initial registrations are diffeomorphic. However, it does not yield much improvement over the best individual registration. On the other hand, LWA, which is seen to improve ADE over all input registrations, meanwhile causes strong image folding as spatial smoothness of the deformations is not considered. MRegFuse, in contrast, leverages such smoothness information to find an optimal partitioning of input registrations. In Tab. 1, it is also seen that the proposed MRegFuseR is able to remove folding completely, as shown exemplary in Fig. 4, without deteriorating registration accuracy as indicated by ADE and average NCC. Jacobian determinants before and after two such sample folding removals are seen in Fig. 4.

Population-Based Registration Fusion. We also evaluated the performance of MRegFuse when registration hypotheses are obtained from indirect paths in a population of images. For the 2D MR dataset, we chose the best performing parametrizations from the previous experiment. For the fusion, we then used the same parameters as in the experiment above, except for λ, which was changed to 0.002 in the 3D experiment to account for the larger physical image spacing. The MRF grid-size was the same as above for the 2D data and was set to $40\times40\times33$ in 3D using the same grid spacing of 4 px. Results on both datasets are reported in Tab. 2. MRegFuse results in lower ADE and TRE compared to averaging-based registration fusion, while generating less folding. For the 3D CT dataset, we also report pairwise post-registration segmentation overlap which was computed using Dice's coefficient. We also compare the results to a typical

Table 2. Fusing registrations obtained by automatic hypothesis generation in sets of mutually registered images. mJD denotes the minimum Jacobian determinant of all pair-wise registrations, while ADE,NCC,TRE and Dice are averaged over the set.

	2D MRI						3D CT					
	Demons			MRF			Demons			MRF		
	ADE	NCC	mJD	ADE	NCC	mJD	TRE	Dice	mJD	TRE	Dice	mJD
Registration	3.5	0.84	0.05	1.92	0.93	0.05	9.62	0.65	-53.51	5.25	0.81	-1.8
+ LWA	2.34	0.94	-65.1	1.83	0.93	-593	7.33	0.78	-70	4.67	0.87	-19
+ MRegFuse	0.78	**0.98**	-2.29	**0.94**	**0.96**	-3.82	6.92	**0.81**	-8.3	**4.31**	**0.88**	-4.6
+ MRegFuseR	**0.71**	**0.98**	$3e^{-4}$	**0.94**	**0.96**	$5e^{-5}$	**6.67**	0.78	$8e^{-6}$	4.33	**0.88**	$1e^{-4}$

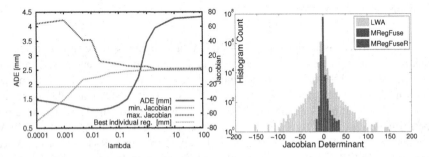

Fig. 5. Left: MRegFuse with different regularization weights λ on the pair-wise fusion experiment for the 2D MR dataset. Right: Histogram of local Jacobian determinants for LWA, MRegFuse and MRegFuseR for all pair-wise registrations on the 2D data.

group-wise registration method, in which all images of a set are iteratively registered to an evolving mean image using residual complexity [21,22]. From the registrations to this mean, we compute pair-wise registrations by inversion and composition. The resulting ADE is then 1.84 mm for the 2D MR dataset, and TRE is 8.1 mm in 3D CT, which are inferior to MRegFuse results. MRegFuseR is seen to succesfully remove folding.

3.1 Discussion

MRegFuse can be seen to result in lower ADE/TRE in all experiments compared to averaging-based fusion. The latter can only improve results when local weights are used, which cannot guarantee that the resulting deformation is smooth even when using large-kernel LNCC weighting. In contrast, the optimization of MRegFuse allows for a trade-off between smooth deformations and local similarity as shown in Fig. 5(left).

We are also very interested in exploring the robustness of MRegFuse with regard to the number and quality of registrations to be fused. As seen in our experimental validation, MRegFuse is more robust with regard to poor input registrations in comparison to averaging-based fusion. One downside of MRegFuse is that it cannot achieve a better performance *locally* than the best of its the input registrations due to its selection-based approach. However, the inputs can be augmented with additional registration hypotheses such as the (weighted) mean of the registrations.

Our MRF fusion is also fast and memory efficient. Average run-time of the MRF-solver for fusing 14 registrations is 30.5 seconds in 3D, while requiring less than 800 MB memory. The local similarity computation is also efficient. The entire process of generating indirect deformations in the group-wise experiment, computing all local similarities, and fusion using the MRF was completed in under two minutes in all cases. Consequently, finer resolution grids or more registrations/parametrizations can be fused in reasonable timeframes, which we will explore in the future.

The employed iterative TRW-S optimizer was stopped when the relative change of the lower bound was small ($1e^{-7}$) or a maximum number of iterations (1000) was reached. We observed that TRW-S was able to find the globally optimal solution in about 69% of the cases for the 2D pair-wise fusion experiment, and the final energy being within 0.5% of the lower bound in all remaining cases of that experiment. For the 3D experiments, the final energy was within 0.03% of the lower bound in all cases.

As can be seen from the experimental results, the fused registrations still exhibit folding as indicated by the negative Jacobian determinants. However, both the minima presented in the tables, as well as the distribution of all such values that can be seen in Fig. 5(right) show that the folding is less severe compared to LWA-fusion. Additionally, the proposed MRegFuseR algorithm can be used to remove folding by fusing the original MRegFuse result with smoothed versions of itself. This process is seen to retain the high registration accuracy of MRegFuse, even with potential (minor) ADE/TRE improvements as seen in the population-based demons experiments in Tab. 2. Using the described kernel pyramid, the folding removal in 3D examples needed on average $K=4.4$ additional smoothed deformation fields and 12 iterations to remove folding entirely. Since the number of graph labels during folding removal is significantly smaller compared to the MRegFuse step, the random field is solved much quicker at 1.5 s on average. The folding removal adds less than one minute on average to the registration fusion process. Potentially, such folding removal can be applied as a post-processing step to any other registration method that may yield non-positive Jacobian determinants.

4   Conclusions

We have presented a novel algorithm for registration fusion, which locally selects displacements from multiple registration hypotheses. An MRF is used to find an optimal solution in terms of local post-registration similarity and registration smoothness. This algorithm can furthermore be used to automatically remove inevitable folding at label seams. The proposed MRegFuse algorithm has been shown to be able to fuse registrations from random parametrizations of different registration algorithms such that the fused registrations exhibit higher accuracy than any of the input registrations. This is a relevant scenario for many image registration applications, where it is typically challenging to choose and parametrize a registration method correctly. We have also demonstrated that registration hypotheses can be obtained automatically within a set of mutually registered images, which allows improving the average pair-wise registration accuracy by using the proposed registration fusion.

References

1. Fischer, B., Modersitzki, J.: Ill-posed medicine - an introduction to image registration. Inverse Probl. 24(3), 1–19 (2008)

2. Glocker, B., Komodakis, N., Tziritas, G., Navab, N., Paragios, N.: Dense image registration through MRFs and efficient linear programming. Med. Image Anal. 12(6), 731–741 (2008)
3. Thirion, J.P.: Image matching as a diffusion process: an analogy with Maxwell's demons. Med. Image Anal. 2(3), 243–260 (1998)
4. Vercauteren, T., Pennec, X., Perchant, A., Ayache, N.: Diffeomorphic demons: efficient non-parametric image registration. Neuroimage 45(1 suppl.), 61–72 (2009)
5. Cachier, P., Ayache, N.: Regularization in Image Non-Rigid Registration: I. Trade-off between Smoothness and Intensity Similarity. Technical report, INRIA (2001)
6. Vercauteren, T., Pennec, X., Perchant, A., Ayache, N.: Symmetric log-domain diffeomorphic Registration: A demons-based approach. In: Metaxas, D., Axel, L., Fichtinger, G., Székely, G. (eds.) MICCAI 2008, Part I. LNCS, vol. 5241, pp. 754–761. Springer, Heidelberg (2008)
7. Avants, B., Epstein, C., Grossman, M., Gee, J.: Symmetric Diffeomorphic Image Registration with Cross-Correlation: Evaluating Automated Labeling of Elderly and Neurodegenerative Brain. Med. Image Anal. 12(1), 26–41 (2008)
8. Keysers, D., Unger, W.: Elastic Image Matching is NP-complete. Pattern Recognition Letters 24, 445–453 (2003)
9. Rueckert, D., Sonoda, L.I., Hayes, C., Hill, D.L., Leach, M.O., Hawkes, D.J.: Nonrigid registration using free-form deformations: application to breast MR images. IEEE Trans. Med. Imaging 18(8), 712–721 (1999)
10. Schapire, R.E.: The strength of weak learnability. Machine Learning 5(2), 197–227 (1990)
11. Heckemann, R.A., Hajnal, J.V., Aljabar, P., Rueckert, D., Hammers, A.: Automatic anatomical brain MRI segmentation combining label propagation and decision fusion. Neuroimage 33(1), 115–126 (2006)
12. Lempitsky, V., Roth, S., Rother, C.: FusionFlow: Discrete-continuous optimization for optical flow estimation. IEEE Comput. Vis. Pattern Recognit., 1–8 (2008)
13. Iglesias, J.E., Karssemeijer, N.: Robust initial detection of landmarks in film-screen mammograms using multiple FFDM atlases. IEEE Trans. Med. Imaging 28(11), 1815–1824 (2009)
14. Santemiz, P., Spreeuwers, L.J., Veldhuis, R.N.J.: Automatic landmark detection and face recognition for side-view face images. In: Int. Conf. Biometrics Spec. Interes. Gr. Lecture Notes in Informatics (LNI) - Proceedings, pp. 337–344 (2013)
15. Gass, T., Székely, G., Goksel, O.: Semi-supervised Segmentation Using Multiple Segmentation Hypotheses from a Single Atlas. In: Menze, B.H., Langs, G., Lu, L., Montillo, A., Tu, Z., Criminisi, A. (eds.) MCV 2012. LNCS, vol. 7766, pp. 29–37. Springer, Heidelberg (2013)
16. Cachier, P., Bardinet, E., Dormont, D., Pennec, X., Ayache, N.: Iconic feature based nonrigid registration: the PASHA algorithm. Comput. Vis. Image Underst. 89(2-3), 272–298 (2003)
17. Cardoso, M.J., Modat, M., Ourselin, S., Keihaninejad, S., Cash, D.: Multi-STEPS: Multi-label similarity and truth estimation for propagated segmentations. In: Math. Methods Biomed. Image Anal., pp. 153–158 (2012)
18. Kolmogorov, V., Zabih, R.: What Energy Functions Can Be Minimized via Graph Cuts. IEEE Trans. Pattern Anal. Mach. Intell. 26(4), 147–159 (2004)
19. Kolmogorov, V.: Convergent Tree-Reweighted Message Passing for Energy Minimization. IEEE Trans. Pattern Anal. Mach. Intell. 28, 1568–1583 (2006)
20. Christensen, G.E., Rabbitt, R.D., Miller, M.I., Joshi, S.C., Grenander, U., Coogan, T.A.: Topological Properties of Smooth Anatomic Maps. In: Inf. Process. Med. Imaging, pp. 101–112. Springer (1995)
21. Myronenko, A., Song, X.: Intensity-based image registration by minimizing residual complexity. IEEE Trans. Med. Imaging 29(11), 1882–1891 (2010)
22. Myronenko, A.: https://sites.google.com/site/myronenko/software

Stepwise Inverse Consistent Euler's Scheme for Diffeomorphic Image Registration

Akshay Pai[1], Stefan Sommer[1], Sune Darkner[1], Lauge Sørensen[1],
Jon Sporring[1], and Mads Nielsen[1,2]

[1] DIKU, University of Copenhagen, Copenhagen, Denmark
[2] Biomediq A/S, Copenhagen, Denmark

Abstract. Theoretically, inverse consistency in an image registration problem can be achieved by employing a diffeomorphic scheme that uses transformations parametrized by stationary velocity fields (SVF). The displacement from a given SVF, formulated as a series of self compositions of a transformation function, can be obtained by Euler integration in the time domain. However in practice, the discrete time integration produces results that are inverse inconsistent, and inverse consistency in the final solution needs to be explicitly ensured. One way of achieving this is to penalize the endpoint displacement offset obtained by evaluating a composition of the transformation with its inverse at an arbitrary point. In this paper, we propose a variation in which the displacement penalization is required only in the first composition step of the transformation thereby bringing down the computational complexity. We compare these two ways of enforcing inverse consistency by applying the registration framework on four pairs of brain magnetic resonance images. We observe that the proposed stepwise scheme maintains both precision and level of inverse consistency similar to the endpoint scheme.

1 Introduction

Inverse consistency is particularly important in studies where voxel-wise statistics are used to characterize anatomical changes over time [1]. Diffeomorphic (differentiable transformation with differentiable inverse) methods in image registration are attractive because they yield transformations that are invertible. However, inverse consistency is in practice achievable only if the discrete integral of the similarity measure and regularization are symmetrically approximated [2]. Several diffeomorphic approaches have been proposed and the two most prominent among them are: large deformation diffeomorphic metric mapping (LD-DMM) [3, 4] and Log-Euclidean framework based on stationary velocity fields (SVFs) [5].

In SVF based image registration, paths of diffeomorphism are generated using one parameter subgroups parameterized by SVFs through the Lie group exponential. The Lie group exponential is realized through a series of self compositions of a transformation function [6]. The generated diffeomorphism paths are geodesic with respect to the canonical Cartan connection [7]. Applications of SVF have found widespread success in image registration [7–9].

S. Ourselin and M. Modat (Eds.): WBIR 2014, LNCS 8545, pp. 223–230, 2014.

Deformations generated by SVFs are invertible. However, due to discretization errors, inverse consistency needs to be explicitly enforced, most often through a regularization. Inverse consistency has been addressed by [10] where both the forward and backward transformations were jointly estimated by minimizing the displacement offset obtained by composing the forward and backward transformations at an arbitrary point. Other methods that enforce inverse consistency (both diffeomorphic and non-diffeomorphic schemes) are, but not limited to, constraining the transformation [11], penalizing the Jacobian [12], symmetrizing every gradient descent step [13], log-average of forward and backward transformations during optimization [14] and finding a mid-space to make sure the transformations are evenly applied [15] .

In this paper, we propose to use a modified version of the inverse consistency term defined in [10] where we will apply the displacement offset penalization only on the first composition of the flow field (or stepwise scheme) as opposed to using the entire flow field (or endpoint scheme) . Section 2 will briefly introduce the concept of SVFs based image registration, followed by an introduction to the inverse consistency enforcing regularization. In Section 3, we will present a comparison of the proposed stepwise regularization and endpoint regularization by applying the framework on four pairs of brain magnetic resonance images (MRIs).

2   Registration

Given an image pair I_1, I_2, registration is formulated as a variational optimization problem, where the cost function that needs to be minimized is represented as,

$$E(I_1, I_2; \varphi) = \int_\Omega M(I_1(\varphi^{-1}), I_2) + \lambda R(\varphi) \; d\boldsymbol{x} \qquad (1)$$

where E is the overall energy, M is the similarity measure, normalized mutual information (NMI) [16] in this study, R is a regularization term, φ is a warp and $\boldsymbol{x} = (x, y, z)$ is a voxel position. Here, we focus on SVF based registration using B-splines where the warp φ is parametrized as

$$\varphi(\boldsymbol{x}) = \phi^1 \text{ where } \begin{cases} \frac{d\phi^t}{dt} = B(\boldsymbol{x}; p) \\ \phi^0 = \boldsymbol{x} \end{cases} , \qquad (2)$$

$$B(\boldsymbol{x}; p) = \sum_{i=0}^{3} \sum_{j=0}^{3} \sum_{k=0}^{3} \beta_i(x)\beta_j(y)\beta_k(z)p_{i,j,k}, \qquad (3)$$

where p is the B-spline parameter and β is a cubic B-spline basis function. A displacement can be realized as an Euler integration with unit time step [6]. For example, given n steps, the Euler integration approximation will be;

$$\phi^{\frac{1}{n}} = \boldsymbol{x} + \frac{B(\boldsymbol{x}; p)}{n}$$

$$\phi^{t+\frac{1}{n}} = \phi^t \circ \phi^{\frac{1}{n}}. \qquad (4)$$

2.1   Inverse Consistency

In [10], inverse consistency was enforced by penalizing the displacement error generated after composing a transformation with its inverse. However, in this method, the computation of inverse is a computationally expensive approximation [13]. We instead combine both the forward and backward registration in the same cost function and explicitly compute the inverse transformation, thus removing the lag due to computing the forward and backward transformations sequentially. With the Euler's scheme, inverse consistency can be achieved in two different ways. The first being the endpoint scheme, where the displacement offset is generated by using the entire flow field,

$$
E_{\text{endpoint}}(I_1, I_2; \varphi) =
$$
$$
\int_{\Omega_b} M(I_1(\phi_b^1), I_2) + \lambda ||\boldsymbol{x} - \phi_f^1(\phi_b^1)||^2 \, d\boldsymbol{x} + \int_{\Omega_f} M(I_1, I_2(\phi_f^1)) + \lambda ||\boldsymbol{x} - \phi_b^1(\phi_f^1)||^2 d\boldsymbol{x}
$$
$$(5)$$

where $\Omega_{f,b}$ are the region of interest in the source and target images and $\boldsymbol{x} \in \Omega_{f,b}$ depending on the direction of registration. Note that $\varphi = \{\phi_f, \phi_b\}$. The advantage of using the Euler's scheme is that, parametrization of the flow field is required only at the first composition. Hence, if the first composition is made inverse consistent, so will their compositions be. Therefore, the cost function (from (5)) for the stepwise scheme can be re-written as,

$$
E_{\text{stepwise}}(I_1, I_2; \varphi) =
$$
$$
\int_{\Omega_b} M(I_1(\phi_b^1), I_2) + n^2 \, \lambda ||\boldsymbol{x} - \phi_f^{\frac{1}{n}}(\phi_b^{\frac{1}{n}})||^2 \, d\boldsymbol{x} +
$$
$$
\int_{\Omega_f} M(I_1, I_2(\phi_f^1)) + n^2 \, \lambda ||\boldsymbol{x} - \phi_b^{\frac{1}{n}}(\phi_f^{\frac{1}{n}})||^2 \, d\boldsymbol{x}
$$
$$(6)$$

where n is the number of compositions used to realize a deformation.

2.2   Scaling and Squaring

The scaling and squaring method [5] speeds up the integration of the SVF. Although B-spline based SVF implementations that use scaling and squaring exist [12], scaling and squaring in this context is limited by the fact that a new B-spline must be fit at each squaring step. As this fitting cannot be exact, the control over the parametrization is lost and folds may occur. Furthermore, if displacement offsets are to be used for ensuring inverse consistency, the entire velocity field needs to be traversed in both directions to measure the offset. Therefore, we focus on inverse consistency only with Euler integration without scaling and squaring.

2.3   Volume Change Computation

Since the transformations are a composition of B-splines and using Jacobian integration might amplify numerical noise in the deformation, we use cube propagation [17] instead to compute local volume changes.

3   Experiments

Four pairs of 1.5T MRIs randomly chosen from the Alzheimer's disease neuroimaging initiative database (2 normal controls and 2 mild cognitively impaired) were co-registered. Bias correction and segmentations were done using the Freesurfer crossectional pipeline. The dimension of the images (both bias corrected and segmentations) was 256^3 mm with 1^3 mm isotropic voxels.

To perform a simple assessment of the methods, only one resolution of control points with a spacing of $\approx$5 mm was used. The images were filtered with a Gaussian kernel of size 0.2 mm. Number of compositions used were $n = 1, 2, 4, 8, 12, 16$ and 24. Registrations were run in 3 variations;

- No IC: Using (5) by setting $\lambda = 0$,
- Endpoint: Using (5) by setting $\lambda = 0.03$,
- Stepwise: Using (6) by setting $\lambda = 0.03$,

3.1   Evaluation Metrics

To evaluate the performance of the registration itself, we will inspect the correlation coefficient between the source and the registered target image [18]. Inverse consistency was checked by computing; the displacement offset (Δx) and atrophy error (AE);

$$\Delta x = \frac{1}{N} \sum_{\Omega} ||x - \phi_b^1(\phi_f^1(x))||, \text{AE} = \frac{1}{N} | \sum_{\Omega} (C_f - \frac{1}{C_b(\phi_f^1(x))}) |$$

where C_f is the forward voxel-wise volume change map computed using cube propgation, $C_b(\phi_f^1(x))$ is the backward change map transformed to the target domain using the forward transformation, x are random $N(25^3)$ points in the image and Ω is a region of interest, whole brain in this case.

4   Results

Figure 1 illustrates the mean correlation coefficient between the source and the registered target image over the 4 image registrations. The correlation coefficient improves with the number of compositions for the non-inverse consistent registration scheme. However, the correlation coefficient tends to remain the same with both the inverse consistent schemes, but better than the non-inverse consistent scheme regardless of the number of compositions used.

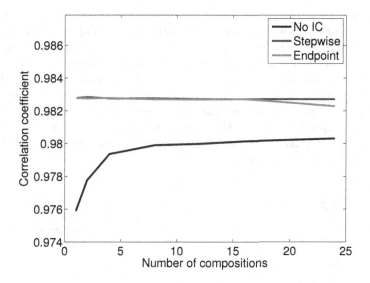

Fig. 1. Mean correlation coefficient between source and registered target image as a function of number of composition

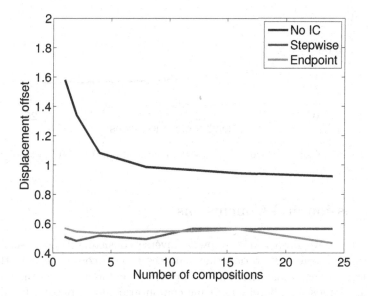

Fig. 2. Δx as a function of number of composition

Initially, we compute displacement offset using the deformations from the inverse inconsistent registration scheme by shooting a set of random points using both the entire flow field and only the first composition of the flow field with the offset multiplied by n^2. We observed that the latter approximates the former well. AE and the displacement offsets can be seen in Figures 2, 3. Both AEs and displacement offsets are quite similar for both stepwise and endpoint schemes.

The runtimes for both stepwise and non-inverse consistent scheme were the same and lower than the endpoint scheme (a scale up factor of ≈3), i.e., for an optimization iteration of a registration (with 8 compositions) run with step-wise/no inverse consistency scheme, the runtime was 10 secs when compared to the 30 secs with the endpoint scheme (single core implementation on a 2.5 Ghz Xeon). It is important to note that the mean numbers presented (correlation coefficient, AE and Δx) were only from the forward runs since the errors were similar with the backward runs.

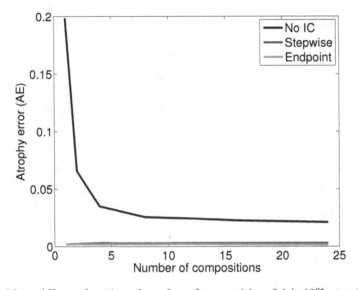

Fig. 3. Mean AE as a function of number of composition. 0.1 is 10% atrophy error

5   Discussion and Conclusions

In this article, we proposed a stepwise inverse consistent Euler's scheme for diffeomorphic image registration that enforces inverse consistency on the first composition of the transformation as opposed to enforcing it on the endpoint of the full composition, hereby reducing computational complexity. In addition, we presented an implementation of SVF based image registration parametrized by B-splines and in conjunction with the Euler's scheme. The proposed regularization is at a discretization level and can enable symmetric realization of large deformations.

We performed a pairwise comparisons of the stepwise and the endpoint inverse consistency scheme. For comparison we report the registration error (intensity correlation coefficient), displacement offset and bidirectional atrophy difference.

The stepwise scheme reduces computational cost while maintaining registration and inverse consistency precision when compared to the endpoint scheme.

This method can be utilized in realizing symmetric large deformations parsimoniously since it parametrizes SVF with the computationally efficient B-splines. In the future, we would like to investigate the impact of this registration scheme in separating diagnostic groups (Alzheimer's disease and normal controls) based on atrophy in both the whole brain and in subcortical structures.

References

1. Miller, M.: Computational anatomy: shape, growth, and atrophy comparison via diffeomorphisms. NeuroImage 23(1), 19–33 (2004)
2. Tagare, H.D., Groisser, D., Skrinjar, O.: Symmetric non-rigid registration: A geometric theory and some numerical techniques. Journal of Mathematical Imaging and Vision 34(1), 61–88 (2009)
3. Beg, M., Miller, M., Trouvé, A., Younes, L.: Computing large deformation metric mappings via geodesic flows of diffeomorphisms. Int. J. Comput. Vis. 61, 139–157 (2005)
4. Sommer, S., Lauze, F., Nielsen, M., Pennec, X.: Sparse multi-scale diffeomorphic registration: the kernel bundle framework. J. of Mathematical Imaging and Vision 46(3), 292–308 (2012)
5. Arsigny, V., Commowick, O., Pennec, X., Ayache, N.: A log-euclidean framework for statistics on diffeomorphisms. In: Larsen, R., Nielsen, M., Sporring, J. (eds.) MICCAI 2006. LNCS, vol. 4190, pp. 924–931. Springer, Heidelberg (2006)
6. Ashburner, J.: A fast diffeomorphic image registration algorithm. NeuroImage 38(1), 95–113 (2007)
7. Lorenzi, M., Pennec, X.: Geodesics, parallel transport and one-parameter subgroups for diffeomorphic image registration. International Journal of Computer Vision 105, 111–127 (2013)
8. Bossa, M., Zacur, E., Olmos, S., for the Alzheimer's Disease Neuroimaging Initiative: Tensor-based morphometry with stationary velocity field diffeomorphic registration: application to adni. NeuroImage 51(3), 956–969 (2010)
9. Hernandez, M., Bossa, M.N., Olmos, S.: Registration of anatomical images using paths of diffeomorphisms parameterized with stationary vector field flows. Int. J. Comput. Vis. 85, 291–306 (2009)
10. Christensen, G.E., Johnson, H.J.: Consistent image registration. IEEE Transactions on Medical Imaging 20, 568–582 (2001)
11. Rueckert, D., Aljabar, P., Heckemann, R.A., Hajnal, J.V., Hammers, A.: Diffeomorphic registration using B-splines. In: Larsen, R., Nielsen, M., Sporring, J. (eds.) MICCAI 2006. LNCS, vol. 4191, pp. 702–709. Springer, Heidelberg (2006)
12. Modat, M., Daga, P., Cardoso, M.J., Ourselin, S.: Parametric non-rigid registration using a stationary velocity field. In: IEEE Workshop on Mathematical Methods in Biomedical Image Analysis (MMBIA), pp. 145–150 (2012)
13. Leow, A., Huang, S.-C., Geng, A., Becker, J., Davis, S., Toga, A., Thompson, P.: Inverse consistent mapping in 3D deformable image registration: Its construction and statistical properties. In: Christensen, G.E., Sonka, M. (eds.) IPMI 2005. LNCS, vol. 3565, pp. 493–503. Springer, Heidelberg (2005)

14. Han, X., Hibbard, L.S., Willcut, V.: An efficient inverse-consistent diffeomorphic image registration method for prostate adaptive radiotherapy. In: Madabhushi, A., Dowling, J., Yan, P., Fenster, A., Abolmaesumi, P., Hata, N. (eds.) MICCAI 2010. LNCS, vol. 6367, pp. 34–41. Springer, Heidelberg (2010)
15. Avants, B.B., Epstein, C.L., Grossman, M., Gee, J.C.: Symmetric diffeomorphic image registration with cross-correlation: Evaluating automated labeling of elderly and neurodegenerative brain symmetric diffeomorphic image registration with cross-correlation: Evaluating automated labeling of elderly and neurodegenerative brain symmetric diffeomorphic image registration with cross-correlation: Evaluating automated labeling of elderly and neurodegenerative brain. Medical Image Analysis 12(1), 26–41 (2009)
16. Darkner, S., Sporring, J.: Generalized partial volume: An inferior density estimator to parzen windows for normalized mutual information. In: Székely, G., Hahn, H.K. (eds.) IPMI 2011. LNCS, vol. 6801, pp. 436–447. Springer, Heidelberg (2011)
17. Pai, A., Sørensen, L., Darkner, S., Mysling, P., Jorgensen, D., Dam, E., Lillholm, M., Oh, J., Chen, G., Suhy, J., Sporring, J., Nielsen, M.: Cube propagation for focal brain atrophy estimation. In: IEEE Symposium on Biomedical Imaging (2013)
18. Rueckert, D., Sonoda, L., Hayes, C., Hill, D., Leach, M.O., Hawkes, D.: Non-rigid registration using free-form deformations: Application to breast MR images. IEEE Transactions on Medical Imaging 18(8), 712–721 (1999)

Registration of Noisy Images
via Maximum A-Posteriori Estimation

Sebastian Suhr[1,4], Daniel Tenbrinck[2], Martin Burger[1,3], and Jan Modersitzki[4]

[1] Institute for Computational and Applied Mathematics,
University of Münster, Münster, Germany
[2] GREYC, UMR 6072 CNRS, École Nationale Supérieure d'Ingénieurs de Caen,
Caen, France
[3] Cells in Motion (CiM) Cluster of Excellence, University of Münster,
Münster, Germany
[4] Institute of Mathematics and Image Computing, University of Lübeck,
Lübeck, Germany
sebastian.suhr@uni-muenster.de

Abstract. Biomedical image registration faces challenging problems induced by the image acquisition process of the involved modality. A common problem is the omnipresence of noise perturbations. A low signal-to-noise ratio – like in modern dynamic imaging with short acquisition times – may lead to failure or artifacts in standard image registration techniques. A common approach to deal with noise in registration is image presmoothing, which may however result in bias or loss of information. A more reasonable alternative is to directly incorporate statistical noise models into image registration. In this work we present a general framework for registration of noise perturbed images based on maximum a-posteriori estimation. This leads to variational registration inference problems with data fidelities adapted to the noise characteristics, and yields a significant improvement in robustness under noise impact and parameter choices. Using synthetic data and a popular software phantom we compare the proposed model to conventional methods recently used in biomedical imaging and discuss its potential advantages.

1 Introduction

Motion estimation using variational methods, e.g., via optical flow [5] or registration [2,11,13], has become a powerful tool in many areas of imaging in the last years. While these methods have originally been designed to be applied on conventional images of relatively high quality, several biomedical imaging devices like ultrasound, PET, SPECT, or low intensity fluorescence imaging have a low signal-to-noise ratio (SNR) and rather lead to significant problems in presence of strong degradations. A common way to suppress noise in biomedical image registration is presmoothing of the given data by image filters. However, filtering can lead to bias and loss of information, in particular small details are canceled out in this process, e.g., in plaque imaging [3]. An appropriate incorporation of statistical noise models into variational methods has gained a lot of interest in several image processing tasks, such as denoising [4] or deconvolution [9].

S. Ourselin and M. Modat (Eds.): WBIR 2014, LNCS 8545, pp. 231–240, 2014.

Until today there are only few approaches that explicitly consider noise in image registration, e.g., in [1] the authors propose a coherent statistical framework for dense deformable templates explicitly assuming an additive Gaussian noise model. In [17] the authors propose a method to adapt an elastic regularization energy for non-rigid image registration to the given data via a hierarchical Bayesian model. Directly incorporating noise information into similarity measures for registration has been investigated by [14]. Without prior information on the motion field the latter authors propose an expectation maximization (EM) framework. In this context for specific classes of transformations (like affine transformations in [16]) several registration criteria have been developed. As these works are designed for a specific transformation or noise model, the aim of this paper is to give a general unified registration framework for dealing with noise for a large set of admissible transformations. Using Bayesian methods we derive a maximum a-posteriori (MAP) estimation in Section 2.1, which allows to incorporate statistical information into the process of image registration. To illustrate the flexibility of this approach we discuss two common noise models for biomedical imaging exemplarily in Section 2.2. We compare the proposed approach to conventional registration methods recently used for biomedical imaging on perturbed synthetic data in Section 3.1 and demonstrate its robustness under image noise and parameter choice. Furthermore, we apply the proposed method on a realistic software phantom for PET imaging in Section 3.2 to investigate its potential in a first experiment. We conclude by a short discussion in Section 4.

2   Methods

In the following we introduce a general unified framework to incorporate statistical noise models in biomedical image registration. For the sake of simplicity we restrict our attention on two consecutive (noisy) images $f_0, f_1 \colon \Omega \to \mathbb{R}$ for which $\Omega \subset \mathbb{R}^N$ denotes the image domain; typically one has $N \in \{2, 3\}$ in biomedical imaging. We interpret the images f_0 and f_1 as stochastic samples of an unperturbed image u in motion. A key observation is that in many imaging devices the noise is generated independently for f_0 and f_1, hence a direct matching of these two would be severely corrupted. Thus, we are interested in estimating the ground truth image u without assuming any additional prior knowledge about its actual form. Using maximum a-posteriori probability (MAP) estimation simultaneously for the unperturbed image u and for the velocity $v \colon \Omega \to \mathbb{R}^N$ with appropriate priors, we are able to deduce a relatively general motion estimation formulation for arbitrary noise models in biomedical imaging.

2.1   MAP Estimation for Image Registration

In order to derive a statistical model for motion estimation we use formal computations with probability densities, implicitly assuming all variables to be finite dimensional as in [14]. An expansion from a derived MAP model to the continuous function space setting can be performed in a straight-forward way.

Given two images $f_0, f_1 \in \mathcal{U}$, we want to estimate an underlying image $u \in \mathcal{U}$ and a motion variable $v \in \mathcal{V}$. Here, $\mathcal{U}$ denotes an appropriate image space and $\mathcal{V}$ the set of admissable transformations. We model the motion of the noise-free image u under v in a general way via a continuous linear operator $T(v) : \mathcal{U} \to \mathcal{U}$. For simplicity we restrict the discussion to forward motion, i.e., f_0 is a noisy version of u and f_1 a noisy version of $T(v)u$. Note that other transformations can also be considered in this setting, e.g., for small motion asymptotics the operators T_i are given by $T_i(v) = I + \tau S(v)$ for a small parameter $\tau > 0$.

The images f_0 and f_1 can be interpreted as independent realizations under a stochastic noise model with probability density $p_0(f_0|u)$ and $p_1(f_1|T(v)u)$, respectively. Hence, one is interested in the posterior distribution of the unperturbed image u and in particular the unknown motion v, given the observation of f_0 and f_1, i.e., by using Bayes' theorem,

$$p(u, v \mid f_0, f_1) = \frac{p(f_0, f_1 \mid u, v)\, p(u, v)}{p(f_0, f_1)} . \tag{1}$$

Using the assumption that the noise is context-free analogously to [14], the likelihood for the data can further be written as

$$p(f_0, f_1 \mid u, v) = p_0(f_0 \mid u)\, p_1(f_1 \mid T(v)u) .$$

Assuming no prior knowledge on the image u, we can set $p(u, v) = p(v)$.

In order to compute the MAP estimate we maximize the posterior density, respectively minimize its negative logarithm. Ignoring terms independent of u and v and denoting with $R(v) = -\log p(v)$ a regularization of the motion field and with $D_i(u, f_i) = -\log p_i(f_i|u)$ the data fidelities, we deduce:

Find a minimizer $(\overline{u}, \overline{v}) \in (\mathcal{U}, \mathcal{V})$ for the energy
$$F(u, v) = D_0(u, f_0) + D_1(T(v)u, f_1) + R(v) . \tag{2}$$

This formulation allows to incorporate statistical noise models for biomedical image registration as well as appropriate regularization functionals to enforce reasonable solutions. Instead of using an alternating minimization scheme to solve (2) as in the EM setting in [12], we choose a different way: assuming the fidelities D_i to be differentiable in the first variable, the first-order optimality condition for a minimizer $\overline{u} \in \mathcal{U}$ for fixed variables v, f_0, and f_1 yields

$$\partial_u D_0(\overline{u}, f_0) + T^*(v)\, \partial_u D_1(T(v)\overline{u}, f_1) = 0 , \tag{3}$$

where $\mathcal{U}$ is an appropriate Lebesgue space for images with its respective standard dot product and T^* is the adjoint operator of T. This equation can be solved uniquely for $\overline{u}$ if the data fidelity terms D_i are strictly convex. Consequently, we are able to define a map

$$U : \mathcal{V} \times \mathcal{U}^2 \to \mathcal{U} , \quad (v; f_0, f_1) \mapsto \overline{u} ,$$

for which $\overline{u}$ solves (3). Inserting this map into the original functional F in (2), we obtain an effective functional J to be minimized only with respect to the unknown motion v,

$$J(v) = F(U(v), v) = D_0(U(v; f_0, f_1), f_0) + D_1(T(v)U(v; f_0, f_1), f_1) + R(v) . \tag{4}$$

2.2   Physical Noise Modeling

In order to give a better understanding of the general framework given in Section 2.1, we discuss specific noise models which are common in biomedical imaging applications, i.e., additive Gaussian noise and multiplicative photon counting noise (Poisson distributed). For the sake of brevity we restrict ourselves to the case $D_0 = D_1 = D$ and omit the dependence of the operator T on the motion v, i.e., $T := T(v)$. However, it is possible to combine different statistical noise models, which is interesting in multi-modal registration settings [14,16].

Additive Gaussian Noise. The most commonly assumed noise model in the literature is additive Gaussian noise since it affects a majority of imaging modalities [1,14]. The image degradation process is given by

$$f = u + \eta , \qquad \eta \sim \mathcal{N}(0, \sigma^2 I) ,$$

for which η is Gaussian random variable with variance $\sigma^2 > 0$. In this case the resulting data fidelity is the popular L^2 fidelity,

$$D(u, f) = \frac{1}{2\sigma^2} \|u - f\|_{L^2(\Omega)}^2 , \qquad \text{and thus} \qquad \partial_u D(u, f) = \frac{u - f}{\sigma^2} .$$

Inserting the derivative into (3) we compute the map U:

$$U(v; f_0, f_1) = (I + T^*T)^{-1} (f_0 + T^* f_1) .$$

The map U is potentially nonlinear in v due the dependence of T on v and the inversion to be carried out but the dependence on f_0 and f_1 remains linear. After some elementary computations we arrive at:

$$J(v) = \langle T f_0 - f_1, (I + TT^*)^{-1}(T f_0 - f_1) \rangle + R(v) , \qquad (5)$$

which is a generalized form of the registration criterion in [16]. Thus, we effectively match f_1 and the transformed image $T(v) f_0$ as in standard models based on an intensity constancy constraint with a norm depending on v.

We can state these relations more precisely for two standard transformation models: the *intensity constancy* T_{ic} and the *mass-preserving* transformation T_{mp},

$$T_{\mathrm{ic}}(v)u = u \circ v , \qquad T_{\mathrm{mp}}(v)u = u \circ v \, \det(\nabla v) . \qquad (6)$$

The respective adjoint operators can be formally computed via the transformation theorem for integrals (cf. [6]) and $w \in \mathcal{U}^*$ (for the case of $\mathcal{U} = L^p$ one has $\mathcal{U}^* = L^q$ with $\frac{1}{p} + \frac{1}{q} = 1$) as,

$$T_{\mathrm{ic}}(v)^* w = w \circ v^{-1} \det(\nabla v^{-1}) , \qquad T_{\mathrm{mp}}(v)^* w = w \circ v^{-1} . \qquad (7)$$

Hence, in both cases $(I + TT^*)^{-1}$ reduces to the multiplication of the image with a factor depending on $\det(\nabla v)$, which leads to the following functionals,

$$J_{\mathrm{ic}}(v) = \frac{1}{2\sigma^2} \int_\Omega \frac{(f_0 \circ v - f_1)^2}{1 + \det(\nabla v)} \det(\nabla v) \, dx + R(v) , \qquad (8)$$

$$J_{\mathrm{mp}}(v) = \int_\Omega \frac{(f_0(v) \det(\nabla v) - f_1)^2}{1 + \det(\nabla v)} \, dx + R(v) . \qquad (9)$$

Poisson noise Another important noise model for biomedical image registration is the Poisson noise model, also known as 'photon counting noise', as used, e.g., in fluorescence microscopy and positron emission tomography [18]. As one counts natural numbers $k \in \mathbb{N}$ of occurring random events, the signal $f(x)$ in each point is modeled as a Poisson random variable with mean $u(x)$. The resulting data fidelity term is given (ignoring terms independent of u and v) by

$$D(u, f) = \int_\Omega u - f \log(u) \, \mathrm{d}x \, , \qquad \text{and thus} \qquad \partial_u D(u, f) = 1 - \frac{f}{u} \, .$$

Inserting the derivative into (3) leads to the optimality condition

$$\left(1 - \frac{f_0}{\bar{u}}\right) + T^* \left(1 - \frac{f_1}{T\bar{u}}\right) = 0 \, . \tag{10}$$

Due to the nonlinearity in $\bar{u}$ we cannot give a solution of (10) for general T. However, it can be computed for T_{ic} and T_{mp} as in the case of additive Gaussian noise above. In the intensity-constancy case we thus have for $f(v) = f_0(v) \det(\nabla v) + f_1$

$$J_{\mathrm{ic}}(v) = \int_\Omega f(v) - f(v) \log \left(\frac{f(v)}{1 + \det(\nabla v)}\right) \, \mathrm{d}x + R(v) \, , \tag{11}$$

while in the case of mass-preservation we find

$$J_{\mathrm{mp}}(v) = \int_\Omega f(v) - f(v) \log \left(\frac{f(v)}{2}\right) \, \mathrm{d}x + R(v) \, . \tag{12}$$

2.3 Hyperelastic Regularization

The MAP estimation in (2) allows to incorporate a-priori knowledge about the expected motion field via a regularization energy. A way to introduce penalizing functionals into the setting above is to use Gibbs probability densities [8] by

$$p(v) \propto e^{-R(v)} \quad \text{and hence} \quad R(v) = -\log p(v) \, ,$$

where usually $R \colon V \to \mathbb{R}$ is a non-negative, convex regularization functional. Since the presented functionals depend on the Jacobian determinant of the transformation we choose hyperelastic regularization for $\det(\nabla v)$ as proposed in [2]:

$$R_{\mathrm{hyper}}(v) = \int_\Omega \alpha_1 \operatorname{len}(\nabla v) + \alpha_2 \operatorname{surf}(\operatorname{cof}(\nabla v)) + \alpha_3 \operatorname{vol}(\det(\nabla v)) \, \mathrm{d}x \, , \tag{13}$$

with $\alpha_i \geq 0, \sum \alpha_i > 0$ for $i = 1, 2, 3$ and the penalty functions

$$\operatorname{len}(s) = \|s - \mathcal{I}\|_{\mathrm{Fro}}^2 \, , \qquad \operatorname{surf}(s) = \left(\|s\|_{\mathrm{Fro}}^2 - 3\right)^2 , \qquad \operatorname{vol}(s) = \frac{(s-1)^4}{s^2} \, .$$

The hyperelastic regularization is a good choice in presence of highly non-rigid motion and simultaneously yields regular (weak) local diffeomorphic deformations, which is a desirable feature in biomedical imaging applications [2].

3   Experimental Results

In the following we demonstrate the validity of the proposed registration framework in Section 2 qualitatively and quantitatively and perform preliminary evaluation experiments on synthetic data. In particular, we compare the MAP estimation approach with hyperelastic SSD registration as realized in the popular FAIR toolbox [2,11] on noisy images as well as presmoothed versions of the latter ones.

For assessing the quality of an estimated transformation between two noisy images we compute the phantom matching error (PME) from [10],

$$\mathrm{PME}(\overline{v}; u_1, u_2) \;=\; \int_\Omega (T(\overline{v})u_1 - u_2)^2 \, \mathrm{d}x \; . \tag{14}$$

Additionally, we evaluate the regularity of the estimated transformation by computing the energy functional value of the regularization from Section 2.3 and validate these observations by visual inspection of the displacement and the associated Jacobian determinants. We choose the regularization parameters as $\alpha_1 = \alpha_3 = \alpha > 0$ and $\alpha_2 = 0$, i.e., the overall impact of the regularization energy in the used multi-level framework is controlled by an adaptive parameter α, which is roughly linked to the noise variance on each level similar to [17].

3.1   Synthetic Noisy Images

We present preliminary experiments on two synthetic images which represent a rather challenging target for image registration. The goal is to estimate the motion of a ring shaped object in a template image (cf. Figure 1b), which contracts towards the image center and thus gets more dense, leading to an increase of signal intensities in the reference image (cf. Figure 1a). However, the integral of the image intensities is constant, thus the mass-preserving model is appropriate in this setting. We added synthetic noise of different levels according to the noise models in Section 2.2, e.g., additive Gaussian noise with $\sigma = 125$ as shown in Figure 1c and 1d, and Poisson noise with a scaling factor of $s = 60$ as shown in Figure 1e and 1f. Note that due to the signal-dependent nature of Poisson noise, the noise characteristics change significantly between the latter two images, hence making physical noise modeling even more important.

First, we quantitatively assess the performance and registration accuracy of the three tested methods by computing the PME in (14) for different noise levels and regularization parameters. Figure 2 plots the results of this test and clearly shows the potential of the proposed general framework for biomedical image registration. In presence of a significant amount of noise the MAP estimation yields the best registration performance with respect to the PME as can be seen in Figure 2a-2b. The standard methods achieve similar results only for a very low regularization parameter α. However, these results can be neglected as the respective regularization energy is larger by magnitudes indicating unreasonable transformations as visualized in Figure 2c-2d. Furthermore, the occurrence of

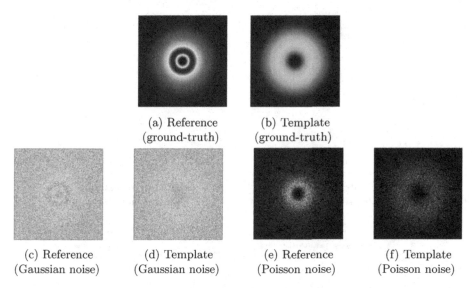

(a) Reference
(ground-truth)

(b) Template
(ground-truth)

(c) Reference
(Gaussian noise)

(d) Template
(Gaussian noise)

(e) Reference
(Poisson noise)

(f) Template
(Poisson noise)

Fig. 1. Ground truth data and noisy images for mass preserving registration: intensity distributed over a wide area (template) and the same amount concentrated in a small circle (reference). Respective image pairs are identically scaled and illustrated in color for better visual comparability.

intersections and overlaps in the computed motion field can be expected for these cases. Additionally, one can observe the high robustness of the proposed registration formulation with respect to the choice of parameters in comparison to the problems of conventional registration methods. A cross validation with a different data fidelity term inserted into the registration formulation shows that choosing the right noise model is crucial for accurate image registration.

Finally, we visualize the magnitude of the Jacobian determinant and transformed ground truth image with respect to the estimated transformations in Figure 3 for the case of additive Gaussian noise. The Jacobian determinants $\det(\nabla v)$ resulting from the proposed method are significantly smoother compared to the FAIR registration result and its presmoothed version (Figure 3a-3c), thus indicating a higher robustness in presence of noise perturbations. This can also be observed for the transformed images $T(v)u$ when applying the estimated motion field in Figure 3d-3f. As can be seen the impact of noise is much lower for the proposed registration formulation.

3.2 XCAT Phantom Data for PET Imaging

In the following we aim to give a proof-of-concept by applying the proposed method on the well-known XCAT software phantom [15]. We use the latter to generate noise corrupted positron emission tomography (PET) images simulating measurements of a human body during a radioactive FDG metabolism study

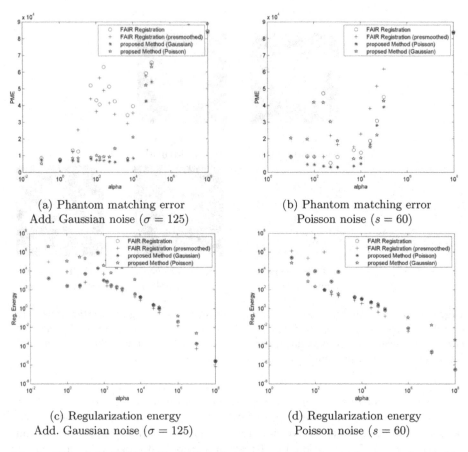

(a) Phantom matching error
Add. Gaussian noise ($\sigma = 125$)

(b) Phantom matching error
Poisson noise ($s = 60$)

(c) Regularization energy
Add. Gaussian noise ($\sigma = 125$)

(d) Regularization energy
Poisson noise ($s = 60$)

Fig. 2. Plot of the PME in Eq. (14) and the values of the hyperelastic regularization energy for different noise levels and regularization parameters α

in data of size $175 \times 175 \times 47$ voxel. The target of interest in this data is the human heart in different phases of the myocardial cycle and we use the end-diastolic phase (reference) and the end-systolic phase (template) in Figure 4a and 4b, respectively. As one can see in Figure 4d for a representative 2D slice, the estimated transformation warps the template image reasonably to the reference image, without matching the noise inherent in the data set. Additionally, one can interpret from the deformation grid in Figure 4c, that the estimated transformation is very smooth and convolution-free. Due to missing ground truth information a evaluation on real biomedical images turns out to be difficult and thus remains an open question for future investigations.

4 Discussion and Outlook

In this paper we proposed a general unified framework for biomedical image registration on noise perturbed images. By incorporating statistical a-priori

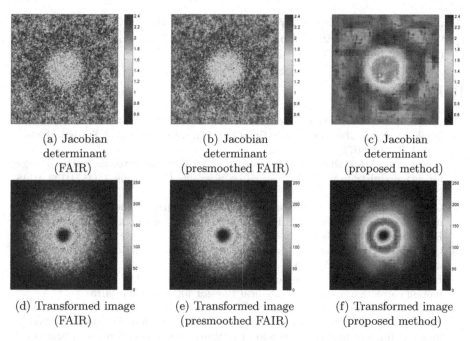

(a) Jacobian
determinant
(FAIR)

(b) Jacobian
determinant
(presmoothed FAIR)

(c) Jacobian
determinant
(proposed method)

(d) Transformed image
(FAIR)

(e) Transformed image
(presmoothed FAIR)

(f) Transformed image
(proposed method)

Fig. 3. Visualization of the Jacobian determinants $\det(\nabla v)$ and the transformed ground truth images $T(v)u$ for the investigated methods in case of additive Gaussian noise as illustrated in Figure 1c and 1d

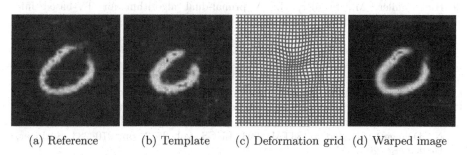

(a) Reference   (b) Template   (c) Deformation grid (d) Warped image

Fig. 4. Registration results for simulated noisy PET images (XCAT phantom)

knowledge into the registration process, we increased both accuracy as well as robustness of image registration. Using a maximum a-posteriori estimation approach we are able to control the regularity of the transformations and thus to enforce reasonable motion fields for biomedical applications. Preliminary experiments on synthetic data showed promising results but a thorough evaluation on real biomedical data and detailed analysis of the proposed model still have to be investigated in the future. Furthermore, the extension of this approach to other noise models, such as speckle noise, will be object of future research as well.

Acknowledgment. This study was supported by the DFG SFB 656 MoBil (project B2), the Cells in Motion (CiM) Cluster of Excellence, both Münster, Germany and by the DFG project MO-1053/2-1.

References

1. Allassonnière, S., Amit, Y., Trouvé, A.: Towards a coherent statistical framework for dense deformable template estimation. Journal of the Royal Statistical Society 69, 3–29 (2007)
2. Burger, M., Modersitzki, J., Ruthotto, L.: A hyperelastic regularization energy for image registration. SIAM Journal on Scientific Computing 35(1), B132–B148 (2013)
3. Cademartiri, F., et al.: Influence of increasing convolution kernel filtering on plaque imaging with multislice CT using an ex-vivo model of coronary angiography. La Radiologia Medica 110(3), 234–240 (2005)
4. Chan, T.F., Shen, J.: Image processing and analysis: variational, PDE, wavelet, and stochastic methods. SIAM (2005)
5. Dawood, M., et al.: A mass conservation-based optical flow method for cardiac motion correction in 3D-PET. Medical Physics 40(1), 012505 (2013)
6. Fremlin, D.H.: Measure theory: broad foundations, vol. 2. Torres Fremlin (2001)
7. Frick, K., Marnitz, P., Munk, A.: Statistical multiresolution Dantzig estimation in imaging: fundamental concepts and algorithmic framework. Journal of Statistical Mechanics: Theory and Experiment 6, 231–268 (2012)
8. Geman, S., Geman, D.: Stochastic relaxation, Gibbs distributions and the Bayesian restoration of images. Journal of Applied Statistics 20, 25–62 (1993)
9. Hintermüller, M., Stadler, G.: A primal-dual algorithm for TV-based inf-convolution-type image restoration. SIAM Journal on Scientific Computing 28(1), 1–23 (2006)
10. Mair, B.A., Gilland, D.R., Sung, J.: Estimation of images and nonrigid deformations in gated emission CT. IEEE Transactions on Medical Imaging 25(9), 1130–1144 (2006)
11. Modersitzki, J.: FAIR: Flexible Algorithms for Image Registration. SIAM (2009)
12. Nicolau, S., Pennec, X., Soler, L., Ayache, N.: Evaluation of a new 3D/2D registration criterion for liver radio-frequencies guided by augmented reality. In: Ayache, N., Delingette, H. (eds.) IS4TM 2003. LNCS, vol. 2673, pp. 270–283. Springer, Heidelberg (2003)
13. Paquin, D.C., Levy, D., Xing, L.: Multiscale deformable registration of noisy medical images. Mathematical Biosciences and Engineering 5(1), 125–144 (2008)
14. Roche, A., Malandain, G., Ayache, N.: Unifying maximum likelihood approaches in medical image registration. International Journal of Imaging Systems and Technology 11, 71–80 (1999)
15. Segars, W.P., et al.: 4D XCAT phantom for multimodality imaging research. Medical Physics 37, 4902–4915 (2010)
16. Sermesant, M., et al.: Deformable biomechanical models: application to 4D cardiac image analysis. Medical Image Analysis 7, 475–488 (2003)
17. Simpson, I.J.A., et al.: Probabilistic inference of regularisation in non-rigid registration. NeuroImage 59, 2438–2451 (2012)
18. Vardi, Y., Shepp, L.A., Kaufman, L.: A statistical model for positron emission tomography. Journal of the American Statistical Association 80, 8–20 (1985)

Author Index